Low Back Pain

Low Back Pain

Edited by **Angus Sanders**

FOSTER
ACADEMICS

New Jersey

Published by Foster Academics,
61 Van Reypen Street,
Jersey City, NJ 07306, USA
www.fosteracademics.com

Low Back Pain
Edited by Angus Sanders

International Standard Book Number: 978-1-63242-261-3 (Hardback)

Printed in the United States of America.

Contents

Preface

The book is a comprehensive compilation of works of different researchers from varied parts of the world. It includes valuable experiences of the researchers with the sole objective of providing the readers (learners) with a proper knowledge of the concerned field. This book will be beneficial in evoking inspiration and enhancing the knowledge of the interested readers.

This book discusses various aspects of low back pain and includes matters related to basic and clinical science, epidemiology, risk factors, evaluation, and the various approaches in exercise therapy. This book will prove beneficial for practitioners like back pain-physiotherapists, osteopaths, chiropractors and doctors of orthopedics, rheumatology, rehabilitation and manual medicine. Furthermore, it will administer guidance and information to the students of movement and to those who are interested in movement exercises such as physiologists, Pilates instructors, yoga teachers, etc.

In the end, I would like to extend my heartiest thanks to the authors who worked with great determination on their chapters. I also appreciate the publisher's support in the course of the book. I would also like to deeply acknowledge my family who stood by me as a source of inspiration during the project.

Editor

Section 1

Basic Science and Evaluation

1

Epidemiology

Akira Minematsu
Kio University,
Japan

1. Introduction

Low back pain (LBP) is a common problem that most people experience at some point in their lifetime. It is reported that the ranges of prevalence of LBP at a point, 1-year and over lifetime were from 4.4% to 33%, from 3.9% to 65% and from 11% to 84%, respectively (Andersson, 1999; Loney et al., 1999; Louw et al., 2007; McBeth et al., 2007; Walker, 2000). The differences of prevalence ranges can be caused by variation in areas, age, lifestyle, social situations and study methodology. In addition, the economic burden of LBP is very heavy (Brooks, 2006; Dagenais et al., 2008). It is, therefore, important for LBP patients to understand LBP and how to prevent LPB.

LBP is a symptom of a pain which can be localised between the twelfth rib and the inferior gluteal folds (low back), with or without leg pain from various causes (Krismer & van Tulder, 2007), but is not a disease. LBP is generally classified as 'specific' or 'non-specific'. Non-specific LBP is defined as symptoms of unknown origin or without identifiable pathology, and specific LBP is defined as that caused by a specific pathophysiological mechanism, such as disc prolapse or herniated nucleus pulposus, infection, inflammatory arthopathy, turmour, osteoporosis or fracture (van Tulder & Waddell, 2005). Most cases are non-specific, but in 5%-10% of cases a specific cause is identified (Krismer & van Tulder, 2007). Though the causes of LBP are varied, these may be classified as spondylogenic, neurogenic, viscerogenic, vascular and psychogenic (Wong & Transfeldt, 2007). These causes can be attributed to non-specific and/or specific factors, and these factors combine with each other in some cases. Moreover, it is necessary to ascertain the factors causing LBP and whether it is primary or secondary LBP. We are able to treat and prevent LBP promptly when we specify the causes of LBP, though most of pathomechanism of LBP is unknown (Nachemson, 1992).

2. Epidemiology of LBP

LBP is an important health problem in both developed and developing countries (Brooks, 2006; Woolf & Pfleger 2003). LBP results in socio-economic losses, health and clinical problems, not only for individuals but also for countries, because LBP causes obstacles to work or work absence and increases economic burden of treatment and compensation. Therefore, epidemiological study holds an important position in understanding LBP.

Epidemiology is the study of the health of human populations. Its functions are:

1. To discover the agent, host, and environmental factors which affect health, in order to provide the scientific basis for the prevention of disease and injury, and the promotion of health.
2. To determine the relative importance of causes of illness, disability, and death, in order to establish priorities for research and action.
3. To identify those sections of the population which have the greatest risk from specific causes of ill health, in order that the indicated action may be directed appropriately.
4. To evaluate the effectiveness of health programs and services in improving the health of the population. (Brownson, 1998).

In the case of LBP, epidemiology investigates the various factors of LBP included in the risk factors for LBP, the effects of prevention measures and interventions on LBP, the interaction of risk factors for LBP, time course changes of LBP, the burden of LBP, associations among this information and so on. Much epidemiological research on LBP has been conducted worldwide. This research is important in understanding the past, present and future of LBP, and epidemiological data provide much information to assist in seeking and solving the various problems related to LBP. Moreover, these data can prevent LBP by avoiding or decreasing risk factors for individuals.

The two most basic concepts of epidemiology are incidence and prevalence. Incidence is defined as the rate at which healthy people develop a new symptom or disease over a specified period of time. In contrast to incident, prevalence is a measure of the number of people in the population who have a symptom or disease at a particular point in time (Manchikanti, 2000). Therefore, it is necessary to note the methodological problems in the study of the epidemiology of LBP.

2.1 Prevalence of LBP in the general population

LBP is more common between the ages of 25 and 64 years (World health organization [WHO], 2001), though it can occur in all age ranges. The prevalence of LBP peaks between ages 35 and 55 (Andersson, 1992). This is considered to reflect the work force and high prevalence in the age between 30 and 50 is reported (European Foundation for the Improvement of Living and Working Conditions [Eurofound], 2007; Japan Industrial Safety & Health Association [JISHA], 1994). The prevalence of LBP has been investigated in many surveys, with point, annual, and lifetime prevalence generally showing that prevalence is widespread among the investigations. This indicates the variety of investigations, especially the methodology such as population (age, gender, race, number and lifestyle), region, time, period, definition of LBP and contents of questionnaires in the investigation. However, the preventive measures for LBP that are suited for regional populations can be found through the epidemiological data.

Cunningham and Kelsey reported that back trouble is a frequent problem and the prevalence of back pain symptoms is estimated to be 17.2% from the data source of The United States (US) Health and Nutrition Examination Survey, 1971-1975 (HANES I) of the US adults aged 25-74 years (Cunningham & Kelsey, 1984). Strine and Hootman reported that from National Health Interview Survey in 2002 the prevalence of LBP increase with aging and the total prevalence of LBP only was 17.0% and the prevalence of both neck and LBP was 9.3% of US adults aged 18 years and over (Strine & Hootman, 2007). In addition, the prevalence of chronic LBP increased from 3.9% in 1992 to 10.2% in 2006 in North Carolina households in those aged21 years and older (Freburger et al., 2009). Cassidy et al. estimated the point and lifetime prevalence of LBP were 28.4% and 84.1% in Canadian aged from 20 to 69 years (Cassidy et al., 1998). In the United Kingdom (UK), Badley and Tennant reported the prevalence of back pain was 10.0% with the prevalence increasing with aging and the highest prevalence was shown in the aged 56-64 years from the survey of Calderdale population aged 16 years and older (Badley & Tennant, 1992). Hillman et al. reported the point and lifetime prevalence of LBP were 19% and 59%, respectively, in the Bradford population aged 25 years and over (Hillman et al., 1996). Ihlebaek et al. reported the prevalence of LBP in Norway and Sweden (Ihlebaek et al., 2006). They showed the point and lifetime prevalence of LBP were 9.9% and 62.4% in men and 16.8% and 59.1% in women in Norway, and 14.6% and 68.9% in men and 20.4% and 69.9% in women in Sweden, respectively (Ihlebaek et al., 2006). In Finland, about one-third of people aged over 30 years experienced back pain during the past month in the early 2000s. Clinical diagnosed back syndrome decreased from 17.6% to 10.4% in men and from 16.5% to 10.6% in women aged over 30 years in 1978-1980 and 2000-2001 (Heliovaara & Riihimaki, 2006).

The prevalence of LBP has been investigated in some systematic reviews. Andersson reported that the lifetime prevalence of back pain as over 70% and 1-year prevalence ranges from 15% to 45%, with point prevalence averaging 30% (Andersson, 1999). Hoy et al. estimated that point and 1-year prevalence of LBP ranged from 1.0% to 58.1%, with a mean of 18.1%, and ranged from 0.8% to 82.5% with a mean of 38.1%, respectively, in their systematic review (Hoy et al., 2010). They estimated the prevalence of LBP to be very widespread. Loney et al. reviewed 18 studies that were conducted 7 countries in Europe, North America and China (Loney & Stratford, 1999). They estimated the average point and 1-year prevalence were 19.2% (ranged from 4.4% to 33.0%) and 32.37% (ranged from 3.9% to 63%), respectively. In high quality studies (over 70 points methodologically), point and 1-year prevalence ranged from 13.7% to 28.7% and from 39% to 44.9%, respectively (Loney & Stratford, 1999). McBeth et al. found that point and lifetime prevalence of LBP ranged from 13% to 30% and from 51% to 84%, respectively, in the investigation using 13 selected studies (McBeth & Jones, 2007). Walker selected 30 studies of 56 studies using methodological examination (75% pass level for methodological acceptable) and reported that point prevalence ranged from 12% to 33%, 1-year prevalence ranged from 22% to 65% and lifetime prevalence ranged from 11% to 84% (Walker, 2000). Louw et al. estimated point, 1-year, and lifetime prevalence of LBP in 27 eligible studies in African countries (Louw et al., 2007). Studies in this review were conducted in 10 countries and they selected 10 South Africa studies, 7 Nigerian, 2 Tunisian and 8 from other countries. They estimated that point prevalence ranged from 16% to 59%, averaging 32% among adults in 9 methodologically sound studies, and 1-year prevalence ranged from 14% to 72%, averaging 50% among adults in 9 studies, and lifetime prevalence ranged from 28% to 74%, averaging 64% among adults in 6 studies. Point, 1-year, and lifetime prevalence of LBP potentially increased with age (Louw et al., 2007). In the study by Volinn in 1995 (Volinn, 1995), it was reported that LBP rates in high-income countries were higher than those in low-income countries. LBP rates among the selected for the high-income countries (Belgium, Germany and Sweden) were approximately twice or even higher than the low-income countries (Nepal, India, Nigeria, China, Indonesia and Philippines), especially in rural areas. Point prevalence of LBP ranged from 29% to 42% in the high-income countries and ranged from 7% to 18% in rural areas in the low-income countries, though point prevalence of LBP was 14% in Britain (Volinn, 1995). In the study by walker (Walker, 2000), the highest point and lifetime prevalence of LBP in developing nations were 16.5% and 50% in Yugoslavia, respectively, excluding unclear information, and the highest point and lifetime prevalence of LBP in other nations were 33% in Germany and Belgium, and 79% in New Zealand, respectively. However, prevalence of LBP in Africa is similar to that of Western countries (Louw et al., 2007). Moreover, Hestbaek et al. reviewed 36 studies (28 observational studies and 8 randomized controlled trials) and reported that point prevalence of LBP in persons with one or more previous episodes of LBP ranged from 14% to 93%, and those without a prior history of LBP ranged from 7% to 39% in 6 studies (Hestbaek et al., 2003). Hillman et al. reported that the annual incidence of LBP was 4.7% (Hillman et al., 1996) and Cassidy et al. reported the cumulative incidence of LBP was 18.6% (Cassidy et al., 2005). Hoy et al. estimated the 1 year incidence of a first-ever episode of LBP ranged from 6.3% to 15.4%, and the 1-year incidence of any episodes of LBP ranged from 1.5% to 36% (Hoy et al., 2010). Manchikanti reported the prevalence of recurrent or chronic LBP at 3, 6 and 12 months to range from 35% to 79% (Manchikanti, 2000).

Study	Studies of number	Range of prevalence (%)		
		Point	Period	Lifetime
Andersson, 1999	12	12.0 - 30.2	25 - 42	51.4 - 69.9
Hestbaek et al., 2003	6	14 - 93		
Hoy et al., 2010	19	1.0 - 58.1	0.8 - 82.5	
Loney et al., 1999	18	4.4 - 33.0	3.9 - 63	13.8 - 84
Louw et al., 2007	27	16 - 59	14 - 72	28 - 74
McBeth, 2007	13	13 - 30	31 - 67	51 - 84
Volinn, 1995	8 (high income countries)	14 - 42		
	6 (low income countries)	7 - 28		
Walker, 2000	30	12 - 33	22 - 65	11 - 84

Table 1. Point, period and lifetime prevalence of LBP in the general population

Point and lifetime prevalence of LBP is estimated to be 6.8% and 13.8%-17.2% in the US, 4.4%-28.7% and 84% in Canada, 14%-19% and 58%-59% in the UK, 19%-33% and 59% in Belgium, 13.7% and 62%-64% in Denmark, and 12%-31% and 31%-70% in Sweden, respectively, according to the systematic reviews (Hoy et al., 2010; Loney et al., 1999; McBeth, 2007; Walker, 2000). The prevalence of LBP decreased from 33% in 2000 to 24.7% in 2005 in Europe (Paoli & Merllie, 2001; Parent-Thirion et al., 2007). Prevalence rates of LBP are difficult to compare because of the time of sampling, the sampling technique and the actual questions asked (Andersson, 1999). Therefore, it is important to know the time-trend of LBP.

2.2 Occupational LBP

In LBP, occupational LBP has been a topic for research for a long time. Occupational LBP is an important problem for workers and nations, and various remedies have been proposed. Occupational LBP will be work-specific when considering the factors causing LBP. Since occupational LBP is caused by work-related factors, which are physical factors (e.g. heavy physical work, manual handling, lifting, bending or twisting, vibration, awkward postures, repetitive work) and psychosocial factors (e.g. work environment, job content, job dissatisfaction, social support, personal relation) (Pope et al., 1991; Andersson, 1992; Burdorf & Sorock, 1997), it can occur in various types of work settings. Therefore, occupational LBP is not only an individual medical problem, but also a social economic problem.

Musculoskeletal disorders (MSDs) are widespread in many countries and they are the single largest category of work-related illness (Punnett & Wegman, 2004). MSDs account for over 50% of occupational diseases in Europe (Eurofound, 2007), and LBP and neck pain are equally a high prevalence in MSDs. The World health organization (WHO) treats occupational and work-related disease separately, and occupational LBP is included in work-related disease (WHO, 2001). WHO defines that occupational diseases are adverse health conditions in a human being, the occurrence or severity of which is related to exposure to factors on the job or in the work environment, and reports that such factors can be physical, chemical, biological, ergonomic, psychosocial stressors and mechanical. WHO characterizes work-related diseases as multifactorial diseases which may frequently be work-related and when such diseases affect the worker they may be work-related in a number of ways: they may be partially caused by adverse working conditions; they may be aggravated, accelerated or exacerbated by workplace exposures; and they may impair working capacity (WHO, 2001). Additionally, Schilling proposed the categories of adverse environmental agents as workplace hazards and the categories of work-related disease and injury as the concept of work-related disorders which has broadened to include those categories with more understanding of the multiple causes of disease (Schilling, 1989). Occupational LBP can occur related to these workplace hazards and under the categories of work-related disorders.

Occupational LBP can be defined as the back pain caused by work-induced and related factors. Generally, physical, psychosocial and personal factors interact with the onset of occupational LBP. In Japan, Aoyama proposed occupational LBP (Aoyama, 1984) as:

1. LBP occurring after working for the first time though there is no incidence of LBP before working, or LBP becoming worse after working even if there is onset of LBP before working,
2. a high prevalence of LBP is seen at the same place of work and the same type of job,
3. LPB improved by measures taken in the place of work, such as improvement of working conditions and environment, absence and reshuffling of personnel.

Also, occupational LBP is defined as work-specific LBP and classified as accidental and non-accidental LBP under regulations related to workmen's compensation (Ministry of Labour, 1976). The former is injury that results from an unexpected event triggering injury during the task, and injuries of muscle, tendon, ligament and soft tissue (strains or ruptures) in the back are found. The latter, where pain arises as a result of normal activities and requirements of the task, and poor body mechanics, prolonged activity, repetitive motions, and fatigue are major contributors to injuries.

It is, however, difficult to determine the relationship between occupational or work-related factors and LBP because:

1. LBP is not easily defined,
2. sickness absence data are influenced not only by pain, but also by physical and psychologic work factors, social factors and the insurance system,

3. the healthy worker effect may bias data,
4. exposure is difficult to determine, and
5. there is poor relationship between tissue injury and disability (Pope et al., 1991).

In Europe, definitions of work-related MSDs are different between countries and there are some nations that lack any definitions of work-related MSDs, nevertheless, the social security institutions in these countries do provide a list of occupational diseases that entitle workers reporting such conditions to compensation (Eurofound, 2007). It is proposed that occupational LBP not be dealt with via compensation or suits, but via prevention and prevention of recurrence through work-related factors, because occupational LBP has become the major cause of work absence causing damage not only to an individual with occupational LBP and his family, but also to a country (Kurihara, 1994). Therefore, it is very important to take measures related to occupational LBP and its recurrence.

2.2.1 Prevalence of occupational LBP

Much epidemiological research on LBP has been conducted worldwide. This research is important to understand the past, present and future of LBP, and in obtaining epidemiological data providing much information in helping to seek and solve various problems of LBP. LBP is more common between the ages of 25 and 64 years (WHO 2001). The lifetime prevalence of back pain is reported as over 70% in industrialised countries, and 1-year prevalence varies between 15% and 45% (Andersson, 1999). The incidence of back pain has been reported to be approximately 5% per year (Hoogendoorn, 1999).

In Europe, MSDs represent more than 50% of serious work-related diseases, with a prevalence rate of over 2.5% among employees (more than 4 million employees), (Eurofound, 2007), and 1 in every 4 workers cites problems with backache (Parent-Thirion et al., 2007). However, prevalence of LBP decreased from 33% in 2000 to 24.7% in 2005 in Europe (Paoli & Merllie, 2001; Parent-Thirion et al., 2007). The trend of backache as a musculoskeletal disorder shows an increase in Spain and stability in the Netherlands and Norway (Eurofound, 2007). In the Netherlands, 12-month period prevalence of low back problems was 44.4% in men and 48.2% in women of the working population; about 12% of them had activity limitation (Picavet et al., 1999) and LBP was the most frequent musculoskeletal pain (point prevalence is 26.9%), (Picavet & Schouten, 2003). In UK, 40% of adults reported back pain in the previous 12 months and 15% of adults suffered from back pain throughout the year. 5% of working people with back pain had taken time off work (Department Health, 1999). In the US, about 2% of the US workers were compensated for back injuries each year (Andersson, 1999). The prevalence of back pain in working people was 17.6% in 1988 (Guo et al., 1995). Ghaffari et al. reported that 1-year prevalence was 20% in men and 27% in women, and 1-year incidence of disabling LBP was 2.1% in Iranian industrial workers (Ghaffari et al., 2006a, 2006b). Guo et al. reported that 1-year prevalence was 18.3% in men and 19.7% in women in workers in Taiwan (Guo et al., 2004). It is estimated that 2%-5% of industrial workers experience LBP each year (WHO 2001). Acute low back pain is usually considered to be self-limiting and 90% of LBP recover within 6 weeks, but 2%-7% of people develop chronic pain (The COST B13 Working Group, 2004b). After an initial episode of LBP, 44%-78% people suffer relapses of pain occur 26%-37%, relapses of work absence (The COST B13 Working Group, 2004a). Therefore, it is considered that many people suffered from chronic LBP and this affected individual and social-economic activities. There is little scientific evidence on the prevalence of chronic non-specific back pain: best estimates suggest that the prevalence is approximately 23%; 11%-12% of population are disabled by LBP (The COST B13 Working Group, 2004a). Recurrent and chronic back pain is widely acknowledged to account for a substantial proportion of total worker absenteeism. About half of days lost due to absenteeism are accounted for by the 85% of people away from work for short periods (<7 days), whilst the other half is accounted for by the 15% who are off work for >1 month; this is reflected in the social costs of back pain, where some 80% of the health care and social costs are for the 10% with chronic pain and disability (The COST B13 Working Group, 2004b).

Occupational LBP can occur in all workers in all types of job, though the prevalence varies according to the type of job. Generally, agricultural workers, construction workers, drivers, mine workers and nursing aids show high prevalence (Behrens et al., 1994; Guo et al., 1995; JISHA, 1994; Parent-Thirion et al., 2007), and the variety of prevalence by job type is considered to depend on the kinds, frequency, time, duration and intensity of occupational exposure. It is considered that many causes of LBP exist in work with a high prevalence of LBP. Table 2 shows the reported backache by sector and gender (Eurofound, 2007).

	A	B	C	D	E	F	G	H	I	J	K	L	total
Men	43.8	28.0	24.7	39.2	21.0	20.0	31.4	9.7	16.6	19.7	19.6	21.1	27.0
Women	54.4	31.2	17.2	17.7	18.7	24.9	17.5	14.6	16.7	19.7	22.4	21.2	23.6
Total	47.0	29.0	23.3	37.0	19.8	22.2	27.9	11.9	16.6	19.7	21.7	21.2	25.6

A: Agriculture and fishing, B: Manufacturing and minig, C: Electricity, gas and water supply,
D: Construction, E: Wholesale and retail trade, F: Hotels and restaurants,
G: Transport and communication, H: Financial intermediation, I: Real estate and business servise,
J: Public administration, K: Education and health, L: Other service.

Table 2. Reported backache by sector and gender (Eurofound, 2007)

It is reported that the ranges of a point or annual prevalence of LBP were from 27% to 75% for farmers (Kumudini & Hasegawa, 2009; Liu et al., 2011; Milosavljevic et al., 2011; O'Sullivan et al., 2009; Taechasubamorn et al., 2011), from 44% to 74% for drivers (Alperovitch-Najenson , 2010; Bovenzi, 2009; Rozali et al., 2009), from 32% to 78% for mine workers (Bio et al., 2007; Sarikaya et al., 2007), from 20% to 23% for construction workers (Inaba et al., 2007, 2009), from 46% to 83% for care workers (Jensen et al., 2009; Minematsu, 2007; Sorensen et al., 2011; Yalcinkaya et al., 2010) in recent studies. Guo et al. reported the highest risk of back pain was among construction workers (22.6%) for men and among nursing aides (18.8%) for women (Guo et al., 1995). It is considered that the prevalence of LBP is highest in workers exposed to many occupational risk factors.

2.2.2 Onset of accidental LBP

Prevalence and incidence of occupational LBP are different according to age, gender, type of job, nations and methods of investigation. High physical and high psychosocial exposures increase the risk of symptoms of back disorder (Devereux et al., 1999). It is considered that long working time or experience increases the risk of LBP because occupational exposure time and occupational impact have a negative effect. It is reported that prevalence of back pain in full-time workers is 25.3% compared with 19.1% in part-time workers, and the prevalence of back pain is more than 23% among workers who worked over 36 hours weekly and more than 38% among workers who worked over 45 hours weekly (Eurofound, 2007). In a study of LBP among drivers, an uncomfortable working station (Alperovitch-Najenson, 2010), long career (Szeto & Lam, 2007), high daily vibration exposure (Bovenzi, 2010), annual driving mileage (Porter & Gyi, 2002) and long daily driving time, and cumulative total hours of exposure (Tiemessen et al., 2008) tended to increase the prevalence of back troubles. Moreover, the prevalence of LBP is significantly higher in those currently or previously exposed to manual material handling and/or tiring postures (20%) compared with those never exposed to these strains (11%) in men below the retirement aged 45-59 (Plouvier et al, 2011). Walsh et al. reported that the incident of LBP was 64.5% in men and 61.4% in women, and the rates of sudden and gradual onset LBP were 32.0% in men and 26.3% in women, and 31.5% in men and 33.0% in women, respectively (Walsh et al., 1989). According to their study, the onset of LBP is similar between sudden and gradual in men, but gradual onset of LBP was higher by 7 points than the sudden onset in women. These factors can help to predict the risk of LBP and the prevention of LBP. However, there are few reports that investigate when LBP is likely to occur. As stated above, occupational LBP is separated into accidental LBP and non-accidental LBP. Since the cause of accidental LBP is clear, accidental LBP is certified as liable for worker accident compensation in many cases, as compared with non-accidental LBP.

At present conditions of the onset of accidental LBP in Japan are mentioned based on the report of a preventive measure of LBP by JISHA (JISHA, 1994) and Kuwashima, et al. (Kuwashima et al., 1997). Accidental LBP has been about 6,000 cases per 1 year, according for more than half of all occupational diseases. The survey studied 13,166 cases that were diagnosed as accidental LBP requiring an absence of 4 days or more. In the results, the number of cases per 10,000 working population is 1.5 for male (85.5%) and 0.4 for female (14.5%), respectively. The number of case per 10,000 of the working population by age-specific groups (under 19 years, every 5 years from 20 to 64 years and over 65 years) is from 1.0 to 1.3 from the age of 25 to 59 years and from 0.2 to 0.9 of the remaining age-specific groups, respectively. The onset rate of accidental LBP was about 90% from the age of 25 to 64 years. The onset of accidental LBP is the highest in July (9.1%, 1,203 cases) and the lowest in December (5.8%, 763 cases), but it is found in every month throughout the year (Figure1). Accidental LBP does not tend to occur frequently in winter season. The onset of accidental LBP by day occurs most on Mondays (20.3%) followed by Tuesdays (16.6%) (Figure 2), therefore, accidental LBP tends to occur frequently at the beginning of the week. Also, the onset rates of accidental LBP by time distinction are 11.2%, 16.6% and 14.9% from 8:01 to 9:00, from 9:01 to 10:00 and from 10:01 to 11:00, respectively (Figure 3). The onset of accidental LBP occurs most often in the morning, the rate being 43.1% between 8:00 and 11:00. Moreover, the onset of accidental LBP is more frequent in non-manufacturers (54.7%) than in manufacturers (31.7%). Specifically, traffic and transportation (22.6%), construction (14.5%), and commerce, finance and advertising (10.4%) in the non-manufacturing account for more than 10% of the onset of accidental LBP, on the other hand, mining (13.9) and cargo handling (12.3) account for more than 10 in the number of case per 10,000 of the working population. The accumulated percentage of cases of LBP by duration of employment shows about half are among those employed for less than 5 years.

It is considered that prevention measures for occupational LBP by type of job have many common parts, as the onset of accidental LBP is similar to prevalence of occupational LBP by type of job in other countries. However, as the incidence of occupational LBP in day and time might be different among countries because of life and working style, it is necessary to take prevention measures in the case of frequent occurrence of occupational LBP.

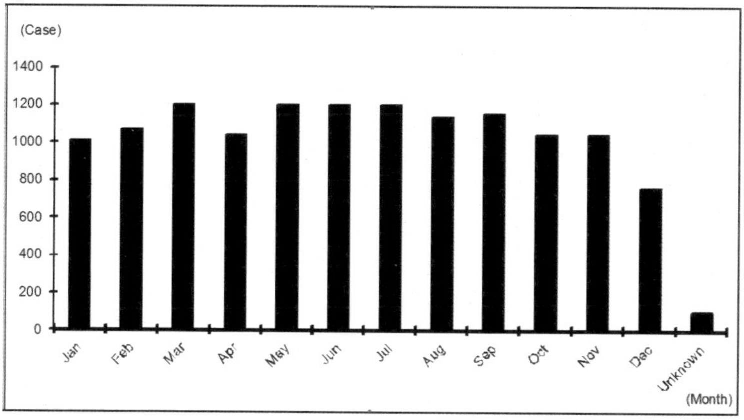

Fig. 1. Onset of LBP by months (JISHA, 1994)

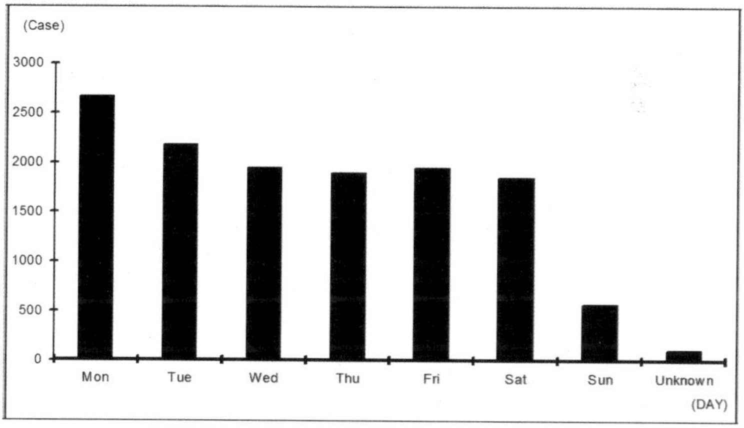

Fig. 2. Onset of LBP by days (JISHA, 1994)

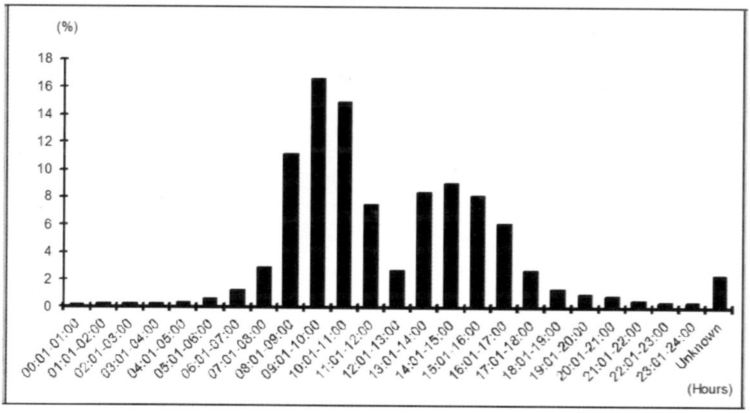

Fig. 3. Onset of LBP by hours (JISHA, 1994)

2.3 Risk factors of occupational LBP

Work-related risk factors in LBP are complex. Physical, psychosocial and personal factors interact in various ways to cause occupational LBP, although the degree of associated with the onset of occupational LBP is different. Namely, these factors have an effect on the incidence of occupational LBP and there is association among these factors (Fig. 4). The influence of these risk factors on LBP are reported, but the results are various.

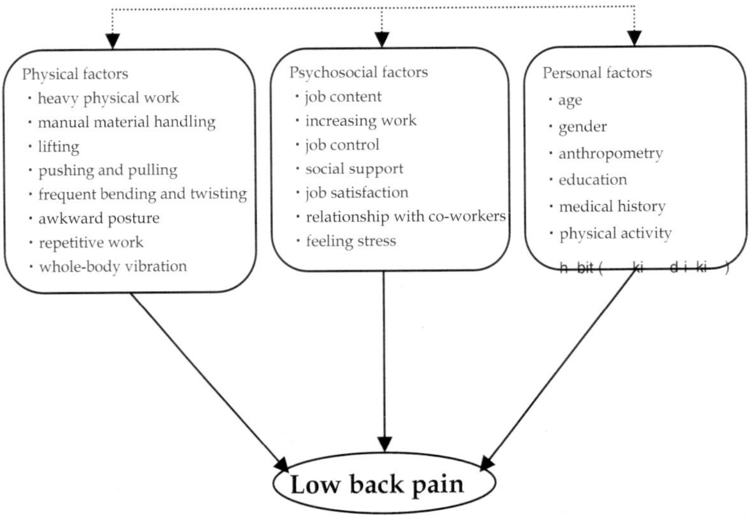

Fig. 4. The relationship of incidence of LBP with physical, psychological and personal factors

Burdorf and Sorock investigated the positive and negative evidence of risk factors for back disorders (Burdorf & Sorock, 1997). They selected 35 studies and estimated the risk of back disorders. Risk estimates of manual material handling, frequent bending and twisting, heavy physical load, static work posture, repetitive movements, and whole-body vibrations for positive associations in physical risk factors at work ranged from 1.12 to 3.07, from 1.29 to 8.09, from 1.54 to 3.71, from 1.30 to 3.29, 1.97, and from 1.47 to 9.00, respectively, and risk estimates of mental stress, job dissatisfaction, work pace, and monotonous work for positive associations in psychological risk factors at work ranged from 1.30 to 2.08, from 1.39 to 2.40, 1.21, and from 1.25 to 2.34, respectively (Burdorf & Sorock, 1997). Thorbjornsson et al., investigated the psychosocial and physical risk factors associated with LBP for over 24 years from 1969 to 1993 (Thorbjornsson et al., 1998). In this study, the prevalence of LBP was 24% among men and 34% among women in 1969, and the cumulative incidence of LBP from 1970 to 1992 were 43% and 38% among men and women, respectively. The prevalence of LBP over the past 12 months in 1993 was 39% among men and 44% among women (Thorbjornsson et al., 1998). Moreover, the highest associations between work related factors and LBP (prevalence ratio adjusted for age) was high physical load (1.4) among men and monotonous work (1.6) among women in 1969, full time work (2.1) among men and high mental load (1.4) among women in 1970-1992, and monotonous work (1.5) among men and poor social support (1.2) among women in 1993, respectively (Thorbjornsson et al., 1998).

These trends of LBP may be caused by the change of the exposure to risk factors and the difference of work by gender.

2.3.1 Physical factors

Physical factors include heavy physical work, manual material handling, lifting, pushing and pulling, frequent bending and twisting, awkward posture, repetitive work, and whole-body vibration (WBV). The one of the causes of LBP by physical factors is the load to disc and back muscles. Disc pressure and muscle activities are changed by posture and way a load is lifted. Fig. 5 and 6 are the figures indicating the change in disc pressure by posture and exercise (Nachemson, 1976).

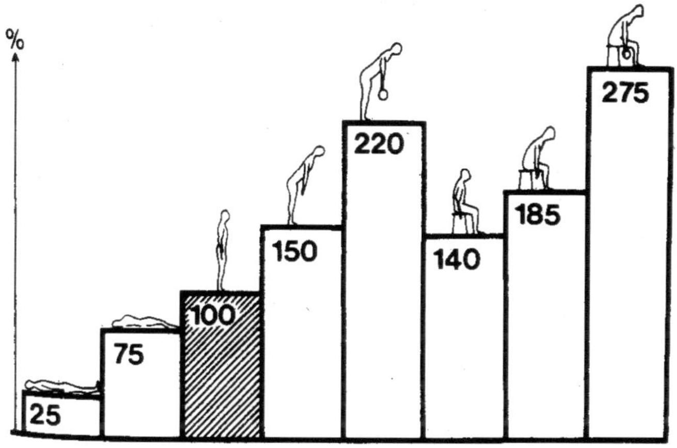

Fig. 5. Relative change in pressure (or load) in the third lumber disc in various positions in living subjects (Nachemson, 1976)

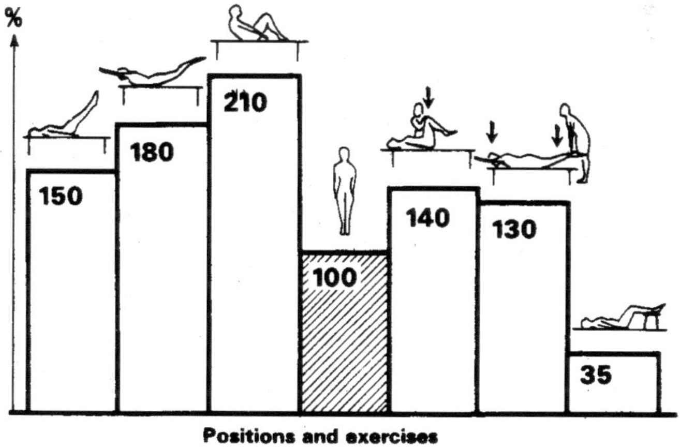

Fig. 6. Relative change in pressure (or load) in the third lumber disc in various muscle-strengthening exercise in living subjects (Nachemson, 1976)

Heavy physical work has been defined as work that has high energy demands or requires some measure of physical strength (Bernard et al., 1997a). The investigation of Bernard et al. provided evidence that low-back disorders are associated with heavy physical work (Bernard et al., 1997a). They selected 18 studies, and odds ratio (OR) and relative risk (RR) in the studies that indicated statistical significance showed the range of 1.2 to 12.1 and 2.2 to 4.3, respectively (Bernard et al., 1997a). Roffey et al. undertook a systematic review of the association of occupational pushing or pulling and workplace manual handling or patient assisting, and LBP (Roffey et al., 2010d, 2010e). Thirteen studies (12,793 participants, 7 countries) that reported a total of 83 estimates of the association between specific categories of occupational pushing or pulling and specific types of LBP outcomes enrolled. The mean prevalence of LBP was 38.1%. Sixteen (19%) were found to be statistically significant and 10 (52%) of which were classified as weak, 4 (24%) were classified as moderate, and 2 (10%) were classified as protective. An equal number of statistically significant estimates were reported in high-quality (50%) versus low-quality studies (50%). They concluded that occupational pushing or pulling does not appear to be independently causative of LBP in workers. There was conflicting evidence for association, though 4 out of 6 high-quality studies did not show any association and only one study with statistically significant weak association indicated a dose-response trend (Roffey et al., 2010d). Additionally, 32 studies (22,143 participants, 16 countries) that reported a total of 329 estimates of the association between specific categories of workplace manual handling or assisting patients, and specific types of LBP outcomes were enrolled (Roffey et al., 2010e). The mean prevalence of LBP was 39.2%. 72 (22%) were reported as statistically significant and of these 72 were statistically significant estimates of association, 49 (68%) were classified as weak, 17 (24%) were classified as moderate, 4 (5%) were classified as strong and 2 (3%) were classified as protective. A difference was noted in the proportion of estimates considered statistically significant from high-quality (38%) versus low-quality studies (62%). They concluded that specific categories of patient assisting could contribute to LBP because of the presence of a combination of strong and conflicting evidence, and assisting patients to ambulate could possibly be associated with disabling types of LBP in the nursing occupation (Roffey et al., 2010e).

Lifting is defined as moving or bringing something from a lower level to a higher one. The concept encompasses stresses resulting from work done in transferring objects from one plane to another, as well as the efforts of varying techniques of patient handling and transfer (Bernard et al., 1997a). Manual materials handling includes lifting, moving, carrying and holding loads. Forceful movements include movement of objects in other ways, such as pulling, pushing, or other efforts (Bernard et al., 1997a). Bernard et al. examined the relationship between back disorders and lifting or forceful movement in 18 studies, and there is strong evidence that low-back disorders are associated with work-related lifting or forceful movement (Bernard et al., 1997a). OR and RR in the studies that indicated statistical significance showed the range of 1.3 to 10.7 and 1.2 to 4.5, respectively (Bernard et al., 1997a). Wai et al. carried out a systematic review of the association of occupational lifting and carrying, and LBP (Wai et al., 2010b, 2010c). Thirty-five studies (88,864 participants, 16 countries) that assessed lifting reported a total of 224 separate estimates of the association between specific categories of occupational lifting and specific type of LBP outcomes were enrolled. The mean prevalence of LBP was 37.2%. 107 (48%) were reported to be statistically significant, and of these 107 statistically significant estimates of association, 33 (31%) were classified as weak, 30 (28%) were classified as moderate, 38 (36%) were classified as strong and6 (5%) were classified as protective. There was noticeable difference in the proportion of estimates considered statistically significant in high-quality (18%) compared with low-quality studies (79%). They concluded that there was some moderate evidence for the association for specific types of lifting and LBP, and some evidence for the association between lifting greater than 25-35kg and LBP (Wai et al., 2010b). Twenty-two studies (27,785 participants, 10 countries) that reported a total of 109 separate risk estimates of the association between specific categories of occupational carrying and specific type of LBP outcomes were enrolled. The mean prevalence of LBP was 33.6%. Twenty-six (24%) were reported to be statistically significant, and of these 26, 15 (58%) were classified as weak, 8 (31%) were classified as moderate and 3 (12%) were classified as strong. There was the marked difference in the proportion of estimates considered statistically significant for high-quality (2%) compared with low-quality studies (35%). They concluded that there was strong and consistent evidence against both an association and temporal relationship between carrying and LBP, and there was no independent causal relationship between carrying and LBP (Wai et al., 2010c).

Bending is defined as flexion of the trunk, usually in the forward or lateral direction. Twisting refers to trunk rotation or torsion. Awkward postures include non-neutral trunk postures (related to bending and twisting) in extreme positions or at extreme angles (Bernard et al., 1997a). Bernard et al. selected 12 studies and investigated the relationship between back disorders and bending, twisting and awkward postures. The evidence of association with low-back disorders and awkward postures was shown (Bernard et al., 1997a). Results were consistent in showing increased risk of back disorder with exposure, despite the fact that studies defined disorders and assessed exposures in many ways. OR in the studies that indicated statistical significance showed the range of 1.2 to 8.1 (Bernard et al., 1997a). In a systematic review of the association of occupational bending or twisting and LBP by Wai et al., 35 studies (44,342 participants, 15 countries) that reported a total of 243 estimates of the association between specific categories of bending or twisting and specific types of LBP outcomes were enrolled. The mean prevalence of LBP was 38.7%. 107 (44%) were reported as statistically significant, and of these 107 statistically significant estimates of association, 61 (57%) were classified as weak, 20 (19%) were classified as moderate and 26 (24%) were classified as strong. No difference was noted in the proportion of estimates considered as statistically significant for high-quality (30%) versus low-quality studies (32%). They concluded that occupational bending or twisting is unlikely to be independently causative of LBP in workers and the strength of association was often rated as weak or moderate, additionally none demonstrated a statistically significant dose response (Wai et al., 2010a).

Static work postures include isometric positions where very little movement occurs, along with cramped or inactive postures that cause static loading on the muscles. These included prolonged standing or sitting and sedentary work. In many cases, the exposure was defined subjectively and/or in combination with other work-related risk factors (Bernard et al., 1997a). Bernard et al. selected 10 studies and resulted that the evidence of association with back disorders and static postures was inadequate though it is not easy to estimate the strength of association for some reasons (Bernard et al., 1997a). OR and RR showed in the studies that indicated statistical significance the range of 1.3 to 24.6 and 1.7 to 2.4, respectively (Bernard et al., 1997a). Roffey et al. carried out a systematic review of the association of 3 factors, awkward occupational postures, occupational sitting, and occupational standing or walking, and LBP (Roffey et al., 2010a, 2010b, 2010c). Twenty seven studies (69,980 participants, 14 countries) that reported a total of 111 estimates of the association between specific categories of awkward occupational postures and specific types of LBP outcomes were enrolled. The mean prevalence of LBP was 47.8%. Fifty-three (48%) were reported as statistically significant, and of these 53 statistically significant estimates of association, 35 (66%) were classified as weak, 9 (17%) were classified as moderate, 4 (7%) were classified as strong and 3 (6%) were classified as protective. There was a difference noted in the proportion of estimates considered statistically significant for high-quality (35%) versus low-quality studies (57%). They concluded that awkward occupational postures do not appear to be independently causative of LBP in workers, and the strength of association was rated as weak, and only one study demonstrated a trend toward a nonstatistically significant dose response. They added that awkward postures could have an association with severe types of LBP in certain working populations, but causal relationship with LBP seems unlikely because of the conflicting or lack of strong evidence identified for the association from their results (Roffey et al., 2010a). Twenty-four studies (75,103 participants, 12 countries) that reported a total of 108 separate estimates of the association between specific categories of occupational sitting and specific types of LBP outcomes were enrolled. The mean prevalence of LBP was 42.2%. Seventeen (16%) were reported to be statistically significant and of these 17 statistically significant estimates, 3 (18%) were classified as weak and 14 (82%) were classified as protective. There was a marked difference in the proportion of estimates considered statistically significant for high-quality (0%) versus low-quality studies (100%). They concluded that occupational sitting does not appear to be independently causative of LBP in workers and the strength of evidence suggesting no association was consistent and rated as strong, with only one study demonstrating a trend toward a nonstatistically significant dose response (Roffey et al., 2010b). Eighteen studies (31,810 participants, 10 countries) that reported a total of 84 estimates of the association between specific categories of occupational standing or walking and specific types of LBP outcomes were enrolled. The mean prevalence of LBP was 43.2%. 21 (25%) were reported to be statistically significant and of these 21 statistically significant estimates, 11 (52%) were classified as weak, 5 (24%) were classified as moderate and 2 (10%) were classified as protective. A difference was noted between the numbers of statistically significant estimates that came from high-quality (19%) versus low-quality studies (81%). They concluded that occupational standing or walking is unlikely to be independently causative of LBP in workers, but if a causal relationship between occupational standing and LBP were to exist, it would likely to be a very weak one and only likely in specific sub categories (Roffey et al., 2010c).

WBV refers to mechanical energy oscillations which are transferred to the body as a whole (in contrast to specific body regions), usually through a supporting system such as a seat or platform. Typical exposures include driving automobiles and trucks, and operating industrial vehicles (Bernard et al., 1997a). Nineteen studies were selected and there is strong evidence of the positive association between exposure to WBV and back disorder though 4 of 19 studies demonstrated no association. OR and RR in the studies that indicated statistical significance showed the range of 1.2 to 39.5 and 1.7, respectively (Bernard et al., 1997). Lis et al. reported that occupational groups exposed to WBV while sitting are at an increased risk of having LBP (OR is over 1.7), and the influence of the duration of the exposure seems more important than the magnitude of the exposure in cumulative effect, though sitting by itself did not increase the association with the present LBP (Lis et al., 2007).

2.3.2 Psychosocial factors

Psychosocial factors are defined as factors influencing health, health services and community well-being stemming from the psychology of the individual and the structure and function of social groups. They include social characteristics such as patterns of interaction within family or occupational groups, cultural characteristics such as traditional ways of solving conflicts, and psychological characteristics such as attitudes, beliefs and personality factors (WHO, 2001). Bongers et al. showed 5 categories of factors that may be associated with musculoskeletal symptoms:

1. psychosocial factors at work - demands and control (monotonous work, time pressure, high concentration, high responsibilities, high work load, few opportunities to take breaks, lack of clarity, and low control and little autonomy),
2. psychosocial factors at work - social support (poor social support from colleagues and poor social support from superiors),
3. individual characteristics (personality type, type A behaviour, extrovert personality, psychological dysfunctioning, coping style, attitude towards own health, low social class and low educational level),
4. stress symptoms (worry, tension, anxiety, physical stress symptoms, fatigue or exhaustion, high perceived work stress, low job satisfaction, and physiological parameters), and
5. physical and behavioural health indicators (poor physician health, respiratory disease or cough, stomach trouble, cardiovascular disease, headache, use of mediation and use of medical service), (Bongers et al., 1993).

Bernerd et al. investigated the association of psychosocial factors with back disorder (Bernard et al., 1997b). 4 of 5 studies that included measures of intensified work load found significant associations between back disorders and perceptions of intensified work load as measured by indices of both perceived time pressure and work load (OR 1.2-2.9). 5 of 7 studies that assess job dissatisfaction also found positive associations with back disorders. One study examined the relationship between social support and back disorders and found only weak evidence for an association.

In a systematic review by Hoogendoorn et al. including 11 cohort and 2 case-control studies, strong evidence was found for low social support in the workplace and low job satisfaction as risk factors for back pain (Hoogendoorn et al., 2000). Also, in the cohort study of 861 workers in Hoogendoorn et al., cumulative incidence of LBP during 3 years follow-up period was 26.6% (Hoogendoorn et al., 2001). The strongest relationships with LBP were found for high quantitative job demands, low supervisory support and low co-worker support (RR 1.3-1.6). However, most of the relationships were not statistically significant. They concluded that low co-worker and supervisory support appeared to be risk factors of LBP.

In a systematic review by Bongers et al. the associations between self-reported work demands (particularly monotonous work), poor social support at work, personality traits and emotional problems, and stress symptoms, and back trouble were reported (Bongers et al., 1993).

It is considered that low job satisfaction and low social support are associated with LBP, but it is unclear as to the associations between psychosocial factors and LBP. Davis and Heaney hypothesized as to the mechanisms of the relationship between psychosocial factors and LBP. First, psychosocial factors are directly related to LBP by influencing the loading on the spine via changes in trunk kinetics, the forces exerted or muscle activity. Second, psychosocial factors influence various chemical reactions in the body that take place during the performance of job tasks. Third, psychosocial factors influence the reporting of an injury by altering tolerance to pain (Davis & Heaney, 2000). They concluded that job satisfaction and job stress (workers reaction to psychosocial work characteristics) are more consistently and more strongly associated with LBP than are psychosocial work characteristics themselves and stated that not only the relationship between job satisfaction and LBP, but also the relationship between physical and psychosocial work characteristics and job satisfaction are needed to investigate in research (Davis & Heaney, 2000).

2.3.3 Personal factors

The common personal factors are age, gender, anthropometry, posture, muscle strength, muscle imbalances, spine mobility, education, medical history, physical fitness, habit (e.g. smoking) and socioeconomic conditions.

Most people experienced their first episode of back pain before 35yeras (Guo et al., 1995). In a European study, a prevalence of 18% was found before 25 years and 24% at 55 years and older (Parent-Thirion et al., 2007). The prevalence is relatively consistent during their working years (Guo et al., 1995). Generally, age and years of work are correlated, as the length of duration of work increases with advancing age. Moreover, the longer the years of work the greater the occupational exposure, additionally the likelihood of disc degeneration and herniation increases with aging. In a systematic review by Burdorf and Sorock, 12 studies reported positive association between age and back disorders, and 15 studies demonstrated no associations out of 30 studies (Burdorf & Sorock, 1997). Though pregnancy (Mogren, 2005) and osteoporotic fractures (Rostom, 2011) which are characteristic of women are causes of LBP, these are not work-related factors. Of course, LBP caused by these factors could possibly lead to leaving work and absence. The prevalence of back pain is equal among men (27%) and women (22%), (Parent-Thirion, 2007), though it is reported that prevalence of LBP is higher in girls than in boys at school age (Jones & Macfarlane, 2009; Mohseni-Bandpei et al., 2007; Watson et al., 2002; Yao et al., 2011). The attributable proportion of occupational LBP was higher for men than women (Punnett, 2005), and the results are very widespread. Occurrence of LBP by gender is considered to be related to differing participation in the various occupations.

It is reported that associations between anthropometry (sitting and standing height, weight, body mass index, trunk asymmetry or kyphosis) and LBP are null or a weak association in children (Kaspiris, 2010; Nissinen, 1994; Poussa, 2005). In adults, Pope et al. reported no associations between anthropometry and LBP (Pope, 1984). However, a weak association is shown between body weight and LBP (Leboeuf-Yde, 2000), and obesity (high body mass index) associated with LBP (Heuch, 2010).

Spine mobility, muscle strength and posture are included in the examination for LBP. Reduction of spine mobility and muscle strength, change of posture and activity, and disable walking are seen in most subjects with LPB due to pain in many cases. However, spine mobility or muscle strength seems to have poor association with the incidence of LBP, as it is considered that these losses are secondary (Andersson, 1992). Hamberg-van Reenen et al. in systematic review found that strong evidence that there was no relationship between trunk muscle endurance and the risk of LBP. Moreover, inconclusive evidence for a relationship between trunk muscle strength or mobility of lumbar spine and the risk of LBP was found (Hamberg-van Reenen et al., 2007). There is the report that sagittal spine mobility, static spinal posture, muscle endurance and spinal repositioning error show no difference between subjects with LBP and without LBP (Mitchell et al., 2009). Conflicting evidence is found for the association between physical activity and LBP in the general population and in school children in 10 high-quality studies (Sitthipornvorakul, 2011). They reported high level physical activity at leisure time related to decreased prevalence of LBP and high level physical activity at work combined with low physical activity in leisure time associated with high prevalence of LBP. Also, Heneweer et al. in systematic review reported that there was strong evidence that intense physical exertion during leisure time (regular home improvement activities and high perceived load in, and regular and high intensity sports, and physical exercise in the upper percentile) was moderately (1.0-2.6) associated with LBP, and everyday physical activities in leisure time and the performance of gardening/yard work were found to be strongly (0.20-0.76) to moderately (0.38-0.80) associated with decreased risk for LBP (Heneweer, 2011).

In the relationship between socioeconomic status and LBP, most studies concluded education is strongly associated with LBP, with a high prevalence and risk of LBP for those with low educational level (Astrand, 1987; Latza et al., 2004; Leclerc et al., 2009; Leino-Arjas et al., 1998). In addition, it is reported that prevalence and risk of LBP is high for those with low-income occupational status and manual workers. Latza et al. also reported that severe current back pain was related to educational level and health insurance status, and members of sick funds for white-collar workers (OR 2.81) and private insurance (OR 2.81) and individuals with intermediate educational level (OR 1.76) utilized more physical therapy for the treatment of back pain (Latza et al., 2004). Severe LBP was less prevalent among adults of higher socioeconomic status (Latza et al., 2000).

It is reported that LBP is associated with smoking in lifestyle factors, though the risk of LBP is depended on smoking history (OR 1.15-1.46 in men), (Leino-Arjas et al., 1998). Smoking is positively associated with both prevalent and future LBP (OR 1.38-6.38), (Hestbaek, 2006). Leboeuf-Yde et al. reported that there was a significant positive association between smoking and LBP that increased with the duration and frequency of the LBP problem, but this association was not appeared in monozygotic twins (Leboeuf-Yde et al., 1998). Leboeuf-Yde also concluded that smoking should be considered a weak risk indicator and not a cause of LBP (Leboeuf-Yde, 1999).

2.4 Prevention of occupational LBP

Both workers and managers should make efforts to prevent occupational LBP. Improvement of work conditions and the working environment leads to workers' understanding of occupational health issues. The three main preventive approaches as concepts are:

1. Designing the job to fit the worker,
2. Selecting the appropriate worker for the job, and
3. Teaching the worker to use the correct work method (Andersson, 1991).

Moreover, prevention measures are different dependent on the stage of occupational LBP i.e. before and after the occurrence of occupational LBP, and acute, sub-acute or chronic LBP. Classic preventive medicine divides prevention into three categories: primary, secondary and tertiary prevention. Primary prevention of occupational LBP is designed to prevent the onset of LBP by avoiding or decreasing as thoroughly as possible the risk factors that are shown by epidemiological study. Therefore, the health care professional should know what constitutes LBP risk. Occupational factors are more important for disability than for disease or injury, and few individual risk factors hold up to scientific scrutiny. The three main alternatives in primary prevention are a pre-employment screening programme, improvements in work habits and changes at the workplace. Secondary prevention is designed to share knowledge about the risks of, or the problems associated with, LBP, with the added problem of early disease (risk) detection. In tertiary prevention, selection of the appropriate therapy to reduce the disability and chronicity of LBP and to prevent recurrence may be the most immediate and practical prevention method. However, this would be totally redundant if primary prevention could be made effective (Andersson, 1991).

In Japan, the guidelines for prevention of LBP (Ministry of Labour, 1994) concretely show how to exclude causes of LBP and how to promote the maintenance and improvement of workers' conditions:

1. work management: a) automation and saving of labour, b) working postures and movements, c) working standards, d) breaks, and e) others,
2. work environmental management: a) temperature, b) lighting, c) flooring conditions for work, d) working space, and e) equipment arrangement,
3. health management: a) pre-employment and periodic medical examination, post-measures, and b) doing exercise before work (warming up) and exercise against LBP,
4. education for occupational health: a) education for occupational health and others.

In addition, the guidelines mention specific measures about 5 types of work (heavy load handling, care work in facilities for severe physically and mentally disabled children, standing work with excessive burden to the back, sitting posture with excessive burden to the back and driving for a long time) where LBP occurs comparatively frequently (Ministry of Labour, 1994). The guidelines demand improvement of working condition and the working environment by the enterprises or employer.

Prevention of occupational LBP is designed to reduce workplace risk at first. This requires the reduction of physical demands by improvement of the workplace (safe working environment such as enough space, arrangement of equipment adapting to workers and temperature), work task (saving of works such as automation, reduction of the weight, shape and size of the load and movement distance), work organization (duration and frequency of loading, rests and supports among workers) and the provision of education and training. The National Institute for Occupational Safety and Health (NIOSH) shows how to improve the workplace (engineering and administrative improvements) in ergonomic guidelines for manual material handling (Cheung et al., 2007). This guideline explains the safety methods for manual material handling in the workplace with pictures.

Carter and Brirrell edited "occupational health guidelines for the management of low back pain at work" (Carter & Brirrell, 2000) and Waddell et al. reported evidence in a review of these guidelines (Waddell & Burrton, 2001). In prevention, there were 3 strong pieces of evidences (provided by generally consistent findings in multiple, high quality studies), 2 limited or contradictory findings (provided by one scientific study or inconsistent findings in multiple scientific studies) and 1 finding with no scientific evidence (based on clinical studies, theoretical consideration and/or clinical consensus) (Carter & Brirrell, 2000; Waddell & Burrton, 2001), (Table 3).

Strong evidence
Traditional biomechanical education based on an injury model does not reduce future LBP and work loss.
Lumbar belts or supports do not reduce work-related LBP and work loss.
Low job satisfaction and unsatisfactory psychosocial aspects of work are risk factors for reported LBP, health care use and work loss, but the size of that association is modest.
Limited or contradictory evidence
Various general exercise/physical fitness programmes may reduce future LBP and work loss; any effect size appears to be modest.
Joint employer-worker initiatives can reduce the number of reported back injuries and sickness absences, but there is no clear evidence on the optimum strategies and inconsistent evidence on the effect size.
No scientific evidence
Educational interventions which specifically address beliefs and attitudes may reduce future work loss due to LBP.

Table 3. Evidences of prevention of LBP (Carter & Brirrell, 2000; Waddell & Burrton, 2001)

Personal preventions of LBP include an exercise programme for improvement of muscle strength, muscle flexibility, muscle balance and spinal movement, back belts and education before onset LBP. Additionally, rest, traction, joint mobilization, acupuncture, physical therapy, hydrotherapy, electrical therapy and behavioural treatment can be used. European guidelines for the prevention of LBP indicate the interventions for prevention of LBP and evaluate the interventions at the evidence level A to D (The COST B13 Working Group, 2004b). The strength of recommendations is based on the 4-level rating: Level A is generally consistent findings provided by (a systematic review of) multiple RCTs, Level B is generally consistent findings provided by (a systematic review of) multiple weaker scientific studies, Level C is one RCT/weaker scientific study or inconsistent findings provided by (a systematic review of) multiple weaker scientific studies and Level D is no RCTs or no weaker scientific studies. The guidelines focus on providing a set of evidence-based recommendations to prevent LBP and/or its consequences in the workforce. Interventions aim at preventing LBP in the workforce can be categorized into 1) individual focus, 2) physical ergonomics, and 3) organizational ergonomics. Recommendation shows in Table 4.

It is difficult to prevent LBP because there are many factors that contribute to LBP and preventive effects can be different according to each individual. Therefore, appropriate prevention of LBP needs to be provided against future LBP, recurrence of LBP, chronic LBP, worsening LBP and so on.

Physical exercise / physical activity Recommendation. Physical exercise may be recommended in prevention of LBP (Level A). Physical exercise may be recommended in prevention recurrence of LBP (Level A) and in prevention recurrence of sick leave due to LBP (Level C). Information / advice / instruction Recommendation. Traditional information/advice/instruction on biomechanics, lifting techniques, optimal postures etc is not recommended for prevention in LBP (Level A). there is insufficient evidence to recommended for or against psychosocial information delivered at the worksite (Level C), but information oriented toward promoting activity and improving coping, can promote a positive shift in beliefs (Level C). Whilst the evidence is not sufficiently consistent to recommend education in the prevention of recurrence of sick leave due to LBP (Level C), incorporating the messages from the accompanying clinical guidelines into workplace information/advice is encouraged. Back belts / lumber supports Recommendation. Back belts/lumber supports are not recommended for prevention in LBP (Level A). Shoe inserts, shoe orthoses, shoe in-soles, flooring and mats Recommendation. Shoe inserts/shoe orthoses are not recommended for prevention in LBP (Level A). There is insufficient evidence to recommend for or against shoe in-soles, soft shoes, soft flooring or antifatigue floor mats (Level D). Physical ergonomics Recommendation. There is insufficient consistent evidence to recommended physical ergonomics interventions alone for reduction of the prevalence and severity of LBP (Level C). There is insufficient consistent evidence to recommended physical ergonomics interventions alone for reduction of [reported] back injuries, occupational or compensable LBP (Level C). There is some evidence that, to be successful, a physical ergonomics programme would need an organisational dimension and involvement of the workers (Level B). There is insufficient evidence to specify precisely the useful content of such interventions (Level C), and the size of any effect may be modest. Organisational ergonomics Recommendation. There is insufficient consistent evidence to recommend stand-alone work organisational interventions alone for prevention in LBP (Level C), yet such interventions could, in principle, enhance the effectiveness of physical ergonomics programmes. Modified work for return to work after sick leave due to LBP Recommendation. Temporary modified work (which may include ergonomic workplace adaptations) can be recommended, when needed, in order to facilitate earlier return to work for workers sick listed due to LBP (Level B)

Table 4. Summary of recommendations of the interventions for prevention of LBP for workers (The COST B13 Working Group, 2004b)

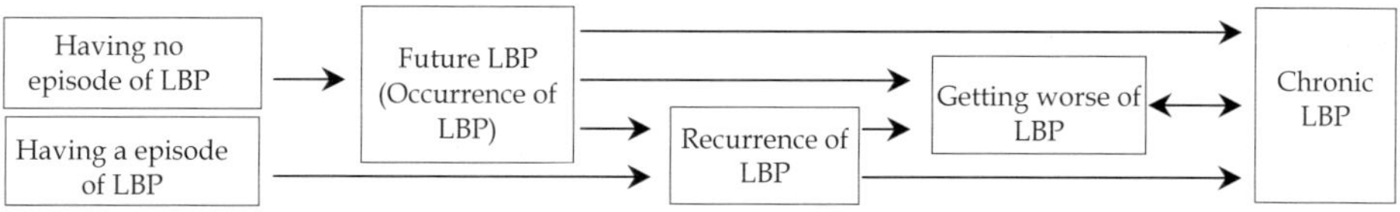

Fig. 7. Prevention and/or intervention of LBP are needed on the every stage (arrows).

3. Conclusion

Many people suffer from LBP. It is considered that the lifetime prevalence of LBP ranged from 50% to 80% and about half of the population experienced LBP in a year. As occupational LBP can occur in most workers in various jobs, it is both an individual and social problems. Accidental LBP tends to occur in the morning (8:00-11:00) at the beginning of week. It is considered that there is the evidence that increased risk of LBP is associated with heavy physical work, manual material handling, awkward posture and whole body vibration among physical factors, and job dissatisfaction and low social support among the psychosocial factors and socioeconomic status (low education and occupational status) among the personal factors. These factors interact with the onset of LBP directly or indirectly. Therefore, employers must take measures to reduce the risk factors for LBP by improvement of the workplace, work task and work-organization designs, and education and training. Workers must take measures to prevent LBP similar to those undertaken by employers. There is evidence that physical exercise may be recommended in the prevention of LBP and the prevention of the recurrence of LBP. It is considered that prevention of LBP can be effective if the exercise programme matches the individuals, as there is contradictory evidence and any effect in reducing LBP by various general exercise programmes. We should take suitable measures fitting the stages (i.e. future LBP, present LBP and continuous LBP) to prevent LBP, disability and so on. Needless to say, it is important to make sure of the causes of LBP in the past, present and future. Therefore, health care professionals should understand the risk factors for LBP and fully understand the subjects with LBP and their circumstances. These should be applied to all workers.

4. Acknowledgment

I borrowed the books of occupational LBP and musculoskeletal disorders from Professor Kurumatani and Dr. Tomioka in the Department of Community Health and Epidemiology, Nara Medical University, School of Medicine. I thank them deeply.

5. References

Alperovitch-Najenson, D., et al. (2010). Low back pain among professional bus drivers: ergonomic and occupational-psychosocial risk factors. *The Israel Medical Association Journal*, Vol.12, No.1, (January 2010), pp.26-31, ISSN 1565-1088

Andersson, G.B.J. (1981). Epidemiological aspects on low-back pain in industry: *Spine*, Vol.6, No.1, (January-February 1981), pp. 53-60, ISSN 0362-2436

Andersson, G.B.J. (1991). Concepts in Prevention. In: *Occupational Low Back Pain: Assessment, Treatment and Prevention*, M.H. Pope, et al. (Eds.), 211-216, Mosby Year Book, ISBN 0-8016-6252-4, St Louis, USA

Andersson, G.B.J. (1992). Factors important in the genesis and prevention of occupational back pain and disability. *Journal of manipulative and physiological therapeutics*, Vol.15, No.1, (January 1992), pp. 43-46, ISSN 0161-4754

Andersson, G.B.J. (1999). Epidemiological features of chronic low-back pain. *The Lancet*, Vol.354, No.9178, (August 1999), pp. 581-585, ISSN 0140-6736

Aoyama, H. (1984). Background of the issue of low back pain in a place of work. In: *Occupational low back pain*, E. Aoyama & K. Akashi (Eds.), Rodo-Chosakai, 17-26, ISBN 4-89782-710-8, Tokyo, Japan (In Japanese)

Astrand N.E. (1987). Medical, psychological, and social factors associated with backabnormalities and self reported back pain: a cross sectional study of male employees in a Swedish pulp and paper industry. *British Journal of Industrial Medicine*, Vol.44, No.5, (May 1987), pp.327-336, ISSN 0007-1072

Badley, E.M. & Tennant, A. (1992). Changing profile of joint disorders with age: findings from a postal survey of the population of Calderdale, West Yorkshire, United Kingdom. *Annals of the Rheumatic Diseases*, Vol.51, No.3, (March 1992), pp. 366-371, ISSN 0003-4967

Behrens, V., et al. (1994). The prevalence of back pain, hand discomfort, and dermatitis in the US working population. *American Journal of Public Health*, Vol.84, No11., (November 1994), pp.1780-1785, ISSN 0090-0036

Bernard, B.P. et al. (1997a). Low-Back Musculoskeletal Disorders: Evidence for Work-Relatedness. In: *Musculoskeletal Disorders and Workplace Factors*, B.P. Bernard (Ed.), National Institute for Occupational Safety and Health, 6.1-6.96, Colombia, USA, Avairable from http://www.cdc.gov/niosh

Bernard, B.P. et al. (1997b). Work-Related Musculoskeletal Disorders and Psychosocial Factors. In: *Musculoskeletal Disorders and Workplace Factors*, B.P. Bernard (Ed.), National Institute for Occupational Safety and Health, 7.1-7.16, Colombia, USA, Avairable from http://www.cdc.gov/niosh

Bio, F., et al. (2007). Low back pain in underground gold miners in ghana. *Ghana Medical Journal*, Vol.41, No.1, (March 2007), pp.21-25, ISSN 0016-9560

Bongers, P.M., et al. (1993). Psychosocial factors at work and musculoskeletal disease. *Scandinavian Journal of Work Environment & Health*, Vol.19, No.5, (October 1993), pp.258-267, ISSN 0355-3140

Bovenzi M. (2009). Metrics of whole-body vibration and exposure-response relationship for low back pain in professional drivers: a prospective cohort study. *International archives of occupational and environmental health*, Vol.82, No.7, (July 2009), pp.893-917, ISSN 0340-0131

Bovenzi, M. (2010). A longitudinal study of low back pain and daily vibration exposure in professional drivers. *Industrial Health*, Vol.48, No.5, (May 2010), pp.584-595, ISSN 0019-8366

Brooks, P.M. (2006). The burden of musculoskeletal disease - a global perspective. *Clinical Rheumatology*, Vol.25, No.6, (November 2006), pp. 778-781, ISSN 0770-3198

Brownson, R.C. (1998). Epidemiology: The foundation of publich health, In: *Applied Epidemiology*. Theory to practice, R.C. Brownson & D.B. Petitti, (Eds.), 3-34, Oxford University Press, ISBN 0-19-511190-7, New York, USA

Burdorf, A. & Sorock, G. (1997). Positive and negative evidence of risk factors for back disorders. *Scandinavian Journal of Work, Environment and Health,* Vol.23, No.4, (August 1997), pp.243-256, ISSN 0355-3140

Carter, J.T. & Brirrell, L.N. (2000). *Occupational Health Guidelines for the Management of Low Back Pain at Work.* Faculty of Occupational Medicine, London, UK, www.Facoccmed.ac.uk

Cassidy, J.D. et al. (1998). The Saskatchewan health and back pain survey. The prevalence of low back pain and related disability in Saskatchewan adults. *Spine,* Vol.23, No.17, (September 1998), pp.1860-1866, ISSN 0362-2436

Cassidy, J.D. et al. (2005). Incidence and course of low back pain episodes in the general population. *Spine,* Vol.30, No.24, (December 2005), pp.2817-2823, ISSN 0362-2436

Cheuing, M.S. et al. (2007). *Ergonomic guidelines for manual material handling,* M.S. Cheuing et al. (Eds), National *Institute for Occupational Safety and Health,* Available from www.cdc.gov/niosh/docs/2007-131/pdfs/2007-131.pdf

Cunningham, L.S. & Kelsey, J.L. (1984) Epidemiology of musculoskeletal impairments and associated disability. *American Journal of Public Health and the Nation's Health,* Vol.74, No.6, (June 1984), pp.574-579, ISSN 0090-0036

Dagenais, S., et al. (2008). A systematic review of low back pain cost of illness studies in the United States and internationally. *The Spine Journal,* Vol.8, No.1, (January-February 2008), pp. 8-20, ISSN 1529-9430

Davis, K.G & Heaney, C.A. (2000). The relationship between psychosocial work characteristics and low back pain: underlying methodological issues. *Clinical Biomechanics,* Vol.15, No.6, (July 2000), pp.389-406, ISSN 0268-0033

Department of Health. (1999). *The prevalence of back pain in Great Britain in 1998.* Available from www.dh.gov.uk/en/Publicationsandstatistics/Publications/PublicationsStatistics/DH_4006687

Devereux, J.J., et al. (1999). Interactions between physical and psychological risk factors at work increase the risk of back disorders: an epidemiological approach. *Occupational and Environmental Medicine,* Vol.56, No.5, (May 1999), pp. 343-353, ISSN 1351-0711

European Foundation for the Improvement of Living and Working Conditions. (2007). *Managing musculoskeletal disorders,* Eurofound, Dublin 2007

Freburger, J.K., et al. (2009). The rising prevalence of chronic low back pain. *Archives of Internal Medicine,* Vol.169, No.3, (February 2009), pp. 251-258, ISSN 0003-9926

Ghaffari, M., et al. (2006a). Low back pain in Iranian industrial workers. *Occupational Medicine,* Vol.56, No.7, (October 2006), pp. 455-460, ISSN 0962-7480

Ghaffari, M., et al. (2006b). Incidence and recurrence of disabling low back pain and neck-shoulder pain. *Spine,* Vol.31, No.21, (October 2006), pp. 2500-2506, ISSN 0362-2436

Guo, H.R., et al. (1995). Back pain among workers in the United States: national estimates and workers at high risk. *American Journal of Industrial Medicine,* Vol.28, No.5, (November 1995), pp.591-602, ISSN 0271-3586

Guo, H.R., et al. (2004). Plevalence of musculoskeletal disorder among workers in Taiwan: a nationwide study. *Journal of Occupational Health,* Vol.46, No.1, (January 2004), pp.26-36, ISSN 1341-9145

Hamberg-van Reenen, H.H., et al. (2007). A systematic review of the relation between physical capacity and future low back and neck/shoulder pain. *Pain*, Vol.130, No.1-2, (July 2007), pp.93-107, ISSN 0304-3959

Heliovaara, M. & Riihimaki, H. (2006). Musculoskeletal diseases. In: *Health in Finland (Koskinen, S., et al eds.)*, 64-65, National Public Health Institute KTL, National Research and Development Center for Welfare and Health STAKES, and Ministry of Social Affairs and Health, ISBN 951-740-631-2, Helsinki, Finland

Heneweer, H., et al. (2011). Physical activity and low back pain: a systematic review of recent literature. *European Spine Journal*. Vol.20, No.6, (June 2011), pp.826-845, ISSN 0940-6719

Hestbaek, L., Leboeuf-Yde, & Manniche, C. (2003) Low back pain: what is the long-term course? A review of studies of general patient populations. *European Spine Journal*, Vol.12, No.2, (April 2003), pp.149-165, ISSN 0940-6719

Hestbaek, L., Leboeuf-Yde, C. & Kyvik, K.O. (2006). Are lifestyle-factors in adolescence predictors for adult low back pain? A cross-sectional and prospective study of young twins. *BMC Musculoskeletal Disords*, Vol.7, (March 2006), pp.27, ISSN 1471-1474

Heuch, I., et al. (2010). The impact of body mass index on the prevalence of low back pain: the HUNT study. *Spine*, Vol.35, No.7, (April 2010), pp.,764-768 ISSN 0362-2436

Hillman, M., et al. (1996). Prevalence of low back pain in the community: implications for service provision in Bradford, UK. *Journal of epidemiology and community health*, Vol.50, No.3, (June 1996), pp.347-352, ISSN 0143-005X

Hoogendoorn, W.E., et al. (1999). Physical load during work and leisure time as risk factors for back pain. *Scandinavian Journal of Work, Environment & Health*, Vol.25, No.5, (October 1999), pp.387-403, ISSN 0355-3140

Hoogendoorn, W.E., et al. (2000). Systematic review of psychosocial factors at work and private life as risk factors for back pain. *Spine*, Vol.25, No.16, (august 2000), pp.2114-2125, ISSN 0362-2436

Hoogendoorn, W.E., et al. (2001). Psychosocial work characteristics and psychological strain in relation to low-back pain. *Scandinavian Journal of Work Environment & Health*, Vol.27, No.4, (August 2001), pp.258-267, ISSN 0355-3140

Hoy, D., et al. (2010). The epidemiology of low back pain. *Best Practice & Research. Clinical Rheumatology*, Vol.24, No.6, (December 2010), pp. 769-781, ISSN 1521-6942

Ihlebaek, C., et al. (2006). Prevalence of low back pain and sickness absence: a "borderline" study in Norway and Sweden. *Scandinavian Journal of Public Health*, Vol.34, No.5, (October 2006), pp. 555-558, ISSN 1403-4948

Inaba, R., Kurokawa, J & Mirbod, S.M. (2009). Comparison of subjective symptoms and cold prevention measures in winter between traffic control workers and construction workers in Japan. *Industrial Health*, Vol.47, No.3, (July 2009), pp.283-291, ISSN 0019-8366

Inaba, R. & Mirbod, S.M. (2007). Comparison of subjective symptoms and hot prevention measures in summer between traffic control workers and construction workers in Japan. *Industrial Health*, Vol.45, No.1, (January 2007), pp.91-99, ISSN 0019-8366

Japan Industrial Safety & Health Association. (1994). Epidemiology of accidental low back pain. In: *Report of a preventive measure of low back pain in the investigation committee (Yamamoto, S., chairman),* 2-21, Japan Industrial Safety & Health Association (In Japanese)

Jensen, J.N., et al. (2009). The predictive effect of fear-avoidance beliefs on low back pain among newly qualified health care workers with and without previous low back pain: a prospective cohort study. *BMC Musculoskeletal Disorders*, Vol.10, (September 2009), pp.117, ISSN 1471-2474

Jones, G.T. & Macfarlane, G.J. (2009). Predicting persistent low back pain in schoolchildren: a prospective cohort study. *Arthritis and Rheumatism*, Vol.61, No.10, (October 2009), pp.1359-1366, ISSN 0004-3591

Kaspiris, A., et al (2010). Nonspecific low back pain during childhood: a retrospective epidemiological study of risk factors. *Journal of clinical rheumatology : practical reports on rheumatic & musculoskeletal diseases*, Vol.16, No.2, (March 2010), pp.55-60, ISSN 1076-1608

Krismer, M. & van Tulder, M. (2007). Strategies for prevention and management of musculoskeletal conditions. Low back pain (non-specific). *Best Practice & Research. Clinical Rheumatology*, Vol.21, No.1, (February 2007), pp. 77-91, ISSN 1521-6942

Kumudini, G. & Hasegawa, T. Workload and awkward posture problems among small-scale strawberry farmers in Japan. *Journal of human ergology*, Vol.38, No.2, (December 2009), pp.81-88, ISSN 0300-8134

Kurihara, A. (1994). Occupational low back pain; Present and future. *Journal of Japanese Society of Lumbar Spine Disorders*, Vol.8, No.1, (October 2002), pp.10-15, ISSN 1345-9074 (In Japanese)

Kuwashima, A., et al. (1997). National survey on accidental low back pain in workplace. *Industrial Health*, Vol.53, No.2, (April 1997), pp. 187-193, ISSN 0019-8366

Latza, U. et al. (2000). Influence of occupational factors on the relation between socioeconomic status and self-reported back pain in a population-based sample of German adults with back pain. *Spine*, Vol.25, No.11, (June 2000), pp.1390-1397, ISSN 0362-2436

Latza, U., et al. (2004). Can health care utilization explain the association between socioeconomic status and back pain? *Spine*, Vol.29, No.14, (July 2004), pp.1561-1566, ISSN 0362-2436

Leboeuf-Yde, C. Kyvik, K.O. & Bruun, N.H. (1998). Low back pain and lifestyle. Part I: Smoking. Information from a population-based sample of 29,424 twins. *Spine*, Vol.23, No.20, (October 1998), pp.2207-2213, ISSN 0362-2436

Leboeuf-Yde, C. (1999). Smoking and low back pain. A systematic literature review of 41 journal articles reporting 47 epidemiologic studies. *Spine*, Vol.24, No.14, (July 1999), pp.1463-1470, ISSN 0362-2436

Leboeuf-Yde, C. (2000). Body weight and low back pain. A systematic literature review of 56 journal articles reporting on 65 epidemiologic studies. *Spine*, Vol.25, No.2, (January 2000), pp.226-237, ISSN 0362-24362436

Leclerc, A., et al. (2009). Level of education and back pain in France: the role of demographic, lifestyle and physical work factors. *International Archives of*

Occuppational Environmental Health, Vol.82, No.5, (April 2009), pp.643-652, ISSN 0310-0131

Leino-Arjas, P., Hänninen, K. & Puska, P. (1998). Socioeconomic variation in back and joint pain in Finland. *European Journal of Epidemiology*, Vol.14, No.1, (January 1998), pp.79-87, ISSN 0393-2990

Lis, A.M. et al. (2007). Association between sitting and occupational LBP. *European Spine Journal*, Vol.16, No.2, (February 2007), pp. 283-298, ISSN 0940-6719

Liu, X., et al. (2012). Back pain among farmers in a Northern area of China. *Spine*, Vol.37, No.6, (March 2012), pp.508-514, ISSN 0362-2436

Loney, P.L. & Stratford, P.W. (1999). The prevalence of low back pain in adults: A methodological review of the literature. *Physical Therapy*, Vol.79, No.4, (April 1999), pp. 384-396, ISSN 0031-9023

Louw, Q.A., Morris, L.D. & Grimmer-Somers, K. (2007). The prevalence of low back pain in Africa: a systematic review. *BMC Musculoskelet Disorders*, Vol.8, (November 2007), pp. 105, ISSN 1471-2474

Luttmann, A., et al. (2003). *Preventing Musculoskeletal Disorders in the Workplace*. WHO, ISBN 92-4-159053X, Geneva, Switzerland

Manchikanti, L. (2000). Epidemiology of low back pain. *Pain Physician*, Vol.3, No.2, (April 2000), pp. 167-192, ISSN 1533-3159

McBeth, J. & Jones, K. (2007). Epidemiology of chronic musculoskeletal pain. *Best Practice & Research. Clinical Rheumatology*, Vol.21, No.3, (June 2007), pp. 403-425, ISSN 1521-6942

Milosavljevic, S., et al. (2011). Exposure to whole-body vibration and mechanical shock: a field study of quad bike use in agriculture. *The Annals of Occupational Hygiene*, Vol.55, No.3, (April 2011), pp.286-295, ISSN 0003-4878

Minematsu, A. (2007). Understanding and prevention of low back pain in care workers. *Journal of The Japanese Physical Therapy association*, Vol.10, No.1, (April 2007), pp.27-31, ISSN 1344-1272

Ministry of Labour (the incumbent Ministry of Health, Labour and Welfare). (1976). *Criterion for the recognition of occupational low back pain*. Circular notice No. 750, Labour Standards Bureau, Japan 1976 (In Japanese)

Ministry of Labour (the incumbent Ministry of Health, Labour and Welfare). (1994). *Guideline for prevention in low back pain in workplace*. Circular notice No. 547, Labour Standards Bureau, Japan 1994 (In Japanese)

Mitchell, T., et al. (2009). Biopsychosocial factors are associated with low back pain in female nursing students: a cross-sectional study. *International Journal of Nursing Studies*, Vol.46, No.5, (May 2009), pp.647-688, ISSN 0020-7489

Mogren, I.M. & Pohjanen, A.I. (2005). Low back pain and pelvic pain during pregnancy: prevalence and risk factors. *Spine*, Vol.30, No.8, (April 2005), pp.983-991, ISSN 0362-2436

Mohseni-Bandpei, M.A., Bagheri-Nesami, M. & Shayesteh-Azar, M. (2007). Nonspecific low back pain in 5000 Iranian school-age children. *Journal of Pediatric Orthopedics*, Vol.27, No.2, (March 2007), pp.126-129, ISSN 0271-6798

Nachemson, A.L. (1976) The lumber spine, An orthopaedic challenge. *Spine*, Vol.1, No.1, (March 1976), pp. 59-71, ISSN 0362-2436

Nachemson, A.L. (1992) Newest knowledge of low back pain. A critical look. *Clinical Orthopedics and Related Research*, Vol.279, (June 1992), pp. 8-20, ISSN 0009-921X

Nissinen, M., et al. (1994). Anthropometric measurements and the incidence of low back pain in a cohort of pubertal children. *Spine*, Vol.19, No.12, (June 1994), pp.1367-1370, ISSN 0362-2436

O'Sullivan, D., Cunningham, C. & Blake, C. (2009). Low back pain among Irish farmers. *Occupational Medicine*, Vol.59, No.1, (January 2009), pp.59-61, ISSN 0962-7480

Paoli, P. & Merllie, D. (2001). Outcomes. In: *Third European Working Conditions Survey*, 31-35, European Foundation for the Improvement of Living and Working Conditions, ISBN 92-897-0130-7, Dublin, Ireland

Parent-Thirion, A., et al. (2007). Impact of work on health. In: *Fourth European Working Conditions Survey*, 61-66, European Foundation for the Improvement of Living and Working Conditions, ISBN 92-897-0974-X, Dublin, Ireland

Picavet, H.S.J., et al. (1999). Prevalence and consequences of low back problem in the Netherlands, working VS non-working population, the MORGEN-study. *Public Health*, Vol.113, No.2, (March 1999), pp.73-77, ISSN 0033-3506

Picavet, H.S.J. & Schouten, J.S. (2003). Musculoskeletal pain in Nethewrlands: prevalence, consequences and risk group, the DMC(3)-study. *Pain*, Vol.102, No.1-2, (March 2003), pp.167-178, ISSN 0304-3959

Plouvier, S., et al. (2011). Low back pain around retirement age and physical occupational exposure during working life. *BioMed Central Public Health*, Vol.11, (April 2011), pp.268, ISSN 1471-2458

Pope, M.H., Andersson, G.B.J. & Chaffin, D.B. (1991). The Workplace. In: *Occupational Low Back Pain: Assessment, Treatment and Prevention*, M.H. Pope, et al. (Eds.), 117-131, Mosby Year Book, ISBN 0-8016-6252-4, St Louis, USA

Pope, M.H., et al. (1985). The relationship between anthropometric, postural, muscular, and mobility characteristics of males ages 18-55. *Spine*, Vol.10, No.7, (September 1985), pp.644-648, ISSN 0362-2436

Porter, J.M. & Gyi D.E. (2002). The prevalence of musculoskeletal troubles among car drivers. *Occupational Medicine*, Vol.52, No.1, (February 2002), pp. 4-12, ISSN 0962-7480

Poussa, M.S., et al. (2005). Anthropometric measurements and growth as predictors of low-back pain: a cohort study of children followed up from the age of 11 to 22 years. *European Spine Journal*, Vol.14, No.6, (August 2005), pp.595-598, ISSN 0940-6719

Punnett, L. & Wegman, D.H. (2004). Work-related musculoskeletal disorders: the epidemiologic evidence and the debate. *Journal of Electromyography and Kinesiology*, Vol.14, No.1, (February 2004), pp. 13-23, ISSN 1050-6411

Punnett, L., et al. (2005) Estimating the global burden of low back pain attributable to combined occupational exposures. *American Journal of Industrial Medicine*, Vol.48, No.6, (December 2005), pp.459-469, ISSN 0271-3586

Roffey, D.M., et al. (2010a). Causal assessment of awkward occupational postures and low back pain: results of a systematic review. *The Spine Journal*, Vol.10, No.1, (January 2010), pp.89-89, ISSN 1529-9430

Roffey, D.M., et al. (2010b). Causal assessment of occupational sitting and low back pain: results of a systematic review. *The Spine Journal*, Vol.10, No.3, (March 2010), pp.252-261, ISSN 1529-9430

Roffey, D.M., et al. (2010c). Causal assessment of occupational standing or walking and low back pain: results of a systematic review. *The Spine Journal*, Vol.10, No.3, (March 2010), pp.262-272, ISSN 1529-9430

Roffey, D.M., et al. (2010d). Causal assessment of occupational pushing or pulling and low back pain: results of a systematic review. *The Spine Journal*, Vol.10, No.6, (June 2010), pp.544-553, ISSN 1529-9430

Roffey, D.M., et al. (2010e). Causal assessment of workplace manual handling or assisting patients and low back pain: results of a systematic review. *The Spine Journal*, Vol.10, No.7, (July 2010), pp.639-651, ISSN 1529-9430

Rostom, S., et al. (2012). The prevalence of vertebral fractures and health-related quality of life in postmenopausal women. *Rheumatology International*, Vol.32, No.4, (April 2012), pp.971-980, ISSN 0172-8172

Rozali, A., et al. (2009). Low back pain and association with whole body vibration among military armoured vehicle drivers in Malaysia. *Medical Journal of Malaysia*, Vol.64, No.3, (September 2009), pp.197-204, ISSN 0300-5283

Sarikaya, S., et al. (2007). Low back pain and lumbar angles in Turkish coal miners. *American journal of industrial medicine*. Vol.50, No.1, (February 2007), pp.92-96, ISSN 0271-3586

Schilling, R.S.F. (1989). Health protection and promotion at work. *British Journal of Industrial Medicine*, Vol.46, No.10, (October 1989), pp. 683-688, ISSN 0007-1072

Sitthipornvorakul, E. et al. (2011). The association between physical activity and neck and low back pain: a systematic review. *European Spine Journal*, Vol.20, No.5, (May 2011), pp.677-689, ISSN 0940-6719

Sorensen, G., et al. (2011). The role of the work context in multiple wellness outcomes for hospital patient care workers. *Journal of occupational and environmental medicine*, Vol.53, No.8, (August 2011), pp.899-910, ISSN 1076-2752

Strine, T.W. & Hootman J.M. (2007). US national prevalence and correlates of low back and neck pain among adults. *Arthritis and rheumatism*, Vol.57, No.4, (May 2007), pp.656-665, ISSN 0004-3591

Szeto, G.P.Y. & Lam, P. (2007). Work-related musculoskeletal disorders in urban bus drivers of Hong Kong. *Journal of Occupational Rehabilitation*, Vol.17, No.2, (January 2007), pp.181-198, ISSN 1053-0487

Taechasubamorn, P., Nopkesorn, T. & Pannarunothai, S. (2011). Prevalence of low back pain among rice farmers in a rural community in Thailand. *Journal of the Medical Association of Thailand*, Vol.94, No.5, (May 2011), pp.616-621, ISSN 0125-2208

The COST B13 Working Group. (2004a). *European guidelines for the management of chronic non-specific low back pain*. European Commission, Research Directorate - General, department of Policy, Co-ordination and Strategy. Available from www.backpaineurope.org

The COST B13 Working Group. (2004b). *European guidelines for prevention in low back pain*. European Commission, Research Directorate - General, department of Policy, Co-ordination and Strategy. Available from www.backpaineurope.org

Thorbjornsson C.O.B., et al. (1998). Psychosocial and physical risk factors associated with low back pain: a 24 year follow up among women and men in a broad range of occupations. *Occupational and Environmental Medicine*, Vol.55, No.2, (February 1998), pp.84-90, ISSN 1351-0711

Tiemessen, I.J., et al. (2008). Low back pain in drivers exposed to whole body vibration: analysis of a dose-response pattrn. *Occupational and Environmental Medicine*, Vol.65, No.10, (October 2008), pp.667-675, ISSN 1351-0711

Van Tulder, M.W. & Waddell, G. (2005). Evidence-based medicine for non-specific low back pain. *Best Practice & Research. Clinical Rheumatology*, Vol.19, No.4, (August 2005), pp. vii-ix, ISSN 1521-6942

Volinn, E. (1997). The epidemiology of low back pain in the rest of world. *Spine*, Vol.22, No.15, (August 1997), pp.1747-1754, ISSN 0362-2436

Waddell, G. & Burrton, A.K. (2001). Occupational health guidelines for the management of low back pain at work: evidence review. *Occupational Medicine*, Vol.51, No.2, (March 2001), pp.124-135, ISSN 0962-7480

Wai, E.K., et al. (2010a). Causal assessment of occupational bending or twisting and low back pain: results of a systematic review. *The Spine Journal*, Vol.10, No.1, (January 2010), pp.76-88, ISSN 1529-9430

Wai, E.K., et al. (2010b). Causal assessment of occupational lifting and low back pain: results of a systematic review. *The Spine Journal*, Vol.10, No.6, (June 2010), pp.554-566, ISSN 1529-9430

Wai, E.K., et al. (2010c). Causal assessment of occupational carrying and low back pain: results of a systematic review. *The Spine Journal*, Vol.10, No.7, (July 2010), pp.628-638, ISSN 1529-9430

Walker, B.F. (2000). The prevalence of low back pain : A systematic review of the literature from 1966 to 1988. *Journal of Spinal Disorders*, Vol.13, No.3, (June 2000), pp. 205-217, ISSN 0895-0385

Walsh, K. et al. (1989). Occupational causes of low-back pain. *Scandinavian Journal of Work, Environment and Health*, Vol.15, No.1, (February 1989), pp.54-59, ISSN 0355-3140

Watson, K.D., et al. (2002). Low back pain in schoolchildren: occurrence and characteristics. *Pain*, Vol.97, No.1-2, (May 2002), pp. 87-92, ISSN 0304-3959

Wong, D.A. & Transfeldt, E. (2007). Classification of low back pain and alerts for different age groups, In : *Macnab's Backache (4th ed.)*, 19-25, Lippincott Williams & Wilkins, ISBN 978-0-7817-6085-0, Philadelphia, USA

Woolf, A.D. & Pfleger, B. (2003). Burden of major musculoskeletal conditions. *Bulletin of the World Health Organization*, Vol 81, No.9, (September 2003), pp.646-656, ISSN 0042-9686

World Health Organization. (2001). Occupational and other work-related diseases, In: *Occupational health*, 39-69, WHO, Cairo 2001

Yalcinkaya, E.Y., et al. (2010). Low back pain prevalence and characteristics in caregivers of stroke patients: a pilot study. *Topics Stroke Rehabilitation*, Vol.17, No.5, (September-October 2010), pp.389-393, ISSN 1074-9357

Yao, W., et al. (2011). A cross-sectional survey of non-specific low back pain among 2083 schoolchildren in China. *Spine*, Vol.36, No.22, (October 2011), pp.1885-1890, ISSN 0362-2436

2

The Treatment of Low Back Pain and Scientific Evidence

E. Latorre Marques
Spanish Working Group of COST B13 Program,
Dep. of Anesthesiology, "Miguel Servet" Hospital, School of Medicine,
University of Zaragoza,
Spain

1. Introduction

Low back pain (LBP) is one of most prevalent and controversial diseases for clinical management by multiple factors: resistance of practitioners to the application of the knowledge based on scientific evidence, limited use of reliable information, excessive and costly radiologic prescriptions either tendency to apply "innovative" technologies and, in some cases, to satisfy wishes patients (Cabana MD, 1999).

There is great variability in medical practice, even within developed countries, which can worsen the outcome of the treatment, unjustifiably increase the risk of iatrogenic, and needlessly increase healthcare costs.

So guidelines are needed to reduce it; clinical practice is defined as: "assertions developed systematically for help to the doctor and the patient to make decisions appropriate in clinical and specific circumstances" (Field MJ & Lohr KN, 1990).

If further complemented by analysis of cost effectiveness, they adapt to local differences, provide for improvement quality systems, are revised and can be summarized and disseminated by various means, we will largely achieve the desired goal.

This chapter aims to disseminate knowledge contrasted on the management of low back pain based on scientific evidence and assist medical personnel in key facets as "Critical analysis", "Evidence-based medicine" "Design of working groups" and "Clinical trials methodology" for the elaboration of a multidisciplinary and improved clinical practice guideline.

2. Costs and scientific evidence of low back pain

In developed countries the prevalence is estimated between 12-33%, In the USA the annual amount are beetwen 22-65% and the 5th most common cause of doctor visits. (Deyo RA, 2006). A quarter of adults reported a duration of episode of at least one week. (Carey TS,1996).

The costs generated are high, medical treatment is estimated between 9000 and 19000 $ per patient per year, and interventions around 19000 (Straus BN, 2002). Approximately 5% of the population with disability, generates 75% of healthcare costs for low back pain (Frymoyer JW, 1991).

Those who attend care doctor however achieve rapid intensity improvements of pain (58%), disability (58%) and ease returning to work (2%) (Pengel LHM, 2003). But relapses are very frequent, 60-75% of patients may present at least one of year (Gatchel RJ, 1995).

On the other hand there are many options for evaluation and treatment of back pain, but little consensus regarding the appropriate use if diagnostic and treatment media, excessive variation for example indication of surgery, in USA is five times higher than Europe (Cherkin DC, 1994). Few technologies have often proved or ineffective and even damaging, some based on studies with few benefits.

There was an increase of 235% between 1997-2006 interventionist techniques in USA between 2002-2006 increased to 22%, this growth was parallel to a rise in the prevalence of pain due to an improvement of diagnostic means, and progress new injection techniques guided by fluoroscopy. Lifetime prevalence of spinal pain was 54-80% (Walker BF, 2000).

There are significant geographic variations, duration and chronicity also disputes, 90% of attacks are resolved in 6 weeks, 5-10% of patients develop persistent pain, however despite believing that there will be more episodes, are frequent relapses (4-10%) (Nachemson A, 2000).

The "Eurobarometer" 2003-2007 analiyze various aspects of European citizens health, is a part of the European Commission Health Strategy. Musculoskeletal problems (bone, muscles and joints) affects 22 per cent population, a third of respondents (32%) had experienced some pain week prior to the survey. Pain most common type was low back,affects 67 million Europeans, became apparent factors demographic. The 55 age group are the most likely to say they experienced restrictive pain (44%) (Special Eurobarometer, 2007).

Each year one in five adults have low back pain, (Cassidy JD, 2005) to the silent suffering back is the second location more frequent of pain (Watkins et al., 2006). However 5-15% of acute cases with an established cause should be identified, chronic pain lasts more than 3 months and affects 10% of cases with high annual costs to 100-200 billion $ (Katz JN, 2006). Few documents provide advantages or outcomes assessment, and the first international guide for prevention and management of chronic cases was published 2006 (Airaksinen O, et al. 2006).

Low back pain is the most common cause and orthopedic, industrial, face of disability of workers under 45. Those who have medical care 25-40% have radiated pain and only 2% have strong findings of good surgical results forecasts for the nerve root decompression (Saal JA et al., 1990).

Those with signs of disk herniation, one in half recover a suitable tolerance of daily activities so dismiss the surgery.

Back is one of the most frequently reasons for primary care visit (Saal JA, 1990), sciatica slows recovery and is considered announcement of a significant loss of tolerance to activities. There is a significant cultural influence on disability appreciation, 20% of Swedes who deny having had problems with his back causing disability, continue the work during episodes, have been visited and treated, and many of them being farmers on their own (Blau Jn. & Logue V, 1978).

In Europe lifetime prevalence reaches 59% (Veerle Hermans, 2000), in working population with up to 85% recurrence (The bone and joint decade Report 2005).

The peril of LBP at work affect more frequently to the agriculture, fisheries, and construction. The most common body location is the back (Eurobarometer 2007) (Figure 1)

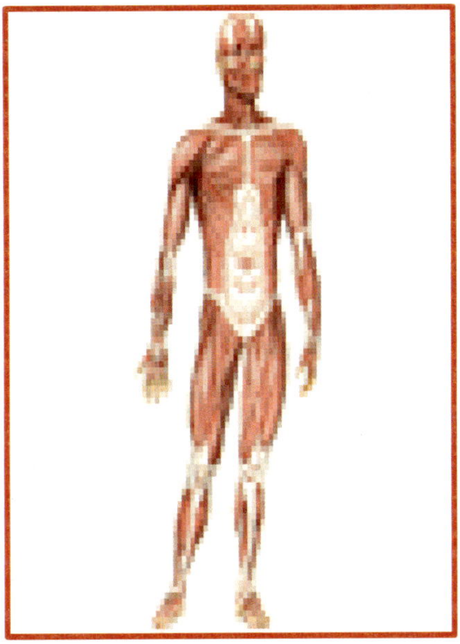

Locations of pain restricting activity

Head 6 %

Neck / Shoulder 7 %

Low back 11 %

Knees 8%

Ankle/Foot 5 %

Fig. 1. Special Eurobarometer 272e/Wave 66.2 requested by Directorate General SANCO of European Commission 2003-2007

2.2 Scientific evidence

Annual scientific production is estimated to be close to 900,000 publications, which nearly 40000 are medical. Exponential growth since 1970, thanks to the development of basic sciences such as mathematics, statistical analysis, computer engineering, the epidemiology and biology amongst others.

The number of systematic reviews and Meta-analysis in Biomedical Sciences published per year, is high and increasing, only in English reaches the 2,500. Despite the efforts made with certain "resources" and "Declarations" that contemplate later, studies show deficiencies in quality and few demonstrate impact of improvement initiatives or inclusion on editorial criteria (Moher D the al., 2007).

Try to standardize clinic practices through diagnostic and therapeutic "protocols" that contemplated management diagrams but were due more to a development consensus and panels of experts; that is why a group of epidemiologists from Mc Master University

(Sackett) published a series of articles on "how to interpret the publications", especially those of a clinical and experimental nature.

Born in 1980s, Canadian Medical Association Journal by proposing term "critical appraisal" to describe application of basic rules that allow to find evidence in scientific literature, converted by Sackett in "appreciation criticism in header of patient", to extend clinical practice.

In 90´s Guyatt coined term "evidence-based medicine" which should apply from University education to clinical practice, to provide efficiency and effectiveness in clinical events and individualized way (Guyatt GH, Renie D, 1991). Emerging entities as Collaboration Cochrane made systematic revisions of scientific literature by extracting truly relevant studies through Meta-analysis and promoting the edition of clinical practice guidelines based on scientific evidence (www.cochrane.org).

Due to variability of medical practice, not consistent with scientific evidence, and profusion of scientific literature with poor quality, emerging entities as CONSORT (1994) which are intended to implement the quality of work and scientific tests in health area. Through global outreach programs that use internet resources developed during the past 25 years (www.consort-statement.org).

2.3 Health economics

Health systems in the West have been developped and consolidated with the hospital network, organization of primary care which began to generate significant economic costs, the European Community adopted a common policy called "System of Social Welfare" which provided for the right to universal and State health care whose costs are loaded to state budgets and they did recover through taxes fairly distinct. Soon will detect need for implementation principles of Economics. Comes the concept of "Clinical Governance"

Within this trend, large companies and institutions begin became interested in the policies of containment of costs and including derivatives of industrial casualties (Spengler D, 1986) and the financial outlay to cover the fees of workers and medical care costs (Frymoyer J, 1991).

So develop epidemiological research on diseases most prevalent in the industry (Bergquist-Ullman M, 1977) in parallel with studies of Biomechanics and ergonomics, with adoption of measures of legislation to limit the burden on labour and improve the productivity and cost.

In 1991 Deyo RA publishes one research and collaborators which examines all aspects related to low back pain and its impact labor, health, economic and social system is entering a crisis.

First Clinical Practice Guidelines (CPG) were developed in order to manage more prevalent diseases; in 1994 the Agency for Health Care Policy Research published the "CPG for management of acute low back pain in adults" based on consensus (Bigos S, 1994).

Subsequently they adapt and develop guides aimed at acute low back pain as "Committee on health of New Zealand" (New Zealand acute low back pain guide 1997) which analyses risk factors for long-term disability and work loss. Improvement of aspects such as diagnosis and treatment as the case of the Guide to Australasia (Bogduk N, 1999).

In Europe from population-based studies on low back pain (Biering Sorensen f., 1983), National cost-effectiveness in Netherlands (Van Tulder MW, 1995) and systematized the Cochrane Cochrane Collaboration reviews, of clinical practice guidelines amounts a step, based on scientific evidence and cost-effectiveness. Articulate local adaptations for all national health systems in European Union, be revised and therefore adaptable to further scientific evidence.

The COST B13 Guide is pan-European, multidisciplinary, based on scientific evidence, publicly funded without participation of the industry or profit institutions. It provides for comprehensive management of acute, chronic low back pain and its prevention (Van Tulder MW, 2002). In the Spanish adaptation recommendations relating to acute and chronic low back pain were merged into a single temporal sequence, in order to improve clinical practice application, ordering implementation of technologies recommended depending on type of patients and scientific evidence, efficacy, effectiveness and efficiency, and safety (Latorre E 2008). Added a declaration of conflicts of interest of its members, and followed the collaboration criteria AGREE applying this instrument to improve quality (www.agreecollaboration.org).

3. Which is Low Back Pain (LBP)?

3.1 Concept and types

In general, Low back pain is "the pain between the costal margins and the inferior gluteal folds, it is influenced by physical activities and postures, accompanied by painful limitation of motion, frequently associated with referred pain".

"Common Low Back Pain is not related to fractures, ankylosis, direct trauma or systemic conditions" (or “Non-Specific”).

Specific low back pain is related to specific pathologies and can be diagnosed early through warning signs (Neoplasm, Infectious,vascular,metabolic,or endocrine related) (Wipf & Deyo RA, 1995).

The distribution of the cause of LBP are by frequency: Common low back pain 90%, symptomatic herniated disk 3-4%, ankylosis 0.3 - 5%, compression fractures 4%, and spinal malignancy 0.7% (Van Tulder, 2006).

Pain can occur in different ways:

Episodes acute last less than 3 months in more than 90% of the cases, which are usually benign, and they can be treated with simple steps, usually this corresponds to the type "Non-specific" but the rest of the cases may be due to other causes and therefore must diagnose and treat "specifically" and quickly (Van Tulder MW & COST B13 working group 2006).

Chronic pain lasts more than 3 months and constitutes about 10% of cases, but which generates higher costs.

This classification may seem simplistic since in many cases the pain yields around 6 weeks, why is has introduced the term subacute to see episodes that reach between 6 and 12 weeks and are warning signs (“Yellow flags”) that requires new evaluations and treatments. (Burton A.K. & COST B13 working group 2006). The key to preventing acute pain occurrence and chronicity is implementation of preventive measures (Burton AK & COST B13 working group 2006).

Can be integrated into low back pain clinical course; diagnostic, therapeutic and preventive actions so optimize long term results (table 1).

Course of LBP	Red Flags	Yellow Flags
Acute (< 6 weeks)) Information Rule out red flags No routine Radiology Stay active + Analgesics Muscle relaxants (optional) Aware Yellow Flags *Subacute (6-12 weeks)* Expectations of patient Regular Re-assessment Active treatments Cognitive behavioral therapy Multidisciplinary Occupational programme for workers? *Chronic (> 12 weeks)* Low disability: simple therapies Severe disability: biopsychosocial	*Systemic disease:* Pain < 20 or > 50 age. Thoracic spine pain Deficit Neurologic Deformity, not flexion of 5th Bad general State, fever Trauma or Neoplasms Use of corticosteroids Addictions Immunodeficiency, AIDS *Surgery* *Urgent* : Paresis, loss of control of sphincters, "saddle" anesthesia *Consultation* : 6 Weeks of treatment, limitation of ambulation. Radicular pain > 6 months + image of spinal stenosis	*Emotional problems* Depression, low morale, and social withdrawal *Use / Abuse of psicho-mimetics* *Inappropriate attitudes and beliefs about pain* "pain is harmful or disabling" "passive, rather than active, treatment will be beneficial" *Inappropriate pain behavior* Fear and reduced activity levels *Social, Financial problems* *Labour disputes*

Table 1. Current status and management of LBP and warning signs changed (Van Tulder & Araksinen 2006)

3.2 Basis of spinal pain

Not only low-back pain is a clinical entity, but also a psycho-social and economic problem.

It seems that relationship exists between adoption of bipedal position and biomechanical changes of musculoskeletal, spine aging, loss of exercise capacity and stamina, working conditions, personal expectations, psychological state, intersocial relationship, with low back pain. These aspects are detailed in other chapters, but introduce variables that increase the complexity of diagnosis management and treatment results.

This multidimensional mechanism has generated different handlings for different specialties for decades producing poor results, however since publication of Bio-psycho-social model in 1977, with adoption of management models based on evidence and cost-effectiveness, has been creating multidisciplinary teams integrating information and improving outcomes (Kovacs FM, 2006).

However he tends in some areas to excessive psycho-social reductionism and based exclusively on this model of treatment, leaving the Neurophysiologic model which based part of the treatment on interventional techniques (Manchikanti L, 2009).

Clinical application of nerve blockade or surgical techniques on the focus and pain pathway, has emerged as response to need for action on physical structures that generate, but arising in many cases studies with poor methodological quality and so not supported Meta-analysis, generating controversy.

Techniques "not recommended" in various guides (COST B13, RCGP UK) are being revised based on improvements in the quality of study design, include studies of cost-effectiveness, and therefore possibly be integrated into new "reviews" (Latorre E., 2008).

4. Critical appraisal & methodology of scientific evidence

The Begining of medicine until today, the concern has been to provide the best possible assistance, applying means proper diagnosis and optimal treatment. The Hippocratic principle is relevant for people with pain.

Since the development of science in the industrial era until today, we have attended to the improvement of the scientific method, and in turn the dissemination of information, which in recent years is massive. However in what affects the biomedical sciences, have originated important defects because at present we do not have instruments of ratification of the veracity of the information and analysis to make checks at the same speed that discovered new treatments or diagnostic applications.

At the moment we have a method, perfected from the 20th century, involving the application of the "Critical Analysis" of the scientific literature, and "Systematic Reviews" & "Meta-Analysis" for development of clinical practice guidelines based on what really is helpful, so try to minimize the variability of medical practice and clinical research.

However this process is expensive, slow and is occasionally provide obsolete results at the time of its publication and dissemination.

The scientific method have been based on the three classical premises (elaboration of hypothesis, experimentation and analysis, and conclusion) to another more complex process that we intend to explain to the reader and allows you to start or improve their skills in the development of strategies for applied research in the clinic practice, following our experiences.

The script indicated below is intended to achieve a systematization to avoid biases that are generated throughout the process and thus increase the reliability of the results:

- Approach to the issue to investigate
- Scope of the topic of research

- Collection and analysis of existing information
- Assessment of the methodological quality of the detected evidence
- Development, review and approval
- Conflicts of interest statements
- External and editorial review
- Dissemination of the results of the research

We understand that they may be useful basic facets as the description of the method of critical analysis of the publications and resources for clinical research provided by various institutions and entities, which have electronic edition of easy access, which includes chapters of methodology and practical aid as well as the possibility of on-line training. Given the limited scope of the chapter we have narrated in the first place a brief description, but we urge strongly are consulted for its value.

4.1 Critical reading

Critical reading is a technique that allows increase effectiveness our reading, acquiring necessary skills to exclude low quality scientific articles and accept others to help our decision-making process for care of patients.

Scientific articles should be evaluated in three aspects:

- Validity:

Confident in validity of results? The criteria of methodological validity articles are different for different questions: treatment, diagnosis, prognosis, economic evaluation... Depending on validity, an article may be classified in evidence levels scale, and grades of recommendation.

- Effects and Precision:

How do results measure the effect? Are results accurate?

- Applicability:

Are these results in my middle applicable?

There are quality scales will help us evaluate job quality in a simple way. In the example before us, we used the "**Jadad quality scale**" to rate on a range of zero to 5 points:

- Does the study random assignment? IF = 1 POINT; NOT = 0; If random assignment was explained and suitable gives 1 point and if wasn't it him remains.
- Meet the study criteria of double-blind? IF = 1 POINT; NOT = 0; If the double blind is unspoken and applied adequately is assigned 1 point and if does not take away.
- Are described withdrawals and dropouts from the study? IF = 1 POINT; NO = 0

There is also a rating system "**Validation Level Pain of Oxford**" (The Oxford Pain Validity Scale: IPOs) with a maximum of 16 points.

This scale has been developed to test internal validity pain trials and their results. The scale assigns points to an essay based on the number of patients in each treatment group, whether or not study satisfies criteria of blind or not and if this is correct, used results, summary test statistics and if these results or evidence were properly employed.

The Evidence-based medicine (on Systematic reviews & Meta-analysis), have become increasingly in health care. They are often used as a starting point for developing clinical practice guidelines (Green S et al., 2007).

A systematic review is a review of to clearly formulated question that uses systematic and explicit methods to identify, select and critically appraise relevant research, and to collect and analyze data from the studies that are included in the review.

Meta-analysis refers to the use of statistical techniques in a systematic review to integrate the results of included studies.

REVIEW	*Attempt of synthesis of findings and conclusions of two or more publications related to a theme.*
SYSTEMATIC	*Review with exhaustive identification of all literature, quality assessment and synthesis of results of a given subject.*
META-ANALYSIS	*Systematic review incorporating a specific statistical strategy bring together results of several studies on a single estimate.*

Table 2. Sackett D et al. Clinical Epidemiology: A basic science for clinical medicine 2nd ed. Little, Brown & Company, 1991.

4.2 Resources

Unfortunately medical reviews are subjective, scientifically unsound, and often inefficient (Group VPC-IRYS, 2005). Strategies for identifying and selecting information are rarely defined. Collected information is reviewed haphazardly with little attention to systematic assessment of quality. Under such circumstances, cogent summarization is an arduous not insurmountable task.

Experts from different areas, such as appropriate specialists, statisticians, and research methodologists, can be used both to help develop standardized appraisal forms and to rank data.Resources used for these purposes have also access program and provide training and support for clinical research, are the following:

4.2.1 Search, bibliographic databases systems.

They are varied and known of published articles (Medline, Lilacs, Embase) and unpublished as recognized research centers internationally accessible through institutional web pages.

4.2.2 QUOROM Statement

To address suboptimal reporting of meta-analysis, an international group developed a guidance called "QUOROM Statement" (QUality Of Reporting Of Meta-analysis), which focused reporting meta-analysis of randomized controlled trials (RCT) (Moher D, 1999).

4.2.3 COCHRANE Collaboration

Stimulus for systematic reviews has come from hand of Cochrane Collaboration. Archie Cochrane was a wake-up call to underline how collected evidence through RCTs could affect medical practice.

Acknowledged that professionals interested in making their decisions based on the best evidence found had no real access to this information and much less elaborate results.

In 2008 changed "Cochrane Handbook Reviewer" version 5, which serves to help authors reviews explicit and systematic development. Collaboration also has interesting possibilities for training and development on its website and is accessible at http://www.cochrane-handbook.org .

Available in Spanish, access is universal and free thanks to the subscription by Ministry of Health and Social Policy.

The edition of the Web site (Cochrane.es) is borne by the Iberoamerican Cochrane Centre located in "Hospital de la Santa Cruz and San Pablo" of the Autonomous University of Barcelona, also contribute to maintenance activities "Instituto de Salud Carlos III", as Ministry of Health.

Handbook Website offers a multitude aid to health professional, investigator or public. Includes resources for users of Cochrane Library plus, design reviews, introduction to authors research methodology in English, manual search and training. Access to finished clinical practice guides, program of skills of reading criticism, the Center for evidence-based medicine and evidence-based health care.

4.2.4 Bandolier

Bandolier is a health resource for physicians, evidence based, available over Internet (http://www.ebandolier.com) print as a monthly magazine, primarily in United Kingdom. The wealth of information based on evidence that contains Bandolier appears mainly in form of short articles and systematic reviews on various conditions and medical interventions. Information submitted in concisely and already performed, mainly in "Number Needed to Treat" (NNT).

From Bandolier home page, is an Oxford Pain link Internet Site, with various systematic reviews summaries previously published on acute and chronic pain.

Another link leads to Pain Research Unit, Oxford, which contains detailed information on current and past research.

4.2.5 PRISMA (PRoposal to Improve the publication of Systematic reviews and Meta-Analysis)

QUORUM statement was published 1999 in order to establish objective standards that improve quality reporting randomized trials meta-analysis. Contains checklist with 18 sections that allow researchers and editors certify work quality that will be published, and a flow diagram describe the process.

PRISMA (2009) statement arises to update and expand aspects of QUORUM which had deficiencies and enable acceptance of editors those standards of quality. Consists of 27 items and a ellaboration process of guidelines as well as 7 tables that explain key aspects of methodology and conduction of systematic reviews. New features in PRISMA are: adoption of COCHRANE collaboration terminology, application extension scope, not only systematic reviews of randomized trials, but also for other study types. 4 new aspects are:

- After publication Protocol to reduce the impact of biases.
- Distinction between driving and research study publication.
- Evaluation risk of bias through studies or outcomes.
- The importance of publication bias.

Detailed tables and diagrams information is available at http://www.Prisma-statement.org.

Main differences between QUOROM (Quality Of Reporting Of Meta-analysis) and PRISMA arethe relating to:

- Flow diagram more detailed and informative. PRISMA based on randomized clinical trials, and have useful for meta-analysis as QUOROM, trials continues with total number of records or unique citations and ends with individual studies included in qualitative synthesis (systematic review) and quantitative (meta- analysis).
- Establishes differences at each stage process between records or references, articles to full and individual studies.
- Includes format peak (description of participants, interventions, comparisons and outcomes).
- Explanation of previous Protocol to review and access medium.
- Strategies for electronic search and evaluation risk bias.
- Extent text increases expense of improving clarity and transparency of information.

4.2.6 EQUATOR Network (Enhancing the QUality and transparency Of Health Research) (Altman & Simera, 2008)

Is a network of resource development aimed at improving the quality of publications in health sciences, this has provided assistance through its website (http://www.equator-network.org/) that allow a single researcher as well as groups, teach design guidelines for developing quality and transparency. (Liberati A, 2009)

4.2.7 CONSORT declaration (Consolidated Standards of Reporting Trials)

This led to clinical trials improve quality methodology and resources publication as CONSORT statement, 25 items checklist set of recommendations and a flow diagram development progress.

Objetives are to assist preparation, transparency, critical review and interpretation of Randomized Controlled Trials (RCT).

The first version of 2001 has been revised and perfected in 2010 and includes on its website (http://www.consort-statement.org/) additional resources such as CONSORT "Explanation and Elaboration" document and CONSORT Library of examples of good reporting.

Pureed both access to Downloads, Evidence Database, Glossary, Related Instruments, and link to Useful sites as for example EQUATOR

Members of CONSORT Group continually monitoring literature. Information gleaned from these efforts provides an evidence base on which to update CONSORT statement. We add, drop, or modify items based on that evidence and recommendations of "CONSORT Group", an international and eclectic group of clinical reserarchers, epidemiologists, statisticians, and biomedical editors. More than 400 journals, published around the world and in many languages, have explicitly supported CONSORT statement. However, there is a significant limitation based on this instrument orientation, which is limited to two-group, parallel randomized, controlled trials (RCT) .The items should elicit clear pronouncements of how and what authors did, but do not contain any judgments on how and what authors should have donate. Moreover, CONSORT 2010 Statement does not include recommendations for designing and conducting randomized trials (Schulz K 2010).

4.2.8 AGREE instrument (Appraisal of Guidelines Research and Evaluation in Europe)

Defines European criteria standards for preparation clinical practice guidelines (GPC). Is available for researchers in http://www.agreecollaboration.org. Assesses both, Information of quality of document provided and some aspects of recommendations. Provides validity guide. Means quality clinical practice guideline confidence that potential biases of the development of the guide have been identified in an appropriate manner and that recommendations are valid both internally and externally, and can lead to practice. Designed to evaluate guidelines developed by local, regional, national or international groups as governmental organizations. Applicable to published guides in paper and electronic format. AGREE consists of 23 key items organized in six areas. Each area tries to cover a dimension differentiated quality of the Guide:

Domains of AGREE Appraisal Instrument II
• **Scope & Purpose (1,2,3)** objective, health question and population specifically described. • **Stakeholder involvement (4,5,6**) Relevant professional groups, Views and preferences of the target population, Target users defined. • **Rigour of Development (7-14)** Systematic search, Criteria, strenghs and limitations, metods of formulating recommendations, health benefits, side effects and risks, explicit link beetwin recommendation and evidences, Externally reviewed by experts, procedure updating provided. • **Clarity of Presentation (15-17)** Recommendations specific / ambiguous, different management options, Key recommendations identifiable. • **Applicability (18-21)** describe barriers/facilitators, Advices/Tools to put in practice, Potential resource implications, Monitoring / Auditing. • **Editorial Independence (22, 23)** Not influence of Publisher, Conflicts of interest group members.

Table 3. Appraisal of Guidelines Research and Evaluation in Europe Instrument AGREE II

Aims and scope (items 1-3) refers to the overall purpose of the Guide to clinical specific questions and target patient population.

Participation of those involved (items 4-7) refers to the degree in which the Guide represents the views of users to which it is intended.

Rigor in drawing up (items 8-14) refers to the process used to gather and synthesize evidence, to formulate recommendations and methods for updating them.

Clarity and presentation (items 15-18) deals with the language and format of the Guide.

Applicability (items 19-21) refers to the possible implications of the implementation of the guidance on organizational aspects, behavior and costs.

Editorial independence (items 22-23) has to do with the independence of the recommendations and the recognition of the potential conflicts of interest by the group.

At the present time there is only another validated scale which assesses the quality of the GPC (Shaneyfelt TM, 1999), but a comparative study between these two instruments (Rich R, 2004) shows that the instrument AGREE, as well as being that in this moment has greater acceptance and provides a more manageable format, manages to make a grouping of criteria more clearly and fully. In recent years he has tried to improve the validity of this instrument and value items that better assess the quality of a guide; as a result is the development of the II AGREE to replace the original version (AGREE, 2009).

4.3 Recommendations for the process of research development

The fundamental steps to be taken in the development process include the sections described as selection of the topic to research, defining the scope of the review of existing scientific evidence and the process of development, revision, and approval of the recommendations. Furthermore today should be added others relating to the integrity of the members of the research team, transparency and editorial independence, utility, and the costs.

4.3.1 Previous guidelines and state of the question

One of the first evidence-based clinical practice guidelines for management of low back pain was published by "The Quebec Task force on spinal Disorders" in 1987.Using an explicit scientific basis found insufficient evidence to support the use of most common diagnostic procedures and treatment modalities.

The U.S. Agency for Health Care and Policy Research (AHCPR) convened a multidisciplinary panel of experts issued recommendations on management of Acute Low Back Pain (LBP) in 1994, however none of the 40 recommendations made for clinical care were viewed as support by strong research evidence, and only 6 by at least moderate quality.

More than eleven international guidelines have been published since 1994, but their diagnostic and therapeutic recommendations are similar. Only there are few discrepancies to recommendations for exercise, spinal manipulation, muscle relaxants and patient information that reflect contextual differences between countries without signification.

The most interesting from a methodologic point of view are the U.S. Guideline issued by the Veterans Affairs/Department of Defense (VA/DoD) in 1999, the Guideline of Royal College of General Practicioners (RCGP) initially released in 1996 and updated in 1999 , and the European COST B 13 Guidelines.

The European Multinational COST B 13 program was developed by The European Commission Directorate General Research Political Co-Ordination and Strategy branch under the title "Low Back Pain: Guidelines for its management". Since 1999 to 2005 were reviewed 74 clinical practice guidelines and 871 Systematic Reviews, Randomized control trials (RCT´) and Prevention studies. Involving a total of 49 experts including Epidemiologists, Public Health, Chiropractors, Psychologists, Physiotherapists, Ergonomists, Physiologists, and Medical Specialists (Primary Care, Anesthesiology, Pain Terapy, Rheumatology, Traumatology, Neurosurgery, Pathology, Rehabilitation, Radiology, Sports Medicine, Emergency Medicine and Occupational Medicine.). The main difference with previous guides is that COST B13 Guide includes recommendations for management Acute, Chronic and prevention of LBP.

In 2009 the American Pain society (APS) has issued a new clinical practice guideline that emphasizes the use of non-invasive treatments over interventional procedures, published of the journal *Spine.* Based on a extensive review of existing research , this review 913 citations for systematic reviews, 265 full text articles for inclusion, of those 186 met inclusion criteria. Identifies 7591 citations from 44 searches for primary studies , from these, 202 primary studies were relevant. For Interventional Therapies and surgery a total of 1331 citations.

However controversy is served because reaffirm previous recommendations (see COST B13 Guide) that avoid invasive therapies and showing benefits of non-invasive (stay active, intensive rehabilitation and cognitive/behavioural emphasis). In contrast the American Society of Interventional Pain Physicians has been published a critical review of Interventional Techniques for chronic and acute LBP (2010) that differs from APS Guidelines including caudal epidural injections, lumbar facet joint nerve blocks, radiofrequency neurotomy, and percutaneous adhesiolysis as appropriate methodology.

Probably better designed studies obtain a balance between non-invasive and interventional therapies.

4.3.2 Key points of systematic reviews and LBP

A systematic review is a complex process, but we want to emphasize the fundamental aspects of methodology.

1. Selection of Topics

Choosing a topic is the first step in development process. We must consider the following criteria: effect of condition on morbidity , mortality , prevalence of back pain , areas of uncertainty evidence , cost, relevance and availability of developed recommendations.

2. Scope of Topics

Address screening , diagnosis and treatment of back pain focus on the effectiveness of interventions , cost and cost-effectiveness.

3. Review of Evidence for Clinical Recommendations

Evaluating Evidence.

The key questions and scope for the evidence-review papers are developed from the Clinical Guidelines Committee. The evidence review paper is a comprehensive systematic review of meta-analysis that address to management of back pain. Specifies the criteria that are used to identify evidence related to each the key questions for inclusion in the review.

Quality of evidence were evaluated using the AHCPR Guide and "The Levels of Evidence" recommended for The Back Group of Cochrane Collaboration (van Tulder 2003). Evidence reviews provide information about whether the studies included are reliable and accurate and provide reasonable assessments of potential adverse effects, information on systematic gaps particularly with respect to areas of clinical importance or relevance.

Statistical Review.

The evidence reviews also go through a statistical peer-review process to staticians during its early stages of development.

A three-stage development process was undertaken. First, recommendations were derived from systematic reviews. Secondly, existing national guidelines were compared and recommendations from these guidelines summarised. Thirdly, the recommendations from the systematic (Cochrane) reviews and guidelines were discussed by the group. A section was added to the guidelines in which the main points of debate are described. The recommendations are put in a clinically relevant order; recommendations regarding diagnosis have a letter D, treatment T. A grading system was used for the strength of the evidence. This grading system is simple and easy to apply, and shows a large degree of consistency between the grading of therapeutic and preventive, prognostic and diagnostic studies. The system is based on the original ratings of the AHCPR Guidelines (1994) and levels of evidence recommended in the method guidelines of the Cochrane Back Review group. Several of the existing systematic reviews have included non-English language literature, usually publications in French, German, and Dutch language and sometimes also Danish, Norwegian, Finnish and Swedish. All existing national guidelines included studies published in their own language. Consequently, the non-English literature is covered for countries that already have developed guidelines.

The group additionally included the Spanish literature, because this evidence was not covered by existing reviews and guidelines.

The Working Group aimed to identify gaps in the literature and included recommendations for future research.

4.3.3 Methodological quality of studies and levels of evidence

A grading system was used for the strength of the evidence. This grading system is simple and easy to apply, and shows a large degree of consistency between the grading of therapeutic and preventive, prognostic and diagnostic studies. The system is based on the original ratings of the AHCPR Guidelines (1994) and levels of evidence used in systematic (Cochrane) reviews on low back pain.

Level of evidence:

1. Therapy and prevention:

Level A:

Generally consistent findings provided by (a systematic review of) multiple high quality randomised controlled trials (RCTs).

Level B:

Generally consistent findings provided by (a systematic review of) multiple low quality RCTs or non-randomised controlled trials (CCTs).

Level C:

One RCT (either high or low quality) or inconsistent findings from (a systematic review of) multiple RCTs or CCTs.

Level D:

No RCTs or CCTs.

Systematic review: systematic methods of selection and inclusion of studies, methodological quality assessment, data extraction and analysis.

2. Prognosis:

Level A:

Generally consistent findings provided by (a systematic review of) multiple high quality prospective cohort studies.

Level B:

Generally consistent findings provided by (a systematic review of) multiple low quality prospective cohort studies or other low quality prognostic studies.

Level C:

One prognostic study (either high or low quality) or inconsistent findings from (a systematic review of) multiple prognostic studies.

Level D, no evidence:

No prognostic studies.

High quality prognostic studies: prospective cohort studies Low quality prognostic studies: retrospective cohort studies, follow-up of untreated control patients in a RCT, case-series

3. Diagnosis:

Level A:

Generally consistent findings provided by (a systematic review of) multiple high quality diagnostic studies.

Level B:

Generally consistent findings provided by (a systematic review of) multiple low quality diagnostic studies.

Level C:

One diagnostic study (either high or low quality) or inconsistent findings from (a systematic review of) multiple diagnostic studies.

Level D, no evidence:

No diagnostic studies.

High quality diagnostic study: Independent blind comparison of patients from an appropriate spectrum of patients, all of whom have undergone both the diagnostic test and the reference standard. (An appropriate spectrum is a cohort of patients who would normally be tested for the target disorder. An inappropriate spectrum compares patients already known to have the target disorder with patients diagnosed with another condition) Low quality diagnostic study: Study performed in a set of non-consecutive patients, or confined to a narrow spectrum of study individuals (or both) all of who have undergone both the diagnostic test and the reference standard, or if the reference standard was unobjective, unblinded or not independent, or if positive and negative tests were verified using separate reference standards, or if the study was performed in an inappropriate spectrum of patients, or if the reference standard was not applied to all study patients.

The methodological quality of additional studies will only be assessed in areas that have not been covered yet by a systematic review or of the non-English literature.

The methodological quality of trials is usually assessed using relevant criteria related to the internal validity of trials. High quality trials are less likely to be associated with biased results than low quality trials. Various criteria lists exist, but differences between the lists are subtle.

Quality assessment should ideally be done by at least two reviewers, independently, and blinded with regard to the authors, institution and journal.

However, as experts are usually involved in quality assessment it may often not be feasible to blind studies. Criteria should be scored as positive, negative or unclear, and it should be clearly defined when criteria are scored positive or negative. Quality assessment should be pilot tested on two or more similar trials that are not included in the systematic review. A consensus method should be used to resolve disagreements and a third reviewer was consulted if disagreements persisted. If the article does not contain information on the methodological criteria (score 'unclear'), the authors should be contacted for additional information. This also gives authors the opportunity to respond to negative or positive scores.

The following checklists are recommended:

4.3.4 Checklist for methodological quality

Checklist for methodological quality of therapy / prevention studies

Items:

1. Adequate method of randomisation,
2. Concealment of treatment allocation,
3. Withdrawal / drop-out rate described and acceptable,
4. Co-interventions avoided or equal,
5. Blinding of patients,
6. Blinding of observer,

7. Blinding of care provider
8. Intention-to-treat analysis,
9. Compliance,
10. Similarity of baseline characteristics.

Checklist for methodological quality of prognosis (observational) studies

Items:

1. Adequate selection of study population,
2. Description of in- and exclusion criteria,
3. Description of potential prognostic factors,
4. Prospective study design,
5. Adequate study size (> 100 patient-years),
6. Adequate follow-up (> 12 months),
7. Adequate loss to follow-up (< 20%),
8. Relevant outcome measures,
9. Appropriate statistical analysis.

Checklist for methodological quality of diagnostic studies

Items:

1. Was at least one valid reference test used?
2. Was the reference test applied in a standardised manner?
3. Was each patient submitted to at least one valid reference test?
4. Were the interpretations of the index test and reference test performed independently of each other?
5. Was the choice of patients who were assessed by the reference test independent of the results of the index test?
6. When different index tests are compared in the study: were the index tests compared in a valid design?
7. Was the study design prospective?
8. Was a description included regarding missing data?
9. Were data adequately presented in enough detail to calculate test characteristics (sensitivity and specificity)?

4.3.5 Inclusion of non-English language literature

Background

There is still an ongoing debate about inclusion in systematic reviews of studies published in other languages than English. Although inclusion of non-English literature is often recommended, it may not always be feasible and may depend on the time and resources available. Some authors suggested that there is empirical evidence that exclusion of trials published in other languages than English might be associated with bias. Positive results by authors from non-English speaking countries are more likely to be published in English and negative results in the authors' language. They found an example of a meta-analysis where inclusion of a non-English language trial changed the results and conclusion.

Authors of German-speaking countries in Europe were more likely to publish RCTs in an English-language journal if the results were statistically significant. On the other hand, Moher et al. (1996) evaluated the quality of reporting of RCTs published in English, French, German, Italian and Spanish between 1989 and 1993 and did not find significant differences. Trials published in some non-English languages (Chinese, Japanese, Russian and Taiwanese) had an unusually high proportion of positive results.

Excluding trials published in other languages than English generally has little impact on the overall treatment effect.

Although the evidence seems to be inconclusive, most authors concluded that all trials should be included in a systematic review regardless of the language in which they were published, to increase precision and reduce bias. The Cochrane Back Review Group recommended in its method guidelines for reviews on low back pain that if RCTs published in other languages are excluded from a review, the reason for this decision should be given. (van Tulder et al 2003) Especially on topics where there are likely to be a significant number of non-English language publications (for example, the Asian literature on acupuncture) it may be wise to consider involvement of a collaborator with relevant language skills. The members of the Working Group acknowledged that a different literature search should be performed for non-English literature than for the English literature. Databases do not exist for most other languages, the reliability and coverage of the databases that do exist is unclear, and sensitive search strategies for these databases may not have been developed.

Most of the systematic reviews used in the European guidelines included trials published in English and some other languages (mostly German, French, Dutch and sometimes Swedish, Danish, Norwegian and Finnish). Obviously, the national guidelines that we have used as basis for our recommendations have included studies published in their respective languages. National committees that developed guidelines in these languages have considered Danish, Dutch, Finnish, French, German, Norwegian and Swedish language studies. Only Italian and Spanish trials have yet not been considered, because guidelines in these countries do not exist.

Because there was no Italian member participating in the WG, we only considered the Spanish literature.

Objectives

To summarise the evidence from the Spanish literature and evaluate if it supports the evidence review and recommendations of the guidelines.

Methods

Literature search

Relevant trials were identified in existing databases: Literatura Latino Americana e do Caribe em Ciencias da Saude (LILACS) and Índice Médico Español (IME). The Iberoamerican Cochrane Centre (Centro Iberoamericano de la Colaboración Cochrane) was contacted for additional trials.

Inclusion criteria are: 1) randomised controlled trials, 2) acute and subacute low back pain (less than 12 weeks), and 3) any intervention.

Quality Appraisal

The abstracts with no English version have been translated from Spanish by a native English speaker. Some papers had an English version of their abstracts. In these cases, the translator has just done a linguistic review of them and, in those cases in which the Spanish and English versions did not match, a translation of the Spanish abstract has been done. Some Spanish journals publish only short reports of the studies (similar to abstracts). In these cases, the entire report has been considered as the abstract. Other Spanish journals have a mandatory structure for the abstracts they publish, which may have changed over time, but most do not. Therefore, there is a considerable difference in the amount of information provided by different abstracts.

Two reviewers assessed the quality of the trials using the checklist for methodological quality of therapy/prevention studies.

Data extraction

Data were extracted regarding characteristics of patients, interventions and outcomes (pain, functional status, global improvement, return to work, patient satisfaction, quality of life, generic functional status and intervention-specific outcomes) and the final results of the study for each outcome measure at each follow-up moment.

Data analysis

The results of the Spanish literature (quality, data and results) were considered by the members of the WG to see if the results do or do not support the recommendations. If not, reasons for these inconsistencies were explored.

4.4 Dissemination and implementation

Clinical guidelines are usually defined as 'systematically developed statements to assist practitioner and patient decisions about appropriate health care' as a vehicle for assisting health care providers in grasping new evidence and bring it into daily clinical routines for improving practice and for diminishing costs.

Implementation of guidelines means putting something (e.g. a plan or an innovation) into use. The process of spreading clinical guidelines implies diffusion, active dissemination and implementation. Diffusion is a passive concept while dissemination is a more active process including launching of targeted and tailored information for the intended audience. Implementation often involves identifying and assisting in overcoming barriers to the use of the knowledge obtained from a tailored message.

Normally implementation procedures mean a multi-disciplinary enterprise.

Effectiveness of interventions

Success in the implementation process requires knowledge about important factors behind general positive and negative attitudes towards guidelines related to usefulness, reliability, practicality and availability of the guidelines. Also the overall individual, team and organisational competence to follow recommended procedures seem to be vital.

Systematic reviews of the effectiveness of interventions to promote professional behaviour or change have shown:

Consistently effective are

- Educational outreach visits (for prescribing in North American settings)
- Reminders (manual or computerised)
- Multifaceted interventions
- A combination that includes two or more of the following: audit and feedback, reminders, local consensus process and marketing
- Interactive educational meetings
- *Participation of health care providers in workshops that include discussions of practice*

Mixed effects

- Audit and feedback
- Any summary of clinical performance
- Local opinion leaders
- Use of providers nominated by their colleagues as 'educationally influential'
- Local consensus process
- Inclusion of participating providers in discussion to ensure that they agreed that chosen clinical problem was important and the approach to managing the problem was appropriate.
- Patient mediated interventions
    - Any intervention aimed at changing the performance of health care providers where specific information was sought from or given to patients.
    - *Little or no effect*
- Educational materials
- Distribution of published or printed recommendations for clinical care, including clinical practice guidelines, audio-visual materials and electronic publications.
- Didactic educational meetings
- Lectures

4.4.1 Barriers and facilitators

A successful implementation of guidelines requires thoroughly performed planning and monitoring of the implementation whereof addressing barriers and facilitators appear to be of vital importance to enhance the implementation process. Before starting the implementation such barriers and facilitators should be systematically recorded among target groups for applying the clinical guidelines.

Potential barriers to change may include:

Practice environment

- Limitations of time
- Practice organisation, e.g. lack of disease registers or mechanisms to monitor repeat prescribing.

Educational environment

- Inappropriate continuing education and failure to link up with programmes to promote quality of care
- Lack of incentives to participate in effective educational activities

Health care environment

- Lack of financial resources
- Lack of defined practice populations
- Health policies which promote ineffective or unproven activities
- Failure to provide practitioners with access to appropriate information

Social environment

- Influence of media on patients in creating demands/beliefs
- Impact of disadvantage on patients' access to care

Practitioner factors

- Obsolete knowledge
- Influence of opinion leaders
- Beliefs and attitudes (for example, related to previous adverse experience of innovation)

Patient factors

- Demands for care
- Perceptions/cultural beliefs about appropriate care

Implementation strategies should be tailored according to recorded identified barriers and facilitators. How to do this is described in detail in *Evidence Based Practice in Primary Care.*

Evaluation

In general it is also recommended to evaluate outcome and result of the implementation process. Outcome measures related to low back pain will often be before and after status of use of health services, for instance x-ray, sickness absence and back related health status of the patient population (e.g. pain, function/quality of life). Types of evaluation may include RCTs, cross-over and semi-experimental trials, before-after study and interrupted time series analyses. An economic evaluation is also required on both the course and the benefits of implementation analysis.

Oxman *et al.* reviewed 102 randomised controlled trials in which changes in physician behaviour were attempted through means such as continuing medical education workshops and seminars, educational materials, academic detailing and audit and feedback. Each produced some change but the authors concluded that a multi-faceted strategy was called for using a combination of methods and that there can be no "magic bullet" for a successful implementation.

4.5 Search strategy for the systematic reviews

Literature search, conducted 11.12.2001

Databases

1. Cochrane
2. Medline
3. Health Star
4. Embase
5. Pascal
6. Psychoinfo

7. Biosis
8. Lilacs
9. IME (Índice Médico Español)

Search Strategy:

1. **Cochrane**: # 1 Back pain.
2. **Medline and Health Star**:

a. **sensitive strategy:**

#1 (back pain) AND systematic[sb]

#2 (back pain) AND systematic[sb] Field: All Fields, Limits:

Publication Date from 1990

b. **specific strategy: Adding:**

#3 (back pain) AND systematic[sb] Field: All Fields, Limits:

Publication Date from 1990, Review

3. **Embase:** #1 Back pain. De (MESH)

#2 Low back pain. De (MESH)

#3 1 OR 2

#4 Systematic

#5 3 and 4 (Limitado por Review y publicaciones desde 1990)

4. **Pascal, Psychoinfo and Biosis:**

#1 Back pain

#2 Low back pain

#3 1 OR 2

#4 Systematic

#5 3 AND 4 (limit to Publication type"Review" and Publication Date since1990)

5. **Lilacs:** #1 dolor de espalda. [DE]

#2 (lumbago) O lumbalgia. [TI]

#3 (dolor) Y espalda. [TI]

#4 #1 O #2 O #3

#5 (revisión) Y sistemática.

#6 #4 Y #5

6. **IME:** #1 (dolor de espalda) O lumbago O lumbalgia. [DE]

#2 (dolor de espalda) O lumbago O lumbalgia 203

#3 revisión sistemática

#4 #1 Y #3

#5 #2 Y #3

RESULTS

Total hits

Cochrane 12

Medline and Health Star

"Specific": 121 5 excluded 20 redundant

"Sensitive" 273 121 redundant with

Medline specific

14 excluded

10 redundant

Embase 13 1 redundant

Pascal, Psychoinfo and Biosis 14 2 redundant

Lilacs 0

IME 0

Typical subgroup search

(e.g. results for physical treatments and exercise)

Embase

No. Records Request

1 9163 back pain

2 74295 randomized trial

3 458 #1 and #2

4 81 exercise and #3

5 44 training and #3

6 14 traction and #3

7 0 bracing and #3

8 29 manipulation and #3

9 14 massage and #3

10 8 heat and #3

11 5 cold and #3

12 4 ultrasound and #3

13 7 tens and #3

14 0 electrotherapy and #3

15 3 diathermy and #3

16 4 laser and #3

17 9 manual therapy and #3

18 4 TNS and #3

19 1 interferential therapy and #3

* 20 163 #4 or #5 or #6 or #7 or #8 or #9 or #10 or #11 or #12 or #13 or #14 or

#15 or #16 or #17 or #18 or #19

Psychinfo

Search History

#20 #3 or #4 or #5 or #6 or #7 or #8 or #9 or #10 or #11 or #12 or

#13 or #14 or #15 or #16 or #17 or #18 or #19 (6 records)

#19 interferential therapy and #3 and (PY=1995-2002) (0 records)

#18 TNS and #3 and (PY=1995-2002) (0 records)

#17 laser and #3 and (PY=1995-2002) (0 records)

#16 diathermy and #3 and (PY=1995-2002) (0 records)

#15 electrotherapy and #3 and (PY=1995-2002) (0 records)

#14 manual therapy and #3 and (PY=1995-2002) (0 records)

#13 tens and #3 and (PY=1995-2002) (0 records)

#12 ultrasound and #3 and (PY=1995-2002) (0 records)

#11 cold and #3 and (PY=1995-2002) (0 records)

#10 heat and #3 and (PY=1995-2002) (0 records)

#9 massage and #3 and (PY=1995-2002) (0 records)

#8 manipulation and #3 and (PY=1995-2002) (0 records)

#7 bracing and #3 and (PY=1995-2002) (0 records)

#6 traction and #3 and (PY=1995-2002) (0 records)

#5 training and #3 and (PY=1995-2002) (0 records)

#4 exercise and #3 and (PY=1995-2002) (2 records)

#3 #1 and #2 (6 records)

#2 randomized trial and (PY=1995-2002) (352 records)

#1 back pain and (PY=1995-2002) (645 records)

5. Elaboration of a CPG based on scientific evidence. The Spanish version of COST B13 European program

It is a long and complex process that must be completed by a method of work explained in part previous sections and follows a basic sequence (figure 3). The systematic reviews were identified using the results of validated search strategies in the Cochrane Library, Medline, Embase and, if relevant, other electronic databases, performed for Clinical Evidence, a monthly, updated directory of evidence on the effects of common clinical interventions, published by the BMJ Publishing Group (www.evidence.org). The literature search covered the period from 1966 to October 2005. A search for clinical guidelines was first performed in Medline. Since guidelines are only infrequently published in medical journals we extended the 5 search on the Internet (using search terms 'back pain' and 'guidelines', and searching national health professional association and consumers websites) and identified guidelines by personal communication with experts in the field.

A three-stage development process was undertaken. First, recommendations were derived from systematic reviews. Secondly, existing national guidelines were compared and recommendations from these guidelines summarised. Thirdly, the recommendations from the systematic (Cochrane) reviews and guidelines were discussed by the group. A section was added to the guidelines in which the main points of debate are described. The recommendations are put in a clinically relevant order; recommendations regarding diagnosis have a letter D, treatment T.

A grading system was used for the strength of the evidence. This grading system is simple and easy to apply, and shows a large degree of consistency between the grading of therapeutic and preventive, prognostic and diagnostic studies. The system is based on the original ratings of the AHCPR Guidelines (1994) and levels of evidence recommended in the method guidelines of the Cochrane Back Review group. The strength of the recommendations was not graded.

Several of the existing systematic reviews have included non-English language literature, usually publications in French, German, and Dutch language and sometimes also Danish, Norwegian, Finnish and Swedish. All existing national guidelines included studies published in their own language. Consequently, the non- English literature is covered for countries that already have developed guidelines.

The group additionally included the Spanish literature, because this evidence was not covered by existing reviews and guidelines.

The Working Group aimed to identify gaps in the literature and included recommendations for future research.

Basic Sequence:

5.1 Constitution of the multidisciplinary working group

Constitution of the multidisciplinary working group through a Management Committee composed of experts in field of low back pain, appointed by the Governments of 14 countries participating in European Union, framed in the Directorate General Research, Political Co-ordination and Strategy (COST) and B13 program "Low back Pain: Guidelines for its management".

To streamline the work plan were drafting chapters on acute low back pain, chronic and prevention, stratified components in 3 sub-working groups. Finally, in our case was working Spanish Group for improvement and adaptation directed by the Spanish representatives of European Management Committee.

5.2 Search and selection of scientific evidence

Search and selection of scientific evidence by means computerized databases and documentary looking time period more comprehensive as possible, with strategies to include those available in languages other than English, particularly in Spanish, but also supplement with contributions of studies which were undergoing investigation or publication, but excluding not accepted.

Explored databases were Cochrane, Medline, Embase, health Star, Pascal, PsycINFO, SPORT ciscos, Biosis, Lilacs and EMI.

5.3 Methodological evidence quality assessment

Methodological evidence quality assessment detected in each systematic review and original studies found according to Oxman and Guyatt methodological criteria (annex 2 GPC COST)

5.4 Levels of evidence for recommendations

Levels of evidence for recommendations arising from number of studies that underlie them, quality methodology and consistency results, according to criteria based on guidance of advice (Bigos1994) and "levels of evidence" recommended by the Cochrane Collaboration back group (van Tulder 2003). (Table 4)

Level A : Results of a systematic¨ review of multiple studies* (high quality). Level B : Results of a systematic¨ review of studies* (low quality). Level C : Results of a single study * (high or low quality), or inconsistent systematic¨ review of multiple studies. Level D : Non-obviousness (lack of studies).

Table 4. Evidence Levels

¨Criterion of "Systematic review": use of systematic methods to select and include studies, assessment of methodological quality and extraction and analysis of data. Are defined as "results consistent to the coincidence in the sense of the results, at least 75% of the studies". Studies: diagnostic, prognosis (prospective), treatment (controlled clinical trial), prevention (controlled clinical trial)*

5.5 Review and approval content of Guide

Review and approval content of Guide once analysed available scientific evidence each group developed recommendations and discussion according to a fixed timetable, by electronic means and meetings seeing them joint the overall content of the Guide, articulating a mechanism of critical inter groups until approval by unanimity.

5.6 Spanish adaptation by the Working Group

Spanish adaptation by the Working Group formed with the aim of:

5.6.1 Help detect and collect evidence in Spanish

Help detect and collect evidence in Spanish might have been forgotten in e-strategies prior.

5.6.2 Critical analysis

Critical analysis:Successive drafts produced by work groups.

5.6.3 Adaptation

To Spanish health system, dissemination and use of GPC elaborated by working groups. The Spanish adaptation is stuck studying organizational aspects necessary for recommendations implementation, definition targets, measurement organization and registration indicators systems, implementation and identification of local barriers to be overcome.

5.6.4 Application of the criteria of the instrument AGREE

Application of the criteria of the instrument AGREE, and detection of gaps in the previous format (International) as: not-identification of target user, lack of tools to facilitate practical application, or establishment methods to make e final recommendations, and non-inclusion of declarations interest conflicts.

5.6.5 Updating of the Guide COST B13

Through following mechanisms: regular meetings of representatives of participating entities, provision of sources of funding for an automated mechanism for detection, analysis and aggregation of results of further studies. Use as a basis for updates Cochrane Collaboration systematic reviews relating to clinical trials on therapeutic technologies, and formation of a network of evaluation teams in studies published in mentioned area.

5.6.6 Declaration of conflicts of interest

Economic, effective type or species, direct or indirect, generic or specific, personal or collective produced or expected, that goes beyond use of technologies which mentioned in a clinical setting or research purposes. Performed in nominal and explicit way by components of the Spanish working group and contained in a table extensive version.

5.7 Guide publication by previously established, varied media

Written in extended version including a management role and through free electronic access algorithm through www.REIDE.org . In GPC said based on scientific evidence, specify all relevant studies for each specific recommendation, analyzes town methodology and are non-technical summary evidence on efficiency, effectiveness, safety and cost/effectiveness and indications of each treatment.

5.7.1 Algorithm

Integrates all information is published on paper and you can print from electronic access, consists of a flow diagram that includes evidence of each recommended technology and designed to take up a minimum space, is Pocket-Guide.

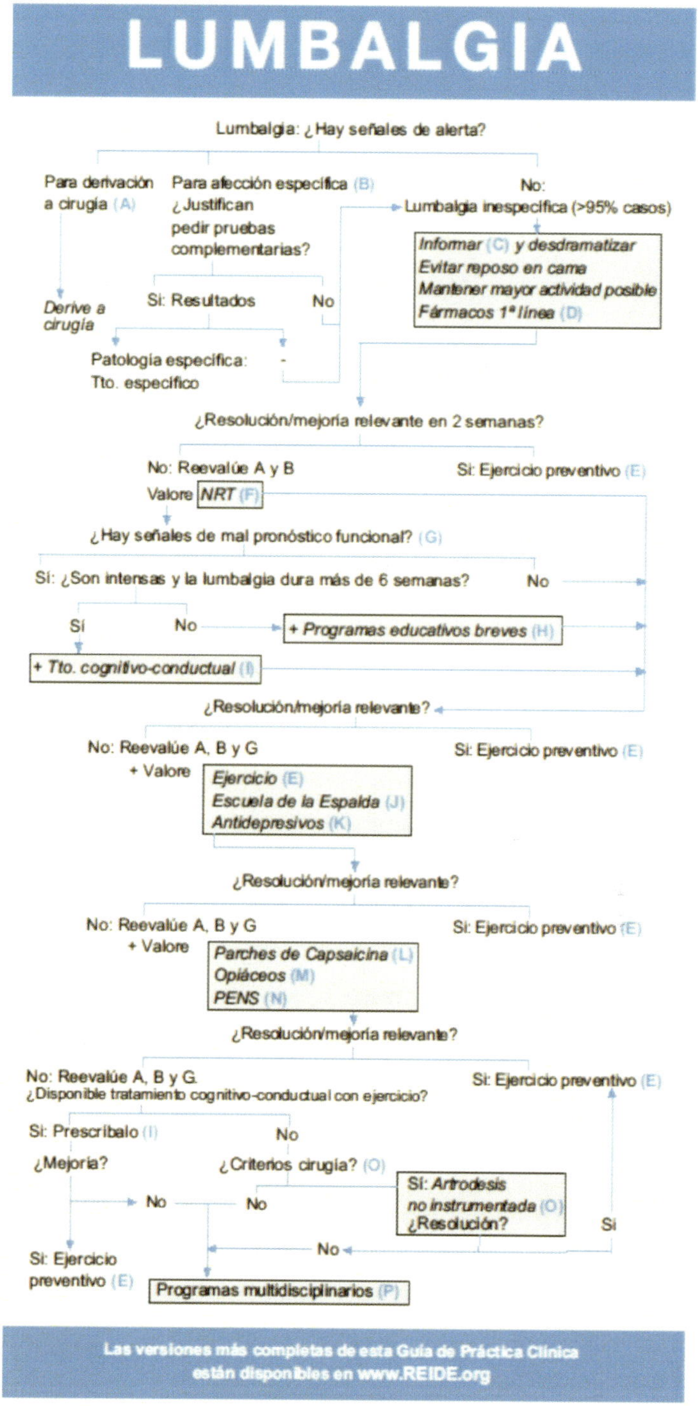
LUMBALGIA
Lumbalgia: ¿Hay señales de alerta?
Para derivación a cirugía (A)
Para afección específica (B)
¿Justifican pedir pruebas complementarias?
No:
Lumbalgia inespecífica (>95% casos)
Informar (C) y desdramatizar
Evitar reposo en cama
Mantener mayor actividad posible
Fármacos 1ª línea (D)
Sí: Resultados
No
Derive a cirugía
Patología específica:
Tto. específico
-
¿Resolución/mejoría relevante en 2 semanas?
No: Reevalúe A y B
Valore
NRT (F)
Sí: Ejercicio preventivo (E)
¿Hay señales de mal pronóstico funcional? (G)
Sí: ¿Son intensas y la lumbalgia dura más de 6 semanas?
No
Sí
No
+ Programas educativos breves (H)
+ Tto. cognitivo-conductual (I)
¿Resolución/mejoría relevante?
No: Reevalúe A, B y G
+ Valore
Ejercicio (E)
Escuela de la Espalda (J)
Antidepresivos (K)
Sí: Ejercicio preventivo (E)
¿Resolución/mejoría relevante?
No: Reevalúe A, B y G
+ Valore
Parches de Capsaicina (L)
Opiáceos (M)
PENS (N)
Sí: Ejercicio preventivo (E)
¿Resolución/mejoría relevante?
No: Reevalúe A, B y G.
¿Disponible tratamiento cognitivo-conductual con ejercicio?
Sí: Ejercicio preventivo (E)
Sí: Prescríbalo (I)
No
¿Mejoría?
¿Criterios cirugía? (O)
Sí: Artrodesis no instrumentada (O)
¿Resolución?
No
No
Sí
No
Sí: Ejercicio preventivo (E)
Programas multidisciplinarios (P)
Las versiones más completas de esta Guía de Práctica Clínica están disponibles en www.REIDE.org

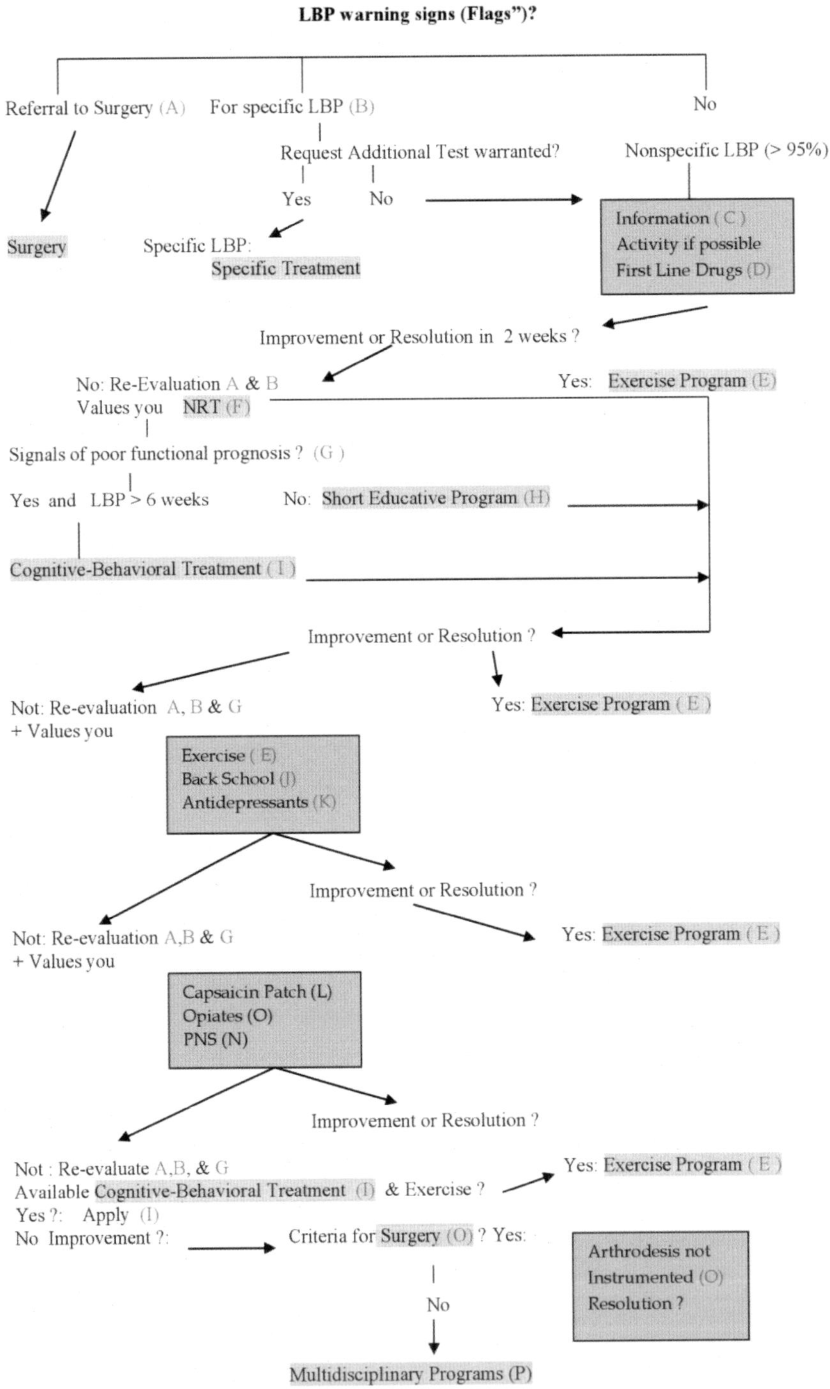
LBP warning signs (Flags")?
Referral to Surgery (A)
For specific LBP (B)
No
Request Additional Test warranted?
Nonspecific LBP (> 95%)
Yes
No
Surgery
Specific LBP:
Specific Treatment
Information (C)
Activity if possible
First Line Drugs (D)
Improvement or Resolution in 2 weeks ?
No: Re-Evaluation A & B
Values you NRT (F)
Yes: Exercise Program (E)
Signals of poor functional prognosis ? (G)
Yes and LBP > 6 weeks
No: Short Educative Program (H)
Cognitive-Behavioral Treatment (I)
Improvement or Resolution ?
Not: Re-evaluation A, B & G
+ Values you
Yes: Exercise Program (E)
Exercise (E)
Back School (J)
Antidepressants (K)
Improvement or Resolution ?
Not: Re-evaluation A,B & G
+ Values you
Yes: Exercise Program (E)
Capsaicin Patch (L)
Opiates (O)
PNS (N)
Improvement or Resolution ?
Not : Re-evaluate A,B, & G
Available Cognitive-Behavioral Treatment (I) & Exercise ?
Yes ?: Apply (I)
No Improvement ?:
Yes: Exercise Program (E)
Criteria for Surgery (O) ? Yes:
Arthrodesis not
Instrumented (O)
Resolution ?
No
Multidisciplinary Programs (P)

Clarification of Algorithm

A For referral to surgery :

a. Emergency Surgery if progresive or bilateral paresis, loss of bladder control or sadle anesthesia.

b. Severe Radicular pain > 6 weeks despite all non surgery treayments (disc herniation). Or only withwalking, needs flexion or sitting, is longer > 6 months and there are images of spinal stenosis.

B For systemic pathology: values X-ray, simple analysis, MRI in early pain in <20 o > 50 years old, dorsal, at night,, neurologic défficit,diffuse, flexion 5° failed, deformation,malaise, loss weigth, fever, neoplasms, corticosteroids, trauma, intranenous addictions, inmunosuppression or AIDS.

C Information patient: Avoid bed rest, nonspecific back pain not due to serious illnes, pain emanating from structures of the spine, spontaneous resolved to 2-6 weeks. To speed recoveryand reduce the risk of recurrence mantainphysical activity including work if possible.

D First line Drugs: Paracetamol 650-1000 mgs each 6-8 hours, AINEs < 3 months, muscle relaxants < 1 week.

E Exercise: Not before 2-6 weeks of episode, as preventive and treatment.

F Neuroreflexotherapy (NRT) : if LBP >2 weeks, moderate to intense (>3 points of 1-10 scale) and there are one acredited unit.

G Signals of Poor functional prognosis

H Brief Educative Programs: Pocket back Manual, chat with patient for positive reinforcement, internet direction with consistent information (www.espalda.org).

I Cognitive-behavioral treatment: Only if LBP > 6 weeks with signals of poor functional prognosis ,potentially active work situation, LBP intense and > 3 months with failure of treatments or with exercise instead of surgery in degenerative spondylosis.

J Back School: Not centered in traditional education but in activity maintenance.

K Antidepressants: Analgesic dosing.

L Capsaicin Patches: If intense pain (>5 points of 1-10 scale)

M Opiates: Patterned and slow-release with strict medical control.

N Peripheral Neuro-Stimulation (PNS)

O Arthrodesis Preferable not instrumented only if disabling pain > 2 years despite all treatments maximum 2 segments of spine.

P Multidisciplinary programs: Intensive and combined D, E, I, K and M , by Psychologist, Physiotherapist and Medical staff in specialized units.

(Based on Figure 1 (Management Algorithm) pg 13-14. And CPG Spanish version pocket guide, disposable in www.REIDE.org

Latorre Marques E., Kovacs F., Gil del Real Mª T., Alonso P., Urrutia G.: Spanish version of COST B13 Guide: A clinical pactical guideline for non-specific back pain based on scientific evidence. *Dolor* 2008; 23: 7-17)

Fig. 2. Management Algorithm of LBP based on Scientific Evidence.

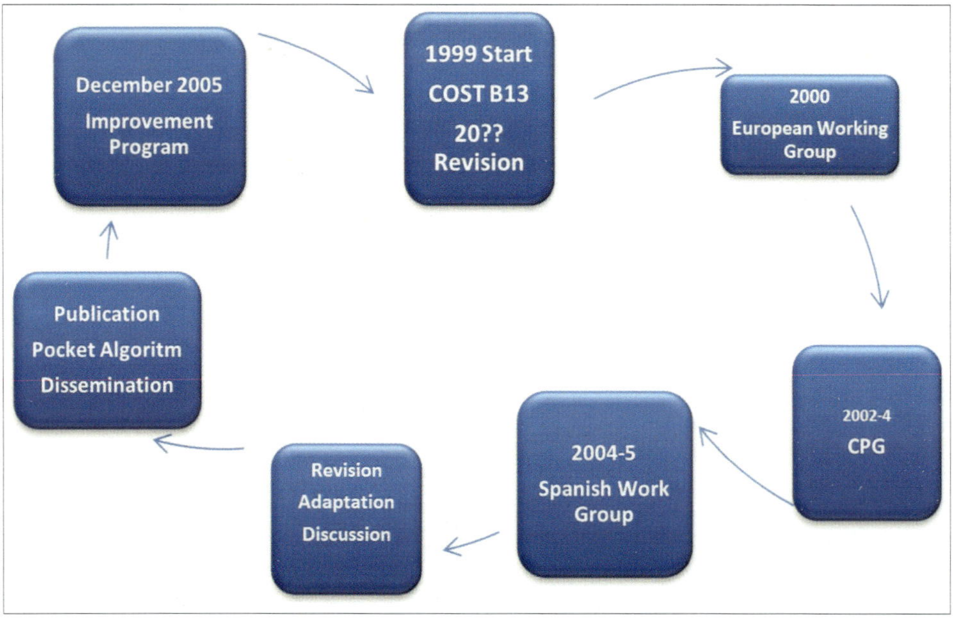

Fig. 3. Development schedule of a CPG based on scientific evidence

Attached and rear face contains explanatory notes of management; as can be seen is integrated into a single temporal sequence low back pain acute, sub-acute and chronic.

5.7.2 Recommendations summary GPC of low back pain

Reflected in a 22 page booklet and contains information relating recommended diagnostic process, recommended treatments based on scientific evidence, technologies not recommended for treatment, prevention of occurrence, or recurrence, and handling algorithm. It can also be downloaded on the internet. Includes authors and reviewers, as well as relevant national entities adopting recommendations.

One of novelties is incorporation of treatments cognitive-behavioral early mode and early detection of signs of poor functional prognosis by simple and specific tests (Table 5).

Signs of poor functional prognosis	Recommended treatments
Mistaken beliefs	Interview training
Misconduct	Written validated information
Occupational factors	Electronic information
Emotional problems	Brief educational program

Table 5. Signs of poor functional prognosis and recommended treatment

6. Discussion

Until the year 2005 revisions and CPG´s served to help primary care to manage only acute low back pain. Few documents provided outcome assessment, until emergence of CPG COST B13 program of European Union.

Inclusion of basic principles management summary and outcome assessment in low back pain, that daily practice medicine, scientific evidence based, makes this CPG a reliable instrument.

Our working group decided include "Criteria to define the evidence needed to develop recommendations":

- For studies considered for each analysis group (builds clinicians, in addition to controlled clinical trials in chronic low back pain and studies on prevention in the corresponding group).
- Referred to non-specific.
- Refer to specific field of each group (acute, chronic low back pain and prevention) and mechanisms of warning mutual between groups given overlapping populations included in systematic reviews or studies.
- Relevant analysis of variable for each field. In case of treatments for acute and chronic low back pain: pain intensity, degree of disability, level of quality of life or absenteeism / return to work.

Numerous adaptations and improvements (Pillastrini P 2011) have been developed. Comparing the quality of the CPG´s from 2004 until today for LBP has improved, however developers need to still increase quality transparency process, especially with regard editorial applicability and independence (Bouwmeester W, 2009).

The process of the CPG´s is still costly in economic resources and time, in best cases for up to 4 years is therefore possible that arise this period new evidence should incorporate, to which review mechanisms should be established involving staff sufficiently prepared both clinical management and analysis of the scientific evidence. For this reason must obtain support of scientific entities and non-profit publishers to remain independent and professionals without conflict of interest.

In our case, was obtained scientific and professional broadest possible support, described favorably by evaluation agencies in health technology, approved by CPG of national health system catalog (GuiaSalud), applied in hospitals and health centers. Its use was recommended by entities as Council official schools of Spain doctors, but unlike other CPG´s included support for consumer organizations in health services. Our version identifies concrete entities of explicit, improving transparency.

However from reading our guide has emerged a contradiction in the meaning of the scientific evidence available at that time because we do not recommended the use of Botulinum Toxin for chronic low back pain treatment, although at that time there was a controlled trial which demonstrated their effectiveness, but after analysis observed low methodological quality and low scale of clinical effects reflected without compensating for the risks of its use. Also our version not recommended vertebral manipulation, while European version was Yes. This is due to the Spanish working group could discuss publications that appeared after first had been released, which showed methodological errors that inclined in negative sense and therefore not apply in daily clinical practice, and still less be taken in National Health Spanish System (Kovacs FM, 2005).

Other technologies that have in Spain anecdotal usage data, such as ozone therapy or drug enforcement anti-TNF (Tumor Necrosis Factor), were discarded for lack of evidence on efficacy, safety or efficiency, after incorporating them by the Spanish working group, to a new analysis of quality whose result was negative.

As evaluated and treatments "not recommended" used in the "treatment of pain unit" also disputes that remain have been (American Pain Society, Chou & Hoyt Huffman, 2009) for the application of nerve blocks in the treatment of low back pain.

Sacroiliac Joint Blockade did not provide evidence that special use, even the infiltration with corticosteroids is no better than placebo (level C), epidural injections were not recommended in non-specific LBP (Level D), however this option can arise in the case of root compression symptomatic herniated disc contained and not extruded, obtaining better results combined with corticosteroid and local anesthesics and is cost-effective (Karpinen J) (2001). Facet injections with corticosteroids were not superior to placebo (level B), and combinations of steroids and local anesthetics were similar to anesthetic alone (level C) effectiveness, therefore not recommended them. Similarly, infiltrations and electrotherapy intra-disc, and facet-joint radiofrequency showed no conclusive data in 2005, probably by the poor quality of the studies, but long series has now been re-designed, with assessment of cost effectiveness and improvement of methodological quality seem to support its use in selected circumstances (Manchikanti L., 2010).

Other low back pain versions CPG´s lack elicitation in relation to the criteria of organizational adaptation to various health services and ensure coordination and efficiency, so the Spanish version includes a process for identification of local variations in story to the applicability and adaptation mechanisms.

Given that the Pan-European version finished his project in 2005, we decided to update mechanisms, based on the detection and analysis of the evidence that arise in the future, marking a timetable for action that also incorporated social and scientific entities to improve adherence and outcomes (Spanish working group program COST B13 2005).

7. Conclusion

Low back pain is a common and potentially disabling condition in adults, and included numerous treatment options. The best available evidence currently suggest that in absence of serious spinal pathology, specific causes of non-spinal origin or progressive neurologic deficit, management should focus on patient education, self-care, common analgesics and exercise.

Short term relief in radiating pain may be obtained with epidural blockade with local anesthetics and steroids, or facet blocks in selected cases. Peripheral Neuromodulation (PNS) and Neuro-Reflex-Therapy (NRT) can offer good results in LBP.

For patients with psychological comorbidities, cognitive-behavioral therapy or multidisciplinary rehabilitation is appropriate. Participation of patient is crucial: patient wish to be taken seriously, give clear and understandable feedback during consultation, and discuss what can be done.

Is needed to improve structuring of multidisciplinary and low cost consultation (Laerum E, 2006), and indicate only surgery treatment in selected cases, by minimally invasive techniques.

The other hand we must improve the procedures for developing clinical trials to make them consistent, and adopt the quality standards in obtaining scientific evidence; for this are emerging tools that help groups and conduct systematic reviews using criteria of quality, transparency and independence. Hope this chapter helps to achieve these objectives.

8. Acknowledgments

Author thanks the Spanish work Group members of COST B13 program *, and Pérez Barrero P. Specialist in Anesthesiology and Plastic/Reconstructive Surgeon, MD of "Miguel Servet Hospital", for suggestions and review of translation style.

*List of members shown in Table 1 (Pg. 10) ; Dolor *Investigacion clinica & terapeutica*. 2008 23: 7-17

9. Potential conflicts of interest

Any financial and nonfinancial conflict of interest of Spanish work group of COST B13 program were declared, discussed, and resolved. Disclosures can be viewed at http:// www.REIDE.org / or the subsequent publication: "Guide to clinical practice of nonspecific low back pain, Spanish version of the Guide to clinical practice of the European program COST B13" Legal deposit M-49781-Madrid, Spain.

10. References

Airaksinen O, et al. On behalf of the COST B13 Working Group on Guidelines for Prevention in low back pain. Chapter 4. European Guidelines for the management of chronic low back pain . Eur Spine J 2006; 15 (suppl 2) :S192-300.

Altman DG, et al. EQUATOR: reporting guidelines for health research. Lancet 2008; 371:1149e50.

Biering Sorensen F. A prospective study of low back pain in a general population. Scand J Rehabil Med 1983; 15 (2): 71-9.

Bigos S, et al. Acute low back pain in adults. Clinical practice guideline. No. 14 , AHCPR publication No. 95-0642. Rockville (MD): Agency of Health Care Policy and Research, Public Health Service, US Department of Health and Human Services ; 1994.

Blau JN, Logue V. A natural history of intermitent claudication fo the cauda equina. Brain 1978; 101: 2111-15.

Bogduk N, on behalf of the Australasian Faculty of Muskuloskeletal Medicine for the Muskuloskeletal Medicine Initiative. Evidence -Based Clinical guidelines for the management of acute low back pain. 1999 November.

Bouwmeester W, van Ernst A, van Tulder M. Quality of low back pain improves. Spine 2009;34 (23):2562-7.

Cabana MD, et al. Why don´t physicians follow clinical practice guidelines? A framework to improvement. JAMA 1999; 282:1458-65.

Cassidy JD, et al. Incidence and course of low back pain episodes in the general population. Spine 2005; 30:2817-23.

Chan AW, Altman DG. Epidemiology and reporting of randomised trials published in PubMed journals. Lancet. 2005;365:1159-62.

Cherkin DC, et al. An international comparaison of back surgery rates. Spine 1994; 19:1201-1206.

Chou R & Hoyt Huffman L. Guideline for the Evaluation and management of Low Back Pain, Evidence Review. American Pain Society 2007/2009. American Pain Society Publisher (Glenview, IL).

Deyo RA, et al. Cost, controversy, crisis: low back pain and the health of the public- annu Rev Public Health 1991; 12:141-145.

Deyo RA, Mirza SK, Martin BI. Back pain prevalence and visit rates. Spine 2000; 31(23):2724-2727.

Field MJ, Lohr KN, eds. Clinical Practice guidelines :Directions for a new program. Wahington (DC): National Academic Press; 1990.

Francisco M Kovacs, & the Spanish Back Pain Research Network. Non-specific low back pain in primary care in the Spanish National Health Service: a prospective study on clinical outcomes and determinants of management BMC Health Services Research 2006, 6:57 doi: 10.1186/1472-6963-6-57.

Frymoyer J, Cats-Baril W. An overview of the incidence and costs of low back pain. Orth clinics of NA 1991:263-9.

Gatchel RJ, Polatin PB, Mayer TG. The dominant role of psychosocial risk factors in the development of chronic low back pain disability. Spine 1995; 20:2702-2709.

Green S et al. Chapter 1: What is a systematic review? In: Higgins JPT, Green Editors. Cochrane handbook for systematic reviews of interventions version 5.0.0. The Cochrane Collaboration 2008. In http://www.cochrane-handbook.org/),

Grupo de variaciones en la Práctica Médica de la Red Temática de Investigación de Resultados y servicios de Salud (Grupo VPC - IRYS). Variaciones de la cirugía ortopédica y traumatología en el Sistema Nacional de Salud . Atlas VPM. Zaragoza: Instituto Aragonés de Ciencias de la Salud; 2005 pg. 17-36.

Guía de Práctica Clínica, Lumbalgia Inespecífica, versión española Guía COST B13. European Commission. Madrid 2005, Depósito Legal N° 49781.

Guyatt GH, Renie D. Evidence - based medicine . ACP J Club 1991;114: A-16

http://www.agreecollaboration.org/

http://www.cochrane.org/

http://www.cochrane-handbook.org /

http://www.consort-statement.org/

http://www.equator-network.org/

http://www.guidelines.gov/

http://www.prisma-statement.org

http://www.REIDE.org , visit December 15 of 2005.

Katz JN. Lumbar disc disorders and low back pain : socio-economic factors and consequences. J Bone Joint Surg Am 2006; 88 (Suppl 2) : 21-24.

Kenneth F. Schulz, Douglas G. Altman, and David Moher, for the CONSORT Group* Ann Intern Med. 2010;152, 11: 1-7.

Kovacs FM, Lázaro P, Muriel A, et al. Does de UK BEAM trial really support the use of maniplulation? URL:www.bmj.com/cgi/content/full/329/7479/1377#responses, (available on line 12 January 2005).

Laerum E, Indahl A, Skouen JS. What is "the good back - consultation? A combined qualitative study of chronic low back pain patient´s interaction with perceptions of consultations with specialist. J Rehabil Med 2006; 38:255-62.

Latorre Marques E, Urrutia G, Alonso P, Kovacs FM, Gil del Real MªT, et al. El manejo de la lumbalgia en la "era del conocimiento": ¿Guías de práctica clínica basadas en la evidencia o en consenso? (Management of low back pain in "The Knowledge Era": ¿clinical practice guidelines based on evidence or in consensus?). Dolor 2008:23:5-6.

Latorre Marques E., Kovacs FM, Gil del Real MªT, Alonso P, Urrutia G, et al. La version española de la Guía COST B13: una guía de práctica clínica basada en la evidencia científica. (The Spanish version of COST B13 Guide: A Clinical Guideline for non-specific back pain based on scientific evidence). Dolor 2008;23:7-17

Liberati A et al.The PRISMA statement for reporting systematic reviewsand meta-analyses of studies that evaluate healthcare interventions : explanation and elaboration. BMJ 2009; 339:b2700, doi:10.1136/bmj.b2700.

Manchikanti L et al. Comprehensive Evidence Based Guidelines for Interventional Techniques in the Management of Chronic Spinal Pain. Pain Phisician 2009; 12: 699-802.

Manchikanti L, et al. A critical review of the American Pain Society clinical practice guidelines for interventional tchniques: part2 . Therapeutic interventions. Pain Physician 2010; 13(4): E215-64.

Memorandum of Understanding, COST ACTION B13: "Low back pain : guidelines for its management". European Commission. Brussels, 1999.

Moher D el al. Epidemiology and reporting characteristics of systematic reviews. PLoS Med. 2007; 4: e78,doi: 10.1371/journal.pmed.0040078.

Moher D, et al. Improving the quality of reports and meta-analyses of randomised controlled trials: The QUOROM statement. Lancet 1999; 354:1896-900.

Nederlandse Vereniging voor Arbeids- en Bedrijfsgeneeskunde. Handelen van de bedrijfsarts bij werknemers met lage rugklachten. Geautoriseerde richtlijn, 2 april 1999. / Dutch Association for Occupational Medicine. Management by the occupational physician of employees with low back pain. Authorised Guidelines, April 2, 1999, ISBN 90 76721 01 7. [the Netherlands]

Owens et al. AHRQ series paper 5: grading the strength of a body of evidence when comparing medical interventions- agency for healthcare research and quality and the effective health-care program. J Clin Epidemiol. 2010; 63:513-23.

Pengel LHM, et al. Acute low back pain: systematic review of its prognosis. BMJ 2003; 327:323-327.

Pillastrini P et al. An updated overview of clinical guidelines for chronic low back pain management in primary care. J Bone Spine 2011; (Epub ahead of print).

Research on work related low back disorders. Luxembourg Office for Official Publications of the European Union (2000), ISBN 92 95007 02 6.

Rico Iturrioz R, Gutiérrez-Ibarluzea I, Asua Batarrita J, Navarro Puerto MA, Reyes Domínguez A, Marín León I, Briones Pérez de la Blanca E. Valoración de escalas y criterios para la evaluación de las Guías de Práctica Clínica Rev Esp Salud Pública 2004;78:457-467

Saal JA, Saal JS, Herzog RJ. The natural history of lumbar intervertebral disc extrusions treated non-operatively. Spine 1990; 683-86.

Saal JA. Natural history and nonoperative treatment of lumbar disc nerniation. Spine 1996; 21:2S-9S.

Sackett, D L et al. Evidence-Based Medicine: How to Practice and Teach EBM. New York: Churchill Livingstone.1997.

Shaneyfelt TM, Mayo-Smith MF, Rothwangl J. Are Guidelines Following Guidelines? The Methodological Quality of Clinical Practice Guidelines in the Peer Reviewed Medical Literature. JAMA 1999:281(20):1900-1905

Simera I, et al. Guidelines for reporting health search: The EQUATOR network´s survey of guideline autors. PLoS Med. 2008; 5:e139, doi: 10.1371/journal.pmed.0050139.

Special Eurobarometer 272/Wave 66.2 - TNS Opinion 6 Social European Commission, September 2007. Health in the European Union. 17-30.

Spengler D, Bigos SJ , Martin NA, et al. Back injuries at industry: a retrospective study. I overview and cost analysis. Spine 1986; 11:141-5.

Straus BN. Chronic pain of spina origin: The costs of intervention. Spine 2002;27:2614-2619.

The AGREE Collaboration. Development and validation of an international appraisal instrument for assessing the quality of clinical practice guidelines: The AGREE proyect. Qual Saf Health Care 2003;12:18-23.

The bone and joint deacade Report, 2005, European Action Towards Better Musculoskeletal Health; European League Against Rheumatism (EULAR), European Federation of Nationa Associations of Orthopaedics and Traumatology (EFFORT) 6 International Osteoporosis Foundation (IOF).

V Encuesta Nacional de Condiciones de Trabajo Octubre 2004 , Instituto Nacional de Higiene y Seguridad en el Trabajo (Fifth National Survey on Working Conditions, INSHT The Spanish National institute of Safety and Hygiene in the Workplace).

Van tulder MW, Koes BW, Bouter JM. A cost-illnes study of back pain in the Netherlands. Pain 1995; 62 (2): 233-40-

Van Tulder MW, Kovacs FM, Mueller G, et al. European commission COST B13 Management Committee: European Guidelines for the management of low back pain. Acta Orthop Sacand 2002; 73 Suppl 305:20-5.

Veerle Hermans, "Research on work-related low backa pain disorders, Institute for Occupational Safety and Health, Brussels.

Walker BF The prevalence of low back pain: a systematic review of the literature from 1966 to 1998. J Spinal Disord 2000; 13(3)205-17.

Watkins et al. Silent pain sufferers. Mayo Clin Proc 2006; 81:167-71.

Wipf JE, Deyo RA. Low back pain. Med Clin North Am 1995; 79(2): 231-46.

3

Low Back Pain in Female Caregivers in Nursing Homes

Hiroharu Kamioka[1] and Takuya Honda[2]
[1]*Department of Physical and Health Education, Faculty of Environmental Science, Tokyo University of Agriculture,*
[2]*Department of Physical and Health Education, Graduate School of Education, The University of Tokyo, Japan*

1. Introduction

In recent years, Japan has become a fast-aging population with the greatest longevity in the world. According to the statistics of Japan, the proportion of the elderly aged 65 years or older reached 20.8% in fiscal, and is estimated to reach 39.6% in 2050 (Japanese Health, Labor, and Welfare Ministry, 2006).

In such an aged society, various health issues occur in caregivers in nursing homes. Particularly in female caregivers, high blood pressure (Hosono et al., 2009) and coronary heart disease (Lee et al., 2003) have been reported to be at high risk. Additionally, caregivers have high prevalence rates of low back pain (LBP) and a high incidence of worker's compensation claims for back injuries (Dehlin et al., 1976; Jorgensen et al., 1994; Fujimura et al., 1995). LBP is common in various occupations, its presence being related to activities requiring repetitive lifting and repeated activities for which anomalous postures tend to be adopted (Josephson et al., 1998). Such work characteristics are common among nursing caregivers. The prevalence of LBP in nursing is high in comparison with other occupations and in relation to other types of work (Ahlberg-Hulten et al., 1995). Risk factors include physical work such as manual lifting and transferring of patients, working conditions such as working time and rest during the night shift, and the working environment (Fujimura et al., 1995). Among these factors, exposures to frequent manual lifting and transferring of patients were widely recognized factors.

On the other hand, for female caregivers, it was reported that dissatisfaction with working conditions and the workplace environment was high (Fujimura et al., 1995), mental stress from work and human relations tended to be high (Ahlberg-Hulten et al., 1995; Failde et al., 2000), and physical fitness elements such as flexibility and muscular strength were low (Kinugasa et al., 1995). Caregivers in nursing homes perform shift work, including night work. In shift workers, a high risk of sleep interruption was reported (Nicholson et al., 1999). A study reported that caregivers who provided care at night suffered from a general sense of fatigue, physical disorders, and reduced mental energy compared with employed women (Tsukasaki et al., 2006). A systematic review indicated that female caregivers had higher levels of burden and depression, and lower levels of subjective well-being and physical health (Pinquart et al., 2006). Therefore, it is necessary that the issue of health in caregivers in nursing homes should include not only low back pain, but also mental and physical health status, and how to interpret these factors.

There are some exercise interventions for the lumbago patient (Cherkin et al., 1996; Frost et al., 1998; Kuukkanen et al., 1998), but so far there are few randomized controlled trials (RCTs) for caregivers in nursing homes. Furthermore, there is no study that assumed mental and physical health status as secondary outcome measurements. In a recent study (Bowen et al., 2009), there was an effort to attach great importance to the feasibility-like accumulation of evidence. Because the possibility of generalization is a serious matter, we needed to examine an intervention program with a few burdens to caregivers in a realistic care scenario. The objective of this review was to summarize the evidence from RCTs on the prevention and curative effects for LBP, and to suggest the concrete strategy as a future agenda.

2. Methods

2.1 Criteria for considering studies included in this review

2.1.1 Types of studies

Studies were eligible if they were RCTs.

2.1.2 Types of intervention, language, and participant

Studies included at least one treatment group in which all therapy was applied. The use of medication, exercise, alternative therapies or lifestyle changes are described, and must have been comparable in the groups studied. There was no restriction on the basis of language. In Japan, nursing is definitely distinguished from care but there are many countries in which this is not the case. Therefore nurses and nursing students were included as search terms. Furthermore, this study established the principal objective in relation to female caregivers, but target articles were included even if they had a small number of male caregivers relative to a majority of female caregivers.

2.2 Search methods for studies identification (Bibliographic database)

We searched the following databases from January 1, 1990 up to July 20, 2011: MEDLINE via PubMed, Web of Science. All searches were performed by a specific searcher (hospital librarian) who was qualified in medical information handling, and who was experienced in searches of clinical trials.

2.3 Review methods

2.3.1 Selection of trials

In order to make the final selection of studies for the review, all criteria were applied independently by two authors to the full text of articles that had passed the first eligibility screening. Disagreements and uncertainties were resolved by discussion.

2.3.2 Summary of studies and data extraction

Two review authors selected the summary from each of the structured abstracts.

2.3.3 Benefit, harm, and withdrawals

The GRADE Working Group (Atkins et al., 2004) reported that the balance between benefit and harm, quality of evidence, applicability, and the certainty of the baseline risk were all considered in judgments about the strength of recommendations. Adverse events, withdrawals, and cost for intervention were especially important information for researchers and users of clinical practice guidelines, and we present this information with the description of each article.

3. Results

The literature searches included 352 potentially relevant articles (Figure 1). Abstracts from those articles were assessed and 11 papers were retrieved for further evaluation (checked for relevant literature). Five publications were excluded because they did not meet the eligibility criteria (see Appendix).

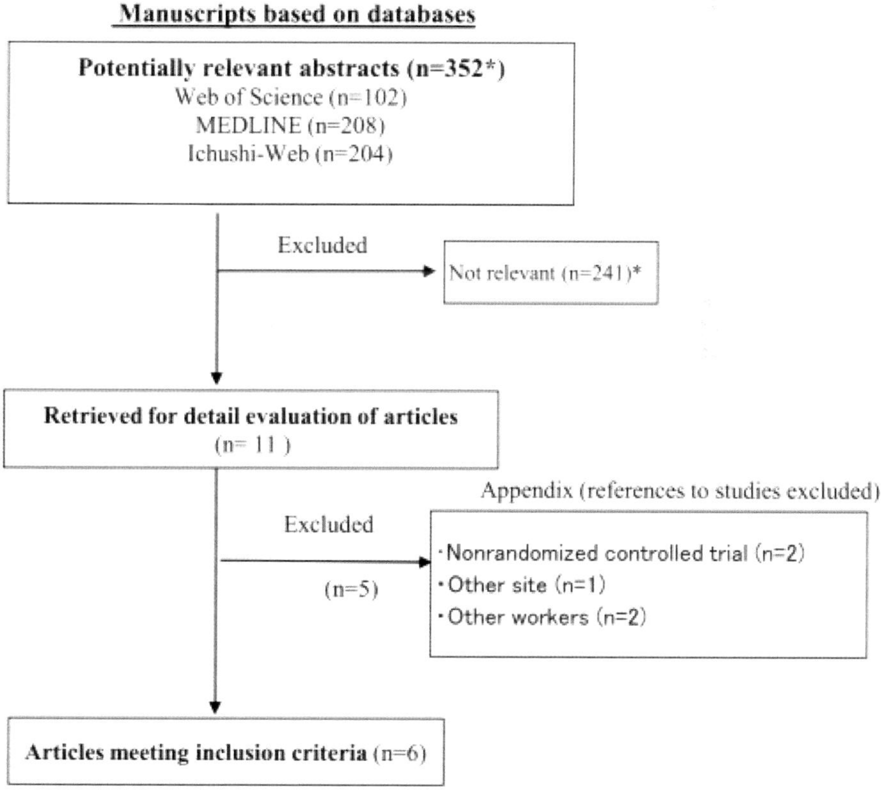

Fig. 1. Flowchart of trial process *reduplication

Six studies met all inclusion criteria, and Table 1 presents the structured abstracts of these six articles. Table 2 provides a brief summary of the six articles. The types of intervention were as follows: multidimensional method (Miyamoto et al., 1998 and Svensson et al., 2008); transfer technique and stress management (Jensen et al., 2006); lumbar support (Roelofs et al., 2007); stretching exercise (Kamioka et al., 2011); and cognitive behavioral theory (Menzel et al., 2006).

Author	Miyamoto M, et al.	Jensen LD, et al.
Citation	Orthop Surg Traumatol 1998; 41: 223-230. (in Japanese with English abstract)	Spine 2006; 31 :1761-1769.
Title	Prospective study for the occurrence of low-back pain in newly-employed nurses educated at the back school	Prevention of Low Back Pain in Female Eldercare Workers: Randomized Controlled Work Site Trial
Aim/Objective	To assess the efficacy of exercise programs for LBP.	To evaluate the effectiveness of an ergonomic and psychosocial intervention in reducing low back pain (LBP) among health care workers.
Setting/Place	Nippon Medical School Hospital	University Hospital of Aarhus
Participants	One hundred and forty-five female nurses (mean 21.7 yrs, range; 20-33yrs) who were newly employed by the hospital.	A total of 234 home care workers, nurses, and nurse's aides from 3 separate eldercare wards were invited to participate in the trial. The invited eldercare workers included all permanent staff engaged in client care at the 3 wards. Of these 234 workers, 210 (90%) agreed to participate. The participation rate in the 3 wards was 85% (mean 44.0 ± 8.5 yrs), 96% (mean 44.6 ± 9.8 yrs), and 89% (mean 44.6 ± 8.4 yrs), respectively.
Intervention	The back school consisted of three courses; a)introductory (lecture on biomechanics and physiology of spine), b) intermediate (lecture on a) + body-mechanics and the trunk muscle exercise for LBP prevention), c) full-course (lecture of a)+b) and exercise of LBP prevention.	The TTI was based on the Stockholm training concept, which aims to reduce the biomechanical load on the back, minimize work in asymmetric postures, and prevent sudden unexpected loads (Figure 2). The SMI was developed to adress the work stress in health care with particular attention to prevention of burnout and development of stategies for stress management (Figure 3). The reference groups had lessons of their own choice in matters unrelated to the intervention programs but of the same duration as the active intervention lessons (*e.g.*, on skin care, proper treatment of a person with diabetes, work, and asthma and safety procedures in chemicals handling).
Main and secondary outcomes*	Habits of trunk muscle exercise and LBP history	The primary outcome was a self-reported rating of the LBP intensity.The implementation of the TTI program was evaluated by comparing ROM values. The SMI program was evaluated by comparing values obtained before and after intervention for each of the 3 dimensions of the SMI program: The Maslach Burnout Inventory, Setterlind's Stress Scores, and rating of social support.
Main results	The adherence of LBP exercise was good in order of c,b,a, but the prevalence of LBP did not have a significant difference among groups. However, in subgroup analysis, high-intensity group(>150days/y) was lower than low-intensity group (149days/y>)in prevalence of LBP.	We found no difference in LBP in any of the intervention arms over the study period.
Conclusion	The adherence of LBP exercise may produce good effects on the prevention of LBP.	The study showed no effect of a transfer technique or stress management program targeting LBP. Thus, there is a need for discussing other priorities in the prevention of LBP among health care workers.

*Two included studies did not distinguish main or secondary outcomes.

Table 1-a. Summary of articles based on structured abstracts

Author	Roelofs PDDM, et al.	Svensson AL, et al.
Citation	Ann Intern Med. 2007; 147: 685-692.	Occupational Medicine 2009; 59: 563-569.
Title	Lumbar Supports to Prevent Recurrent Low Back Pain among Home Care Workers	Multidimensional intervention and sickness absence in assistant nursing students
Aim/Objective	To determine the effectiveness of lumbar supports in the secondary prevention of low back pain.	To ascertain if a multidimensional prevention programme combining psysical training, patient transfer technique and stress management prevents sickness absence and LBP in NA students.
Setting/Place	Home care organization in the Netherlands	Two schools of health and social care in Copenhagen
Participants	360 home care workers with self-reported history of low back pain. The lumbar support group (n=183) was mean 41.8 ± 9.7 yrs. and control group (n=177) was 41.5 ± 9.8 yrs.	The study population comprised 766 female NA students from two schools of health and social care in Copenhagen,Denmark. In all, 668 NA students from 38 classes participated in the study. Students were randomly allocated to the control or intervention group, resulting in 389 students being assigned to the intervention group (20 clusters; mean 26 ± 5yrs.) and 279 students to the control group (18 clusters; mean 25 ± 5 yrs.).
Intervention	Short course on healthy working methods, with or without patient-directed use of 1 of 4 types of lumbar support. Participants could select 1 of 4 types of lumbar supports, supplied by Bauerfeind B.V., Haarlem, the Netherlands. LumboTrain and LumboTrain Lady are individually adjustable, hook-and-loop fastening, fully elastic supports that are available in 5 sizes for men or women.	The LBP prevention programme consisted of an integrated approach of three preventive measures; physical training (48 h), patient transfer technique education (20 h) and stress management with personal development (22 h).
Main and secondary outcomes*	Primary outcomes were the number of days of low back pain and sick leave over 12 months. Secondary outcomes were the average severity of low back pain and function (Quebec Back Pain Disability scale) in the previous week.	Sickness absence was self-reported. The question was phrased 'how many days during the last 12 months have you been absent due to your own sickness?' [17]. Questions concerning LBP were taken from the Standardisd Nordic Musculoskeletal Questionnaire [18,19].
Main results	Over 12 months, participants in the lumbar support group reported an average of -52.7 days (CI, -59.6 to -45.1 days) fewer days with low back pain than participants who received only the short course. However, the total sick days in the lumbar support group did not decrease (-5 days [CI, -21.1 to 6.8 days]). Small but statistically significant differences in pain intensity and function favored lumbar support.	Of 766 female NA students, 668 (87%) completed the baseline questionnaire. Sickness absence during the study period increased in both groups but the increase was significantly lower in the intervention group than the control group, mean (standard deviation) number of days 12 (20) versus 18 (34), $P < 0.05$. The intervention group reported no change in the mean level of general health perception, energy/fatigue or psychological well-being at follow-up, while the control group reported a decline on those scales. There were no significant differences in the prevalence of LBP at follow-up between the intervention and control group.
Conclusion	Adding patient-directed use of lumbar supports to a short course on healthy working methods may reduce the number of days when low back pain occurs, but not overall work absenteeism, among home care workers with previous low back pain. Further study of lumbar support is warranted.	Compared to the control group, the intervention group had significantly less sickness absence. The intervention had no preventive effect on LBP prevalence.

*Two included studies did not distinguish main or secondary outcomes.

Table 1-b. Summary of articles based on structured abstracts

Author	Kamioka H, et al.	Menzel NN, et al.
Citation	Environ Health Prev Med (2011); 16: 97-105.	Pain Management Nurs 2006; 7: 53-63.
Title	Effectiveness of intervention for low back pain in female caregivers in nursing homes: a pilot trial based on multicenter randomization	Back pain in direct patient care providers: early intervention with cognitive behavioral therapy
Aim/Objective	To evaluate the intervention effect of a lecture and stretching exercise on caregivers in nursing homes.	To assess the feasibility and effect size of a cognitive behavioral therapy (CBT) intervention to reduce the measures of back pain, stress, and disability in direct care providers working with back pain.
Setting/Place	The intervention program and the evaluation were carried out in each nursing home, the locations of which were as follows: nursing home A (Setagaya-ku, Tokyo), nursing home B (Koshigaya City, Saitama Prefecture), nursing home C (Konosu City, Saitama prefecture), and nursing home D (Tomi City, Nagano prefecture).	The University of Florida Health Sciences Center Institution
Participants	Of the 88 female caregivers (mean 36.2±13.0 yrs) in the target population, all (100%) consented to participate when provided with enough explanation. 44 were randomly assigned by lottery to the intervention group and 44 to the control group.	The participants included 27 female and 5 male nurses or nursing assistants at 550-bedtertiary care academic medical center in Florida. The mean age of participants was 40.3 years.
Intervention	The intervention program consisted of a lecture and stretching exercise (Table 1). The lecture, which lasted for 30 min, was given by an orthopedist with extensive clinical experience (20 years). The stretching exercise program consisted of classical exercises aimed at the reduction and prevention of lumbago. The program contained the original eight elements of stretching based on the William and Mackenzie exercises utilized widely in the kinesitherapy of rehabilitation (Table 1).	The cognitive behavioral therapy intervention was a weekly stress and pain management session over 6 weeks led by a clinical psychologist. The sessions were held at the medical center and offered one day per week either mid-afternoon (before the evening shift began) or late afternoon (before day shift ended). The topics covered were in relaxation techniques, activity rest cycle, distraction techniques, cognitive restructuring mini-relaxation on the job, on-the-job stress management, assertiveness training, and sleep hygiene/nutrition/exercise.
Main and secondary outcomes*	A 10-cm visual analogue scale (VAS) for low back pain was the main outcome measurement. It was evaluated whether the fingers of both hands could reach the floor (finger-floor distance: FFD) from a standing position during anteflexion.	Visual analogue scale (VAS) for low back pain was the main outcome measurement. It evaluated whether the fingers of both hands could reach the floor (finger-floor distance: FFD) from a standing position during anteflexion.
Main results	A total of 29 (33%) participants withdrew by 12 weeks. Regarding the reasons for withdrawal, 28 participants resigned, and one took a leave of absence due to exacerbation of lumbago. Adherence to the stretching exercises was 2.3 ± 1.3 (mean ± SD) times per week. No significant differences were seen for any outcome measurements. The high adherence group (≧3 times per week) did not show a change in the VAS, but the low adherence group (<3 times per week) and control group showed a tendency towards an increased score ($p = 0.068$).	Pain intensity scores declined in the intervention group, indicationg a large effect ($p=0.06$). However, stress scores increased. Depression scores accounted for one-third of the variance on hours absent because of back pain.
Conclusion	Even with the conduct of one OJT, and exercises of only 6 min every day, the adherence of caregivers was low, and there appeared to be few effects of the OTJ.	Although there was a high dropout rate in the intervention group, a cognitive-behavioral intervention shows promise as a secondary prevention intervention.

*Two included studies did not distinguish main or secondary outcomes.

Table 1-c. Summary of articles based on structured abstracts

Author	Miyamoto M, et al.	Jensen LD, et al.	Roelofs PDDM, et al.	Svensson AL, et al.	Kamioka H, et al.	Menzel NN, et al.
Type of intervention	Multidimension	Transfer technique (TTI) and stress management (SMI)	Lumbar support	Multidimension	Stretching exercise	Cognitive behavioral theory
Effects noted*						
Main outcome (for pain)	No effect	No effect	Effect	No effect	No effect	No effect
Secondary outcomes	Habits of exercise; effect	All items; no effects	Severity and function; effect	Sickness absence; effect	All items; no effects	Stress; no effect
Withdrawals rate**	No description	TTI; 21%, SMI; 19%	22%	36%	14%	50%
Adverse event	No description	No description	No description	No description	No event	No description
Cost of intervention	No description	No description	50–70 euros/participant's support	No description	2,000 dollars/all intervention	17 dollars/h/participant

* 'Effect' is in case of statistical signifinance ($p<0.05$).
** For main outcome measurement

Table 2. Brief summary of six articles

In the main outcome measurement (for pain-relieving), it was only lumbar support that was statistically significantly effective (Svensson et al., 2008). For the multidimensional interventions, it was only sick absence (Svensson et al., 2008) and exercise habits (Miyamoto et al., 1998) were statistically significantly effective in the secondary outcomes. Withdrawal rates were described in 5 articles, and tended to be high (14-50%). Adverse events were not described in most articles.

Three articles did not provide information on the costs of intervention. For lumbar support, it cost 50-70 euros per one unit (Roelofs et al., 2007). For stretching exercise, it cost 2,000 dollars as an overall training expense (Kamioka et al., 2011). And, for cognitive behavioral intervention, the compensation to a participant of one hour was shown to be 17 dollars (Menzel et al., 2006).

We could not perform a meta-analysis due to the heterogeneity of the RCTs.

4. Discussion

4.1 Overall evidence

We did not use the CONSORT 2010 (Moher et al., 2010), example of an extension for trials assessing nonpharmacologic treatments (Boutron et al., 2008), and CLEAR-NPT checklists

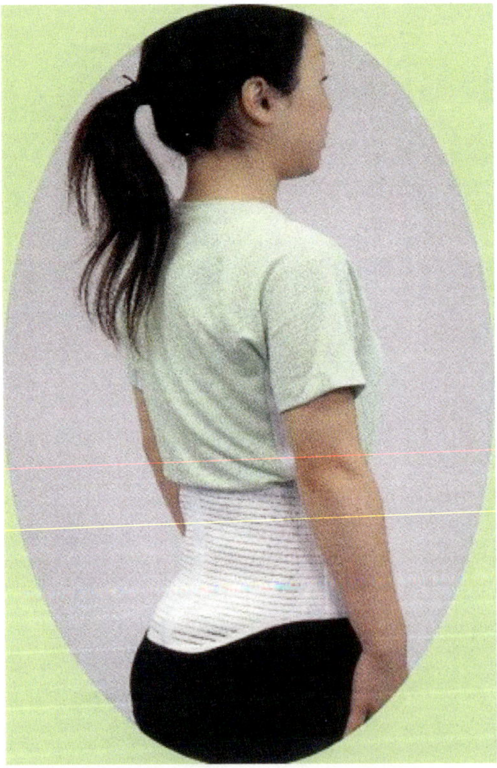

Fig. 2. A sample of lumber support for caregivers (made in Hakujuji corporation, Japan)

(BoutronI et al., 2005) as quality assessments of articles. However, all studies had acceptably clear descriptions. Our study was able to clarify that coping with LBP was extremely difficult for female caregivers (nurses).

For LBP, it was a surprising fact that only lumbar support showed significant effect (Roelofs et al., 2007). The authors suggested that the experienced benefit (overall good adherence of wearing; 78%) most likely outweighs the discomfort of the device (Figure 2). This device stabilizes the low back directly by letting the trunk work more. However, there is a concern that the muscular strength of the abdominal and back muscles will decrease when subjects continually use the device. Unfortunately, it is not known if this problem could be avoided by regulating the timing and duration of use of this device.

4.2 Why other interventions were ineffective

Five RCTs did not show the effects of interventions. A well designed RCT (Jensen et al., 2006) tried to evaluate the effectiveness of the Trans Technique Intervention (TTI; Table 3) and the Stress Management Intervention (SMI; Table 4) in reducing LBP, but both program had no effect on LBP status after 2 years. The authors suggested that the important question remain as to whether the lack of improvement in low back health in the active intervention arms is caused by insufficient implementation of the interventions or if it is the intervention itself that failed to produce better low back health. The authors also described a need for discussing other priorities in the prevention of LBP. Female caregivers always have a tight schedule in the workplace, which may be the main reason they are often not able to use the techniques that they learned. Therefore, we assume that even if an intervention program produces a lasting effect, continuous reinforcement is necessary.

In another well designed RCT (Svensson et al., 2008), a multidimensional program combining physical training, patient transfer technique and stress management had no preventive effect on LBP prevalence (sickness absence). The authors explained that it was sometimes hard to motivate patients to participate in the multidimensional program. We assume that the lack of motivation and readiness of the participants for the program produced a negative result. The authors emphasize that future studies for LBP should focus on the implementation of intervention programs in order to obtain precise information on participation and adherence.

In a RCT based on cognitive behavioral therapy (Menzel et al., 2006), a statistically significant effect was not observed. There was a high dropout rate (50%) in the intervention group. The authors described that the participants either found attending a session at a specific time and day of week difficult or they judged the intervention to be not helpful. We assume this result was caused by a lack of motivation of the participant.

In our RCT (Kamioka et al., 2011), we evaluated the intervention effect of on-the-job training (OJT; a lecture by an orthopedist and stretching exercise) on caregivers in Japanese nursing homes. Unfortunately, even with conducting one OJT and exercising only six minutes every day, adherence of caregivers was low and there appeared to be few effects of the intervention. In the subgroup analysis for the high adherence group (>3 times per week), lumbago tended to be reduced, but in the low adherence group (3 times per week>) and the control group, it tended to be worse ($p=0.068$). This overall ineffectiveness could be attributed to poor adherence by the participants, which was also a problem in other trials.

The TTI was based on the Stockholm training concept. The main principles in the concept are:

1. To reduce the biomechanical load on the back
2. To reduce asymmetric postures
3. To reduce the risk of sudden unexpected load

The technique can be used in all person transfers no matter whether the need is slight support or a transfer of totally dependent person. Lifting and sliding devices, adjustable bed, turntables and slings must be available. Transfer of disabled persons is performed according to the following guidelines

1. Rolling and dragging instead of lifting
2. Work without rotation
3. As little flexion as possible
4. Reduced friction
5. Use of the person's natural movement pattern
6. Close contacts with the aim of making the person to be transferred participate as much as possible in the transfer.

Four supervisors from the project were introduced and trained in the concept during a 3-day work shopby members of the Stockholm training group. The original Swedish manual was translated into Danish and provided the main contents of the education.

After the randomisation, all members of the 7 TTI groups received 2x4 hours of introduction in the basic principles of the training concept, mainly classroom education where each person was trained in about 30 transfer situations. One or two persons from each of the 7 TTI groups volunteered to become instructors, 11 altogether. The instructors were trained for 30 hours in a combination of practical and theoretical lessons in accordance with the concept at the start of the Intervention period. The following 2-6 months focused on implementation of the concept where the instructors had the floor responsibility for supervising their colleagues by observation and bedside education. Besides this ongoing task, the instructors took part in educating the newly employed and formed the link to the occupational health service in matters concerning ergonomics. The instructors established a network and met every second month during the study period to maintain and develop their competence.

Table 3. Contents of the Transfer Technique Intervention (TTI) (Jansen et al., 2006)

The purpose of the SMI programme was to reduce work stress by enhancing coping with stress, preventing burn out and strengthening communication skills. An experienced occupational psychologist developed the program and instructed two fellow psychologists to ensure that the process and the education became similar in the 6 SMI groups. The training took place over 20 weeks with group sessions every fortnight, each session lasting 2 hours. Between sessions, the participants were given assignments concerning implementation of the themes of the session in their daily practice. In addition, every person had her own developing project based on her personal answers from the baseline questionnaire.

Contents of the SMI programme:

1. Analysis of the organisation with the aim of establishing a collective understanding of the resources and weaknesses of the group. This analysis was used to define the developing project for the group with the goal of reducing the psychosocial strain at work.
2. Work with feed back, introduction of criticism and praise as a model of development. Group task concerning self-care.
3. Prevention of burn out, use of tools to recognise connection of one's own demands and others' expectations.
4. Introduction of a model for collegial supervision, establishing ethical rules and selection of subject for collegial supervision.
5. Practical collegial supervision training, examples of stress in different work situations. Introduction of a method to appraise stress.
6. Further work with stress reduction and conflict solving.
7. Behavior related stress and coping strategies, working with personal strategies for coping with stress.
8. Roles and group dynamics. Negotiation of new roles. Internal dialogue about stress.
9. Practicing stress management
10. Status of the personal and collective developing projects and planning of future activities.

A representative from each group volunteered to become a instructor with responsibility for maintaining the process and solving upcoming problems. Like in the TTI, the instructors formed a network with meetings every second month.

Table 4. Contents of the Stress Management Intervention (SMI) (Jansen et al., 2006)

4.3 Future educational program and research agenda

4.3.1 Educational program agenda

Figure 3 shows the educational program for prevention of LBP in nursing facility. First, based on transtheoretical model, identification of the stage of the participant is necessary. Second, before the main interventions, researchers should perform a thorough orientation to promote understanding of the program. Included in the contents of the program should be loss and profit for oneself by participating and protecting one's body, and success and failure samples that are easy to understand. However, unfortunately, in spite of such efforts, it is assumed that there are a few caregivers who will be indifferent or refuse to participate. It is important to the orientation to transfer caregivers to more progressive behavior stages. Greater effects from performing main interventions can be expected when a participant is ready and has enough understanding of the program. In addition, the intervention program should be performed repeatedly and continuously. However, in this concept model, cost-benefit is not considered.

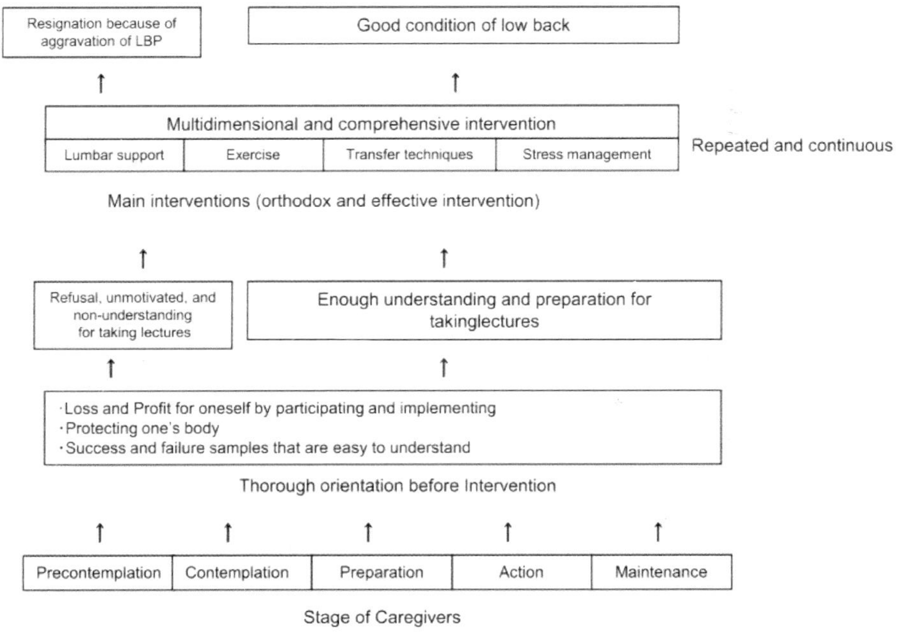

Fig. 3. Concrete educational program for prevention of LBP in nursing facility (Kamioka & Honda, 2011)

4.3.2 Research agenda

Table 5 shows the current evidence (strength of effect) and future research agenda for various interventions. Researchers should present not only the efficacy data, but also any adverse events or harmful phenomena. In particular, they should clarify problems such as muscle weakness caused by wearing lumbar support too often. In various intervention methods, the re-inspection of an effect by an appropriate study design is necessary. It is essential to scientifically explain the mechanism of effect at the same time. Furthermore, in the exercise intervention, it is necessary to make the details of at exercise kind (contents), frequency, time and the period clear. Researcher must judge whether caregiver can enforce them as adherence practically.

Type of intervention	Evidence of effects	Research agenda
Lumbar support	Strong	Study about the timing of the use Study on adverse event such as muscle weakness
Transfer technique	Weak or poor	Can the person whom a skill is high in prevent LBP?
Stress management	Weak or poor	For stress-relieving the degree of effect? The mechanism of effect of LBP prevention by stress-relieving?
Exercise	Weak or poor	The combination of exercise that effect is high in? The degree of effect of a person having high adherence?
Cognitive behavioral theory	Weak or poor	For cognitive befavior the degree of effect? The mechanism of effect of LBP prevention by cognitive befavior?
Multidimension	Weak or poor	The most suitable combination of intervention methods?

Table 5. Current evidence and future research agenda

4.4 Study limitations

This study was based on the PRISMA statement (Liberati A et al., 2009) except for the meta-analysis. However, there were several limitations to the study. Some selection criteria were common across studies, as described above, but bias remained due to differences in eligibility for participation in each study. Publication bias was also a limitation. Although there was no linguistic restriction in the eligibility criteria, we searched studies with only English and Japanese key words. Furthermore, we could not check the references by a hand search. In addition, a nursing job (in a hospital) is essentially different from a care job (in a nursing facility), but, depending on the country, these are approximately similar working institutions. Therefore, an information bias by having included both may exist.

5. Conclusions

For LBP, it was a surprising fact that only lumbar support showed a significant effect. Female caregivers are always on a tight schedule in the workplace, which may be the main reason they are often not able to use the techniques that they learned. Therefore, we assume that even if an intervention program produces a lasting effect, continuous reinforcement is necessary. Initially, based on a transtheoretical model, identification of the stage of the participant is necessary. Then, prior to the main interventions, researchers should perform a thorough orientation to promote understanding of the program. Contents of the program should include loss and profit for oneself by participating and protecting one's body, and success and failure samples that are easy to understand.

In various intervention methods, re-inspection of the effect from an appropriate study design is necessary. It is essential to scientifically explain the mechanism of the effect at the same time.

6. Acknowledgments

We would like to express our appreciation to Ms. Makishi M. and Ms. Higashino R. for their cooperation in this study.

7. Appendix

References to studies excluded in this review

Excusi-on no.	Author. Journal (Year)	Title	Reason of exclusion
1	Rossignol M, et al. Spine (2000)	Coordination of primary health care for back pain	Not nurse or caregivers
2	Dahl JC, et al. Eur J Pain (2001)	Evaluation of a randomized preventive behavioural medicine work site intervention for public health workers at risk for developing chronic pain	Pain of neck, shoulder, and back
3	Maul I, et al. Eur Spine J (2005)	Long-term effects of supervised physical training in secondary prevention of low back pain	All employees of a large hospital
4	Pedersen MT, et al. Spine (2007)	Back muscle response to sudden trunk loading can be modified by training among healthcare workers	Nonrandomiz ed controlled trial
5	Porru S, et al. Med Lav (2009)	Prevenzione dei disturbi del rachide nei lavoratori di un ospedale: intervento multidisciplinare e valutazione di efficacia	Nonrandomiz ed controlled trial

8. References

Ahlberg-Hulten, G.K.; Theorell, T. and Sigala, F. (1995). Social support, job strain and musculoskeltal pain among female health care personnel. Scand J Work Environ Health, Vol. 21, pp.435-439

Atkins, D.; Best, D.; Briss, P.A.; Eccles, M. et al. (2004). Grading quality of evidence and strength of recommendations. BMJ, Vol. 328, pp.1490-1497

Boutron, I.; Moher, D.; Tugwell, P. et al. (2005). A checklist to evaluate a report of a nonpharmacological trial (CLEAR NPT) was developed using consensus. J Clin Epidemiol, Vol. 58, pp.1233-1240

Boutron, I.; Moher, D.; Altman, D. et al. (2008). Methods and processes of the CONSORT group: example of an extension for trials assessing nonpharmacologic treatments. Ann Inter Med, Vol.148, pp.W60-66

Bowen, D.J.; Kreuter, M.; Spring, B. et al. (2009). How we design feasibility studies. Am J Prev Med, Vol. 36, pp. 452-457

Cherkin, D.C.; Deyo, R.A.; Street J.H. et al.(1996). Pitfalls of patient education: limited success of a program for back pain in primary care. Spine, Vol.21, pp. 345-355

Dehlin, O.; Hedenrud, B. and Horal, J. (1976). Back symptoms in nursing aides in a geriatric hospital. Scand J Rehab Med, Vol.8, pp. 47-53

Failde, I.; Gonzalez, J.L.; Novalbos, J.P. et al. (2000). Physical and occupational predictive factors for back pain among employees of a university hospital in southern Spain. Occup Med, Vol.50, pp.591-596

Frost, H.; Lamb, S.E.; Moffett, J.A.K.; et al. (1998). A fitness programme for patients with chronic low back pain: 2-year follow-up of a randomized controlled trial. Pain, Vol.75, pp.273-279

Fujimura, T.; Yasuda, N. and Ohara, H. (1995). Work-related factors of low back pain among nursing aides in nursing homes for the elderly. J Occup Health, Vol.37, pp.89-98

Health & Welfare Statistics Association of Japan. (2006). Annual Statistical Report of National Health Conditions. pp.8-24 (in Japanese)

Hoshino, J.; Hori, Y.; Kondo, T. et al. (2009). Physical and mental health characteristics of female caregivers. Jpn J Public Health, Vol.56, pp.75-86 (in Japanese with English abstract)

Jensen, L.D.; Gonge, H.; Jors, E. et al. (2006). Prevention of low back pain in female eldercare workers: randomized controlled work site trial. Spine, Vol.31, pp.1761-1769

Jorgensen, S.; Hein, H.O. and Gyntelberg, F. (1994). Heavy lifting at work and risk of genital prolapse and herniated lumbar disk in assistant nurses. Occup Med,Vol. 44, pp.47-49

Josephson, M. and Vingard, E. (1998). Workplace factors and care seeking for low-back pain among female nursing personnel: MUSIC-Norrtalje Study Group. Scand J Work Environ Health,Vol.24, pp.465-472

Kamioka, H.; Okuizumi, H.; Okada, S. et al. (2011). Effectiveness of intervention for low back pain in female caregivers in nursing homes: a pilot trial based on multicenter randomization. Environ Health Prev Med, Vol.16, pp.97-105

Kinugasa, T.; Nagasaki, H.; Ito, H. et al. (1995). Effect of physical fitness, sports activities, and aging on low back pain for women working in nursing home. Jpn J Phys Educ, Vol.40, pp. 151-160 (in Japanese with English abstract)

Kuukkanen, T. and Malkia, E. (1998). Effects of a three-month active rehabilitation program on psychomotor performance of lower limbs in subjects with low back pain: a controlled study with a nine-month follow-up. Perceptual Motor Skills, Vol.87, pp. 739-753

Lee, S.; Colditz, G.A.; Berkman, L.F. and Kawachi, I. (2003). Caregiving and risk of coronary heart disease in U.S. women. Am J Prev Med, Vol.24, pp.113-119

Liberati, A.; Altman, D.G.; Tetzlaff, J. et al. (2009). The PRISMA statement for reporting systematic reviews and meta-analyses of studies that evaluate health care interventions: explanation and elaboration. Ann Intern Med, Vol.151, pp.W65-94

Menzel, N.N. and Robinson, M.E. (2006). Back pain in direct patient care providers: early intervention with cognitive behavioral therapy. Pain Manag Nurs, Vol.7, pp.53-63

Miyamoto, M.; Shirai, Y.; Takeuti, T. et al. (1998). Prospective study for the occurrence of low-back pain in newly-employed nurses educated at the back school. Orthop Surg Traumatol, Vol.41, pp.223-230 (in Japanese with English abstract)

Moher, D.; Hopewell, S.; Schulz, K.F.; et al. (2010). CONSORT 2010 explanation and elaboration: updated guidelines for reporting parallel group randomized trials. BMJ, Vol.340, c869

Nicholson, P.J. and D'Auria D.A.P. (1999). Shift work, health, the working time regulations and health assessments. Occup Med, Vol.49, pp. 127-137

Pinquart, M. and Sorensen, S. (2006). Gender differences in caregiver stressors, social resources, and health: an updated meta-analysis. J Gerontol Psych Sci, Vol.61B, pp. P33-45

Roelofs, P.D.; Bierma-Zeinstra, S.M.; van Poppel, M.N. et al. (2007). Lumbar supports to prevent recurrent low back pain among home care workers: a randomized trial. Ann Intern Med, Vol.147, pp.685-692

Stensson, A.L.; Stroyer, J.; Ebbehoj, N.E. et al. (2009). Multidimensional intervention and sickness absence in assistant nuring students. Occup Med, Vol.59, pp.563-569

Tsukasaki, K.; Kido, T.; Makimoto, K. et al. (2006). Naganuma R, Ohno M, Sunaga K. The impact of sleep interruptions on vital measurements and chronic fatigue of female caregivers providing home care in Japan. Nurs Health Sciences, Vol.8, pp.2-9

4

Occupational and Environmental Risk Factors for Development of Low Back Pain in Hospital Nursing Personnel

Jadranka Stričević[1], Zvone Balantič[2], Zmago Turk[3], Dušan Čelan[3] and Majda Pajnkihar[1]
[1]*Faculty of Health Sciences, University of Maribor, Maribor,*
[2]*Faculty of Organisational Sciences, University of Maribor, Kranj,*
[3] *University Clinical Center Maribor, Maribor, Slovenia*

1. Introduction

Nursing was in the past identified as an occupation whose practitioners were at risk of developing low back pain (LBP) (Engkvist et al., 1998; Hoogendoorn et al., 1999; Goldman et al., 2000). Providing nursing care is related to frequent flexion and extension of the body, including manual lifting (Cromie et al., 2000; Elford et al., 2000; Hui et al., 2001; Daynard et al., 2001). Activities connected to lifting and transferring patients represent major physical demands for nursing personnel, which in many cases result in injuries (Marras et al., 1999; Retsas & Pinikahaba, 2000). Some European countries calculate costs related to LBP treatment at around 1% of yearly gross domestic product (van Tulder et al., 1995; Hansson & Hansson, 2005). Among the musculoskeletal disorders, LBP represents the most frequent incident and the most expensive treatment (Balantič & Zupan, 2003, Whiting & Zernicke, 2008). In a German research the cost for a single episode of LBP was estimated to amount approximately to EUR 1300 in medical costs and loss of production (Wenig et al., 2009). The literature estimates that among adults in the general population, 70-85% are believed to experience at least one episode of low back pain at some time during their lifetime (Andersson, 1999; Croft et al., 1999).

The problem of LBP in nursing has been thoroughly researched and the main risks are known, and measures have been suggested for its prevention. Success was in most cases reported as adhering to a 'zero lift policy' by using assistive devices (Zhuang et al., 1999, 2000; Nelson et al., 2003a; Collins et al., 2004; Menzel et al., 2004, Nelson et al., 2006). However, the problem of awkward body postures remains, as it is difficult to avoid these altogether (Smedley et al., 1995; Elford et al., 2000). Biomechanical research revealed the human effort in manual lifting, change of patient position in bed, patient transfer from bed to wheelchair or stretcher, patient transfer from wheelchair to toilet and vice versa as major risks for developing LBP (Owen & Garg, 1989; Owen et al., 2002). Therefore it seems reasonable that nursing personnel should remain in good physical condition, not being overweight, with a supple and firm body. Although body mass index (BMI) was not clearly associated with LBP in the past, research has since shown that low BMI may also represent a risk (Lagerstrom et al., 1995; Kerr et al., 2001; Smedley et al., 2003). Older research also examined smoking and alcohol consumption and concluded that this might represent some risk (Frymoyer et al., 1980; Kelsey et al., 1984; Bigos et al., 1986; Heliovaara et al., 1987). Following literature reviews by Ferguson and Marras (1997) and Rubin (2007), these authors summarised the risk factors for developing LBP in advanced age as being female, having a lower economic standard, lower education, smoking, frail health, physical work, repeated tasks, awkward body postures, lower job satisfaction, depression, spinal structure and visible spinal anomalies.

The international literature suggested four major solutions to prevent LBP in nursing personnel. While the 'zero lift policy' is the most promising among the four strategies, unfortunately it is also the most expensive, because technical equipment needs to be purchased (Nelson et al., 2006). Technical equipment in nursing care provision is only useful if the amount of needed force to handle the equipment does not exceed the forces that are developed by manual handling and lifting (Santaguida et al., 2005). The other three solutions introduced were manual lifting techniques (Larese & Fiorito, 1994; Daltroy, 1997; Lagerstrom & Hagberg, 1997; Hye-Knudsen et al. 2004; Karahan & Bayraktar, 2004), forming nursing personnel or special workforces into so called 'lift teams' (Charney, 1997) and introducing regular prevention exercising (Linton & van Tulder, 2001; Rainville et al., 2004; Burton et al., 2005; Byrne et al., 2006).

Several studies that researched improvements in LBP development by applying manual lifting techniques showed no positive long-term effects (Larese & Fiorito, 1994; Daltroy, 1997; Lagerstrom & Hagberg, 1997; Nelson et al., 2003b). Many older Asiatic traditional motion techniques are currently revived, introducing new manual lifting techniques to best overcome physical burden. Marras et al. (1999) concluded that the essential problem in using manual lifting techniques is the human factor, where stressful working conditions and unexpected situations may eventually lead to failures. From a financial aspect manual, lifting techniques are most popular as a prevention strategy because they cost least.

Heavy lifting became a legislative issue in the 1970s and 1980s to prevent occupational activities that might harm workers' health. In the USA the National Institute on Safety and Health recommended the maximum spinal compression force should be 3400N for heavy manual lifting or manual transfer (NIOSH, 1981, 1994). Zhuang et al. (1999) showed that in performing manual patient transfer, specifically turning a patient in bed and lifting the patient to a sitting position in bed on average exceeds this recommended limit. This was especially evident in care activities of overweight patients. Additional research on different manual lifting techniques in team work in patients weighing more than 75kg resulted in spinal compression forces over the recommended threshold of 3400N (Winkelmolen et al., 1994). Nursing personnel are by their occupational duties regularly exposed to burdens that exceed these limits.

The International Labour Organisation (ILO) issued two conventions that are more closely connected to nursing care provision, (1) (Maximum Weight Convention) and (2) C155 (Occupational Safety and Health Convention). The Maximum Weight Convention was adopted on 28 June 1967 and states that no worker shall be required or permitted to engage in the manual transport of a load which, by reason of its weight, is likely to jeopardise the worker's health or safety. In addition, the employer shall take appropriate steps to ensure that any worker assigned to manual transport of loads other than light loads receives, prior to such assignments, adequate training or instruction in working techniques, with a view to safeguarding health and preventing accidents. The Occupational Safety and Health Convention, adopted 22 June 1981, aims to prevent accidents and injury to health arising out of, linked with or occurring in the course of work, by minimising, so far as is reasonably practicable, the causes of hazards inherent in the working environment (European Agency for Safety and Health at Work, 2008).

The European community mandates certain directives in connection with occupational safety, with each member country having the right to implement the directives according to their own means. Member countries can adopt more intense regulations within individual directives, although this is seldom the case due to economic interests to remain competitiveness with Eastern countries. In general, adopted directives are not intended for certain economic branches and are also not directly connected to musculoskeletal disorders; they give general guidelines to improve occupational health and. Council directive 89/391/EEC obligates employers to introduce measures to encourage improvements in the health and safety of workers at work, whereas information, dialogue and balanced participation on health and safety at work must be developed between employers and workers (Council Directive 89/391/EEC, 1989).

Council directive 90/269/EEC was adopted on 29 May 1990 and supplements the general council directive about measures for occupational health and safety (89/391/EEC) on the minimum health and safety requirements for the manual handling of loads where there is a risk, particularly of back injury, to workers. The general provision states that the employer shall take appropriate organizational measures, or shall use the appropriate means, in particular mechanical equipment, in order to avoid the need for the manual handling of loads by workers. In addition, wherever the need for manual handling of loads by workers cannot be avoided, the employer shall organize workstations in such a way as to make such handling as safe and healthy as possible. Assessment must be made, in advance if possible, of the health and safety conditions of the type of work involved, and in particular examinations of the characteristics of loads. Employers must ensure that workers and/or their representatives receive general indications and, where possible, precise information on the weight of a load, and the centre of gravity of the heaviest side when a package is eccentrically loaded. Employers must ensure that in addition workers receive proper training and information on how to handle loads correctly and the risks they might be open to, particularly if these tasks are not performed correctly (Council directive 90/269/EGS, 1990).

Several studies have indicated that LBP may contribute to nursing personnel turnover. For example, Owen (2000) found that 20% of nursing personnel had changed jobs at least once due to LBP problems. In a survey conducted with over 43,000 members of nursing personnel in five countries, 17% to 39% reported that they planned to leave their job in the next year due to the physical and psychological demands of the profession (Aiken et al., 2001). These findings are especially alarming given the current shortage of nursing personnel and the increasing need for nursing care projected over the next decades (Massey et al., 2009; DiMattio et al., 2010).

To contribute to the above knowledge, the aim of this research was to examine to which extent the occupational and environmental risk factors influence the development of LBP in hospital nursing personnel. According to literature review our research included some occupational risk factors and also some personal characteristics about life style, which were designated as environmental risk factors. Among the risk factors included were also some that were expected to act as prevention for developing LBP. Potential risk or prevention factors were included in a multivariate statistical analysis to conduct factors that best predict development of LBP. In the discussion and conclusion sections we introduce some ideas, suggestions and considerations how our results could be implicated in clinical practice. We also provide some suggestions for future research.

To search in the international literature for similar research strategies as we had applied, we conducted a very general search of electronic databases about LBP and nursing personnel or occupation, followed by a subsequent review of abstracts to find more specific literature. The search in the electronic databases Medline, CINAHL and ScienceDirect resulted in 144 non-overlapping hits. Search terms 'nursing' and 'low back pain' were used by selecting the period from 1990 to 2010. The inclusion criteria for the literature search were for terms to be found in the title, abstract or keywords. The larger group of hits was related to LBP occupational risks and four articles only included recreation or exercise as potential LBP prevention. Occupational and environmental components of nursing personnel have rarely been analysed at the same time, and Feng et al. (2007) was identified as the only contribution where recreation was considered in the statistical analysis in conjunction with other LBP risks. The literature search was extended beyond 2007 (till end of 2010), where our research design was initial made and also the data gathering concluded, in order to find any up to date scientific advances.

2. Methods

As a research method a non-experimental approach with a cross-sectional survey and statistical analysis was used.

2.1 Instrument

A structured questionnaire about LBP included basic demographic and anthropometric characteristics: age, gender, body height and body weight. The second part of the instrument included occupational risk factors: duration of employment in years, duration of employment in the current position in years, frequent manual weight lifting above 10 kg, manual patient transfer and material handling, patient transfer and material handling with assistive devices, availability of height adjustable beds in nursing care provision, treatment of patients in the highest patient classification system category, and hours of daily work at the computer. The third part included physical activities and habits (environmental risk factors): regular exercises to prevent LBP, recreation and sports in youth, recreation and sports at present, and hours of watching television. The question representing the depended variable was how many episodes of LBP respondents experienced during their working career. A list of all measured characteristics is included in table 1. Duration of employment, work at the computer and watching TV were split into two groups by median value. BMI was calculated as quotient of body weight in kilograms and square of body height in metres. Overweight was marked as BMI ≥ 25 kg/m^2 (WHO, 2006).

The structured questionnaire was developed according to literature review about occupational risks connected to development of LBP in nursing personnel, for example, as manual patient transfer, frequent lifting and nursing care provision without the use of assistive devices (Ando et al., 2000; Fairbank & Pynsent, 2000; Davidson & Keating, 2002; Trinkoff et al., 2003; Bot et al., 2004). Included were personal characteristics that were considered to have positive or negative effects on LBP, such as being female, physical condition, BMI, preventive exercising, watching TV (Lahad et al., 1994; Ferguson & Marras, 1997; Maher et al., 1999; Trinkoff et al., 2003; Rainville et al., 2004; Burton et al., 2005; Shehab & Al-Jarallah 2005; Rubin, 2007).

2.2 Sample

The sample consisted of nursing personnel from the University Clinical Center Maribor, the second largest Hospital in Slovenia, with 2800 employees and 1500 members of nursing personnel among them. Hospital nursing personnel in Slovenia involves nursing assistants and registered nurses. Nine hundred questionnaires were distributed among the nursing personnel in 2007, 663 (73.7%) were returned and 581 (64.6%) were considered for analysis. Eighty-two (12.4%) returned questionnaires were excluded due to missing data. Data were collected by convenience sampling. The sample size was selected according to stratification of 40 hospital departments. The strategy in general was to survey 30-40% of nursing personnel from each hospital department to achieve better reliability of results. Gender distribution was 489 (84.2%) women and 92 (15.8%) men, mean age was 37.5±8.9 of years. Frequent LBP was reported in 458 (78.8%) of cases.

The sample size was determined by exemplars from international cross-sectional survey studies, which tend to gather a sample of approximately 500 participants. These sample sizes generally suffice for the needs of the statistical analysis and also give better representation of the researched population. For the statistical relevance, according to alpha level (p-value) of 0.05, the number of predictors (degrees of freedom) of 15 and the anticipated medium effect (f2) size of 0.15, in order to achieve desired statistical power level of 0.8, a sample size of n=139 would be needed (Polit, 1996).

2.3 Statistical analysis

Sample data was presented by frequency and percentage for categorical variables or by mean value and standard deviation for numerical variables. Median values were calculated to split numerical variables into two groups. Univariate and multivariate statistics for LBP risk was calculated by binary logistic regression. The chi-square (χ^2), odds ratio (OR), 95% confidence interval (95%CI) and P-value were calculated. Multivariate binary logistic regression was calculated without a method to omit insignificant variables. Statistical analysis was performed with SPSS 15.0 software (SPSS Inc., Chicago, IL). P-value < 0.05 was marked as statistically significant.

2.4 Ethical considerations

Approval for the study was obtained locally from the Nursing Care Office of the University Clinical Center Maribor. The research participants were informed about the nature of the study and what participation would entail for them, by receiving a printed information sheet (Puotiniemi & Kyngäs, 2004). Participants were also asked to contact head nurses of the hospital departments for further questions. Participation in the research was voluntary and anonymous. By applying the stratification by hospital departments, anonymity was to some extend compromised or contracted, nevertheless it was still not possible to recognise the individual participants. Items in the questionnaire were very general; they did not included private items, provoke feelings or address intimate relationship. Items that may potentially harm participants or the University Clinical Center Maribor were also not included in the questionnaire.

3. Results

Fifteen variables in the form of risk factors were included in the analysis (Table 1).

Risk factor	LBP (in %)		χ^2	OR	95%CI	*P-value*
	rare (n=123)	frequent (n=458)				
Age ≥40 y	26.0	53.9	28.4	3.3	2.1-5.2	*<0.001*
Female gender	75.6	86.5	8.3	2.1	1.3-3.4	*0.004*
Duration of employment ≥20y	26.8	54.6	28.1	3.3	2.1-5.1	*<0.001*
Duration of employment in current position ≥15y	32.5	51.7	14.0	2.2	1.5-3.4	*0.001*
Frequent manual lifting >10kg	43.1	63.5	16.3	2.3	1.5-3.4	*<0.001*
Manual patient transfer and material handling	10.6	16.2	2.3	1.6	0.8-3.1	*0.126*
Patient transfer and material handling with assistive devices	15.4	6.6	9.4	0.4	0.2-0.7	*0.002*
Height adjustable beds in nursing care provision	28.5	21.8	2.4	0.7	0.5-1.1	*0.124*
Treatment of patients in the highest patient classification system category	4.1	11.8	5.8	3.2	1.2-8.1	*0.016*
Work with the computer ≥2h per day	40.7	24.7	12.0	0.5	0.3-0.7	*0.001*
Regular exercises to prevent LBP	27.6	52.0	21.9	2.8	1.8-4.4	*<0.001*
Recreation and sports in youth	60.2	44.3	9.6	0.5	0.4-0.8	*0.002*
Recreation and sports at present	37.4	20.3	15.1	0.4	0.3-0.7	*<0.001*
Watching TV ≥2h per day	52.8	51.7	<0.1	1.0	0.6-1.4	*0.829*
BMI ≥25	*25.2*	*39.3*	*8.2*	*1.9*	*1.2-3.0*	*0.004*

Table 1. Univariate analysis of risk factors for development of LBP

The results of univariate statistics show that three risk factors were not significantly connected to development of LBP. These were manual patient transfer and material handling, height adjustable beds in nursing care provision and watching TV ≥2h per day. LBP incidents were marked as rare if respondents reported none, one or two incidents while employed as nursing personnel (n=123 or 21.2%).

Results of the follow-up multivariate analysis are presented in Table 2. Three risk factors were calculated as independent predictors for development of LBP. Other significant risk factors on the univariate level failed to achieve statistical significance. The prediction quality of the calculated regression model also resulted in statistical significance (χ^2 =99.577, df=15, p<0.001). The regression model explained 24.5% of the original variance.

Risk factor	LBP (in %)		χ^2	OR	95%CI	*P-value*
	rare (n=123)	frequent (n=458)				
Age ≥40 y	26.0	53.9	2.0	2.3	0.7-7.2	*0.152*
Female gender	75.6	86.5	3.0	1.7	0.9-3.0	*0.084*
Duration of employment ≥20y	26.8	54.6	0.0	1.1	0.4-3.6	*0.847*
Duration of employment in current position ≥15y	32.5	51.7	0.6	0.8	0.4-1.4	*0.453*
Frequent manual lifting >10kg	43.1	63.5	14.4	2.4	1.5-3.9	*<0.001*
Manual patient transfer and material handling	10.6	16.2	1.9	1.6	0.8-3.3	*0.166*
Patient transfer and material handling with assistive devices	15.4	6.6	1.5	0.6	0.3-1.3	*0.219*
Height adjustable beds in nursing care provision	28.5	21.8	0.2	0.9	0.5-1.5	*0.638*
Treatment of patients in the highest patient classification system category	4.1	11.8	1.9	2.0	0.8-5.5	*0.164*
Work with the computer ≥2h per day	40.7	24.7	3.3	0.6	0.4-1.0	*0.071*
Regular exercises to prevent LBP	27.6	52.0	16.8	2.8	1.7-4.6	*<0.001*
Recreation and sports in youth	60.2	44.3	0.4	0.9	0.5-1.4	*0.539*
Recreation and sports at present	37.4	20.3	7.1	0.5	0.3-0.8	*0.008*
Watching TV ≥2h per day	52.8	51.7	0.6	0.8	0.5-1.3	*0.447*
BMI ≥25	*25.2*	*39.3*	*2.9*	*1.6*	*0.9-2.6*	*0.091*

Nagelkerke R^2=0.245

Table 2. Multivariate analysis of risk factors for development of LBP (model χ^2 =99.577, df=15, p<0.001)

According to χ^2 values in Table 2, regular exercises to prevent LBP represented the highest risk for development of LBP (OR 2.8, 95%CI 1.7-4.6). This result shows that nursing personnel started with preventive exercises when it was too late and LBP was already developed. In case of rare LBP problems, 72.4% of nursing personnel without frequent LBP problems were not performing any preventive exercises. The second ranked risk factor was frequent manual lifting >10 kg (OR 2.4, 95%CI 1.5-3.9). Of the nursing personnel who developed LBP on a frequent basis, 63.5% reported that their care activities are connected to frequent manual lifting of considerable weight. The third ranked risk factor was conducted in better physical condition by regular recreation and sports, which reduced the risk for frequent development of LBP (OR 0.5, 95%CI 0.3-0.8). Only 20.3% of the nursing personnel who reported frequent LBP were regularly engaged in recreation and sports; this percentage was considerably lower compared to nursing personnel without recreational and sporting interests.

4. Discussion

Frequent LBP was reported in 78.8% of cases, which was similar to results in previous studies (Karahan & Bayraktar, 2004). The strongest risk factor for development of LBP was found in the absence of preventive exercises to strengthen back muscles. Nursing personnel may not be aware of LBP risks and start with preventive exercises when it is already too late and LBP episodes become frequent. Exercises to prevent LBP are considered useful although there is little scholarly agreement on the kind of preventive exercising that should be undertaken or which intensity leads to best possible results (Burton et al., 2005; Byrne et al., 2006). In addition, our results indicate that recreation and sports may reduce risk of developing LBP, although the odds ratio was not as evident. Similar results were obtained by Linton and van Tulder (2001) and Burton et al. (2005).

Manual lifting is the best known risk for development of LBP, especially if the weight is considerable, of frequent nature, or both (Marras et al., 1999; Retsas & Pinikahaba, 2000; Bongers et al., 2002). For many years now, the international literature called to implement working rules for reduction of physical stressors on the human body. The best solution to the problem may be the 'zero lift policy' by using assistive devices when providing nursing care (Collins et al., 2004; Nelson et al., 2006). When considering that the manual lifting hazard grows with advancing age and that the retirement age is increasing, reaching retirement without developing LBP may become a challenge for nursing personnel (Engkvist, 2008). Surprisingly, our results did not significantly confirm this, although odds ratio of 2.3 for higher age (≥40) pointed in the same direction. The financial costs of LBP treatment should not be considered only during employment, because in retirement problems usually increase and become chronic (Turk, 2005). In such cases the financial costs for health insurance may turn out to be considerable for the rest of the person's life due to the need for analgesic drugs and physiotherapy.

Improved physical conditions for nursing personnel is not something that the public directly connects with the purpose of nursing care, which is primarily to offer physical and psychosocial help and care to sick and frail people. Society connects nursing care primarily with virtues like solace, attentiveness, empathy etc., and less with physical strength. It is therefore odd to expect from nursing personnel to expose their low backs far beyond recommended thresholds when manually transferring patients. In that manner, the proposal to reduce workload by grouping nursing personnel or employing specialists as lift teams would considerably reduce exposure to low back problems (Charney, 1997), but due to lack of staff or additional staff costs it is difficult to consider either organisation or employment of such teams. Yet, Charney (1997) argued that if sick leave, subsequent insurance and medical costs, staff turnover and other possible negative side effects of LBP development are taken into account, then this equation should turn out positive in the long run.

Regular prevention exercises to strengthen back and abdominal muscles lead to improved physical strength and relief to the musculoskeletal when lifting manually or needing to use force (Linton & van Tulder, 2001; Burton et al., 2005). Some other studies, however, only partially confirmed that such an approach prevents developing LBP (Lahad et al., 1994; Maher, 2000; Rainville et al., 2004). Nevertheless, improved physical condition is popular and represents a modern life style to reduce the daily stress. LBP prevention should be incorporated in the regular daily working schedule of nursing personnel in particular. There are several possible ways to realise this, but the most important is to gain the support of legislation and employers. In our opinion it would be best if employees could decide on their own which prevention strategy is most suitable for them, considering their abilities and expectations, and in this way employers, for example, would show their contribution with time subsidies (approximately 15-30 minutes daily). It is also very important to consider that prevention activities and especially sports activities can also lead to health contraindications (Burton et al., 2005).

Members of the nursing personnel who are not interested in recreation and sports should not be forced to improve their physical condition in such a way. Nevertheless, only a small effort is needed for significant improvement (Feng et al., 2007). It is our belief that exercises to prevent LBP should be clearly promoted. Employees in Slovenia must participate in various trainings to keep their working licence, but there is no obligation to train how to maintain vitality. The orientation should be on education about physical stressors and routines how to strengthen the musculoskeletal system to at least try to keep the lifelong resistance. Mitchell et al. (2009) suggested that lifestyle and psychological factors associated with LBP should begin to be addressed during undergraduate study.

4.1 Suggestions for future research

The results conducted in this research are much as expected, yet in some cases also surprising, especially that the frequent manual lifting >10kg was the only significant occupational risk factors for development of LBP. Our expectations were oriented towards duration of employment and age as two typical risk factors for any kind of health risk. We also expected that patient transfer and material handling with assistive devices would reduce the risk for developing LBP. At the University Clinical Center Maribor, for example, surgical departments have better technical equipment then internal medical departments. Surgical departments are housed in new buildings with wide corridors and also in patients' rooms there is more space between beds, although conditions differ according to circumstances; usually in winter time there are more injuries. The typical problem in nearly all hospital departments is lack of space around toilet bowls and bath tubs, doors are not wide enough for easy access with wheelchairs or stretchers. These architectural barriers make solutions for a 'zero lift policy' for nursing personnel a far dream. Engkvist et al. (1995) exposed some of these problems scientifically.

Further research is needed, including the risk factors involved in this research and more precise details about specific manual patient transfer or manual material handling (patient transfer to wheelchair, stretcher or bath tub, repositioning in bed, washing, toileting etc.).

We also propose that future research should include specific types of recreation and sports activities (running, cycling, fitness, hiking etc.) and types of regular exercises to prevent LBP (yoga, Pilates, aerobics, abdominal training, traditional morning exercises etc.). Non-inclusion of this data represents some justified self-criticism of our research design and criticism of other similar studies. Results about risk factors are primarily too general and seldom offer precise information which manual lifting activities should be avoided and which recreational, sporting and preventive activities should be fostered.

4.2 Study limitations

The sample in our research was gathered from a single hospital. However, our literature review showed that several international hospitals face similar problems to those in Slovenia, primarily because of inadequate staffing levels and occupational stress (time distress, physical and psychological fatigue), that consequently cause pain and injuries to nursing personnel (Hollingdale & Warin, 1997; Vasiliadou et al., 1997; Aiken et al., 2001; Smedley et al., 2003; Videman et al., 2005). We believe that the University Clinical Center Maribor represents typical European and international hospitals supplying comprehensive health care services and disease treatments. Therefore, our research sample included nursing personnel from all areas or departments that are determined by international medicine.

A concern represents a possible non-response. From 900 distributed questionnaires, 237 or 26%, remained unevaluated. There is a possibility of impact on the results because we could not included variance of nursing personnel who did not respond to the research. Nevertheless, the response rate of 74% was, according to international literature, very good (Trinkoff et al., 2003).

Given the cross-sectional study design and the collection of data by self-report, these findings must, however, be interpreted with caution, because self-report may reflect denial, deception, or difficulty in recall (Trinkoff et al., 2003).

5. Conclusion

Because of various health problems in relation to LBP, which may result in absence from work and consequently increased pressure from employers, it seems reasonable that nursing personnel pay more attention how to maintain a healthy spine. Awkward body postures and manual lifting may be difficult to avoid due to the nature of nursing. Little interest from employers to purchase assistive devices and improve working conditions means that it is important for nursing personnel to find their own suitable LBP prevention strategy. For example, preventive exercises can be more physically oriented, such as abdominal training, or be more vigorous like aerobics, yoga or Pilates. Each prevention strategy may lead to some improvement and if there is dissatisfaction it is easy to stop and to try something else.

The international literature is alarmed about the occupational tasks of nursing personnel that involve a heavy physical burden connected to manual patient and material handling. Nursing personnel are pushed into these risky tasks without much consideration about their health risks. Manual patient transfer and lifting of heavy burden is not defined as an occupational duty or task of nursing personnel. The current shortage of nursing personnel who avoid this ever more physically and psychological stressful occupation, and the increasing need for nursing care of a frail older population must lead to legislation, and to employers to search for solutions to improve working environment.

The LBP problem is very complex one. The battle against spine diseases should include several professions and multidirectional approaches. We see two crucial points where the most important work against LBP in nursing personnel must be executed. First the nursing schools should include the knowledge about spine problems, risk factors and prevention strategies in their educational programme. Second the employers should be aware of cost-benefit of LBP prevention and take care of optimal work organisation and ergonomics with proper technical equipment for diminution of heavy physical work of nursing personnel.

6. References

Aiken, L.H.; Clarke, S.P.; Sloane, D.M.; Sochalski, J.A.; Busse, R.; Clarke, H.; Giovannetti, P.; Hunt, J.; Rafferty, A.M. & Shamian, J. (2001). Nurses' reports on hospital care in five countries. *Health affairs,* Vol.20, No.3, (May 2001), pp. 43-53, ISSN 0278-2715

Andersson, G.B. (1999). Epidemiological features of chronic low-back pain. *Lancet,* Vol.354, No.9178, (August 1999), pp. 581-585, ISSN 1470-2045

Ando, S.; Ono, Y.; Shimaoka, M.; Hiruta, S.; Hattori, Y.; Hori, F. & Takeuchi, Y. (2000). Associations of self estimated workloads with musculoskeletal symptoms among hospital nurses. *Occupational and Environmental Medicine,* Vol.57, No.3, (March 2000), pp. 211-216, ISSN 1351-0711

Balantič, Z. & Zupan, A. (2003). Measurements of respiratory capacity in patients with neuromuscular diseases. *Experimental Lung Research,* Vol.29, No.8, (December 2003), pp. 537-548, ISSN 0190-2148

Bigos, S.; Spengler, D.; Martin, N.; Zeh, J.; Fisher, L.; Nachemson, A. & Wang, M.H. (1986). Back injuries in industry: A retrospective study. II, Injury factors. *Spine,* Vol.11, No.3, (April 1986). pp. 246-241, ISSN 0362-2436

Bongers, P.M.; Kremer, A.M. & ter Laak, J. (2002). Are psychosocial factors, risk factors for symptoms and signs of the shoulder, elbow, or hand/wrist?: A review of the epidemiological literature. *American Journal of Industrial Medicine,* Vol.41, No.5, (May 2002), pp. 315-342, ISSN 0271-3586

Bot, S.D.M.; Terwee, C.B.; van der Windt, D.A.W.M.; Feleus, A.; Bierma-Zeinstra, S.M.; Knol, D.L.; Bouter, L.M. & Dekker, J. (2004). Internal consistency and validity of a new physical workload questionnaire. *Occupational and Environmental Medicine,* Vol.61, No.12, (December 2004), pp. 980-986, ISSN 1351-0711

Burton, A.K.; Balagué, F.; Cardon, G.; Eriksen, H.R.; Henrotin, Y.; Lahad, A.; Leclerc, A.; Müller, G.; van der Beek, A.J. & COST B13 Working Group on European Guidelines for Prevention in Low Back Pain, (2005). How to prevent low back pain. *Best Practice & Research Clinical Rheumatology,* Vol.19, No.4, (August 2005), pp. 541-555, ISSN 1521-6942

Byrne, K.; Doody, C. & Hurley D.A. (2006). Exercise therapy for low back pain: A small-scale exploratory survey of current physiotherapy practice in the Republic of Ireland acute hospital setting. *Manual Therapy,* Vol.11, No.4, (November 2006), pp. 272-278, ISSN 1356-689X

Charney, W. (1997). The lift team method for reducing back injuries: a 10-hospital study, AAOHN Journal, Vol.45, No.6, (June 1997), pp.300-304, ISSN 0891-0162

Collins J.W.; Wolf, L.; Bell, J. & Evanoff, B. (2004). An evaluation of a "best practices" musculoskeletal injury prevention program in nursing homes. *Injury Prevention*, Vol.10, No.4, (August 2004), pp. 206-211, ISSN 1353-8047

Council Directive 89/391/EEC. (1989). The introduction of measures to encourage improvements in the safety and health of workers at work, Brussels, 5.9.2011, Available from http://eur-lex.europa.eu/LexUriServ/LexUriServ.do?uri=CELEX:31989L0391:en:HTML

Council Directive 90/269/EEC. (1990). the minimum health and safety requirements for the manual handling of loads where there is a risk particularly of back injury to workers, Brussels, 15.9.2011, Available from http://eur-lex.europa.eu/LexUriServ/LexUriServ.do?uri=CELEX:31990L0269:en:HTML

Croft, P.R.; Papageorgiou, A.C.; Thomas, E.; Macfarlane, G.J. & Silman, A.J. (1999). Short-term physical risk factors for new episodes of low back pain. Prospective evidence from the South Manchester back pain study. *Spine*, Vol.24, No.15, (August 1999), pp. 1556–1561, ISSN 0362-2436

Cromie, J.E.; Robertson, V.J. & Best, M.O. (2000). Work-related musculoskeletal disorders in physical therapists: prevalence, severity, risks, and responses. *Physical Therapy*, Vol.80, No.4, pp. 336-351, ISSN 0031-9023

Daltroy, L. (1997). A controlled trial of an educational program to prevent low back injuries. *The New England Journal of Medicine*, Vol.337, No.5, (July 1997), pp. 322-328, ISSN 0028-4793

Davidson, M. & Keating, J.L. (2002). A comparison of five low back disability questionnaires: reliability and responsiveness. *Physical Therapy*, Vol.82, No.1, (January 2002), pp. 8-24, ISSN 0031-9023

Daynard, D.; Yassi, A.; Cooper, J.E.; Tate, R.; Norman, R. & Wells, R. (2001). Biomechanical analysis of peak and cumulative spinal loads during simulated patient-handling activities: a substudy of a randomized controlled trial to prevent lift and transfer injury of health care workers. *Applied Ergonomics*, Vol.32, No.3, (June 2001), pp. 199-214, ISSN 0003-6870

DiMattio, M.J.K.; Roe-Prior, P. & Carpenter, D.R. (2010). Intent to Stay: A Pilot Study of Baccalaureate Nurses and Hospital Nursing. *Journal of Professional Nursing*, Vol.26, No.5, (September-October 2010), pp. 278-286, ISSN 8755-7223

Elford, W.; Straker, L. & Strauss, G. (2000). Patient handling with and without slings: an analysis of the risk of injury to the lumbar spine. *Applied Ergonomics*, Vol.31, No.2, (April 2000), pp. 185-200, ISSN 0003-6870

Engkvist, I.-L.; Hagberg, M.; Wigaeus-Hjelm, E.; Menckel, E.; Ekenvall, L. & PROSA Study Froup. (1995). Interview protocols and ergonomics checklist for analysing overexertion back accidents among nursing personnel. *Applied Ergonomics*, Vol.26, No.3, (June 1995), pp. 213-220 ISSN 0003-6870

Engkvist, I.-L.; Hagberg, M.; Hjelm, E.W.; Menckel, E.; Ekenvall, L. & PROSA study group. (1998). The accident process preceding overexertion back injuries in nursing personnel. *Scandinavian Journal of Work, Environment and Health*, Vol.24, No.5, (October 1998), pp. 367-375, ISSN 0355-3140

Engkvist, I.-L. (2008). Back injuries among nurses - A comparison of the accident processes after a 10-year follow-up. *Safety Science,* Vol.46, No.2, (February 2008), pp. 291-301, ISSN 0925-7535

European Agency for Safety and Health at Work. (2008). European legal requirements relating to work-related musculoskeletal disorders, Brussels, 05.09.2011, Available from http://osha.europa.eu/en/topics/msds/legislation_html

Fairbank, J.C.T. & Pynsent, P.B. (2000). The Oswestry Disability Index. *Spine,* Vol.25, No.22, (November 2000), pp. 2940–2953, ISSN 0362-2436

Feng, C.-K.; Chen, M.-L. & Mao, I.-F. (2007). Prevalence of and risk factors for different measures of low back pain among female nursing aides in Taiwanese nursing homes. In: *BMC Musculoskeletal Disorders,* 8:52, (June 2007), Available from http://www.biomedcentral.com/1471-2474/8/52.

Ferguson, S. & Marras, W. (1997). A literature review of low back disorder surveillance measures and risk factors. *Clinical Biomechanics,* Vol.12, No.4, (June 1997), pp. 211-226, ISSN 0268-0033

Frymoyer, J.W.; Pope, M.H.; Costanza, M.C.; Rosen, J.C.; Goggin, J.E. & Wilder, D.G. (1980). Epidemiologic studies of low-back pain. *Spine,* Vol.5, No.5, (September-October 1980), pp. 419-423, ISSN 0362-2436

Goldman, R.H.; Jarrard, M.R.; Kim, R.; Loomis, S. & Atkins, E.H. (2000). Prioritizing back injury risk in hospital employees: application and comparison of different injury rates. Journal of Occupational and Environmental Medicine, Vol.42, No.6, (June 2000), pp. 645-652, ISSN 1351-0711

Hansson, E.K. & Hansson, T.H. (2005). The costs for persons sick-listed more than one month because of low back or neck problems. A two-year prospective study of Swedish patients. *European Spine Journal,* Vol. 14, No.4, (May 2005), pp. 337-345, ISSN 0940-6719

Heliovaara, M.; Knekt, P. & Aromaa, A. (1987). Incidence and risk factors of herniated lumbar intervertebral disc or sciatica leading to hospitalization. *Journal of Chronic Diseases,* Vol.40, No.3, (March 1987), pp. 251-258, ISSN 0021-9681

Hollingdale, R. & Warin, J. (1997). Back pain in nursing and associated factors: a study. *Nursing Standard,* Vol.11, No.39, (June 1997), pp. 35-38, ISSN 0029-6570

Hoogendoorn, W.E.; van Poppel, M.N.; Bongers, P.M.; Koes, B.W. & Bouter, L.M. (1999). Physical load during work and leisure time as risk factors for back pain. *Scandinavian Journal of Work, Environment and Health,* Vol.25, No.5, (October 1999), pp. 387-403, ISSN 0355-3140

Hui, L.; Ng, G.Y.; Yeung, S.S. & Hui-Chan, C.W. (2001). Evaluation of physiological work demands and low back neuromuscular fatigue on nurses working in geriatric wards. *Applied Ergonomics,* Vol.32, No.5, (October 2001), pp. 479-483, ISSN 0003-6870

Hye-Knudsen, C.T.; Schibye, B.; Hjortskov, N. & Fallentin, N. (2004). Trunk motion characteristics during different patient handling tasks. International Journal of Industrial Ergonomics, Vol.33, No.4, (April 2004), pp. 327-337, ISSN 0169-8141

Karahan, A. & Bayraktar, N. (2004). Determination of the usage of body mechanics in clinical settings and the occurrence of low back pain in nurses. *International Journal of Nursing Studies,* Vol.41, No.1, (January 2004), pp. 67-75, ISSN 0020-7489

Kelsey, J.L.; Githens, P.B.; White, A.A. 3rd; Holford, T.R.; Walter, S.D.; O'Connor, T.; Ostfeld, A.M.; Weil, U.; Southwick, W.O. & Calogero, J.A. (1984). An epidemiological study of lifting and twisting on the job and the risk for acute prolapsed lumbar intervertebral disk. *Journal of Orthopedic Research,* Vol.2, No.1, (January 1984), pp. 61-66, ISSN

Kerr, M.S.; Frank, J.W.; Shannon, H.S.; Norman, R.W.K.; Wells, R.P.; Neumann, W. P.; Bombardier, C. & Ontario Universities Back Pain Study Group (2001). Biomechanical and psychosocial risk factors for low back pain at work. *American Journal of Public Health,* Vol.91, No.7, (July 2001), pp. 1069-1075, ISSN 1741-3842

Lagerstrom, M.; Wenemark, M.; Hagberg, M. & Hjelm, E.W. (1995). Occupational and individual factors related to musculoskeletal symptoms in five body regions among Swedish nursing personnel. *International Archives of Occupational and Environmental Health,* Vol.68, No.1, (January 1995), pp. 27-35, ISSN 0340-0131

Lagerstrom, M. & Hagberg, M. (1997). Evaluation of a 3 year education and training program for nursing personnel at a Swedish hospital. *AAOHN Journal,* Vol.45, No.2, (February 1997), pp. 83-92, ISSN 0891-0162

Lahad, A.; Malter, A.D.; Berg, A.O. & Deyo, R.A. (1994). The effectiveness of four interventions for the prevention of low back pain. *Journal of American Medical Association,* Vol.272, No.16, (October 1994), pp. 1286-1291, ISSN 0098-7484

Larese, F. & Fiorito, A. (1994). Musculoskeletal disorders in hospital nurses: a comparison between two hospitals, *Ergonomics,* Vol.37, No.7, (July 1994), 1205-1211, ISSN 0014-0139

Linton, S.J. & van Tulder, M.W. (2001). Preventive interventions for back and neck pain problems: What is the evidence? *Spine,* Vol.26, No.7, (April 2001), pp. 778-787, ISSN 0362-2436

Maher, C.; Latimer, J. & Refshauge, K. (1999). Prescription of activity for low back pain: What works? *The Australian Journal of Physiotherapy,* Vol.45, No.2, (June 1999), pp. 121-132, ISSN 0004-9514

Maher, C.G. (2000). A systematic review of workplace interventions to prevent low back pain. *The Australian Journal of Physiotherapy,* Vol.46, No.4, (December 2000), pp. 259-269, ISSN 0004-9514

Marras, W.S.; Davis, K.G.; Kirking, B.C. & Bertsche, P.K. (1999). A comprehensive analysis of low-back disorder risk and spinal loading during the transferring and repositioning of patients using different techniques. *Ergonomics,* Vol.42, No.7, (July 1999), pp. 904-926, ISSN 0014-0139

Massey, L.; Esain, A. & Wallis, M. (2009). Managing the complexity of nurse shortages: A case study of bank and agency staffing in an acute care Trust in Wales, UK. *International Journal of Nursing Studies,* Vol.46, No.7, (July 2009), pp. 912-919, ISSN 0020-7489

Menzel, N.N.; Brooks, S.M.; Bernard, T.E. & Nelson, A. (2004). The physical workload of nursing personnel: association with musculoskeletal discomfort. *International Journal of Nursing Studies,* Vol.41, No.8, (November 2004), pp. 859-867, ISSN 0020-7489

Mitchell, T.; O'Sullivan, P.B.; Smith, A.; Burnett, A.F.; Straker, L.; Thornton, J. & Rudd, C.J. (2009). Biopsychosocial factors are associated with low back pain in female nursing students: A cross-sectional study. *International Journal of Nursing Studies,* Vol.46, No.5, (May 2009), pp. 678-688, ISSN 0020-7489

Nelson, A.; Lloyd, J.; Menzel, N. & Gross, C. (2003a). Preventing nursing back injuries: redesigning patient handling tasks. AAOHN Journal, Vol.51, No.3, (March 2003), pp. 126-134, ISSN 0891-0162

Nelson, A.; Fragala, G. & Menzel, N. (2003b). Myths and facts about back injuries in nursing. *American Journal of Nursing,* Vol.103, No.2, (February, 2003), pp. 32-40, ISSN 0002-936X

Nelson, A.; Matz, M.; Chen, F.; Siddharthan, K.; Lloyd, J. & Fragala, G. (2006). Development and evaluation of a multifaceted ergonomics program to prevent injuries associated with patient handling tasks. *International Journal of Nursing Studies,* Vol.43, no.6, (August, 2006), pp. 717-733, ISSN 0020-7489

NIOSH - National Institute for Occupational Safety and Health. (1981). *Work Practices Guide for Manual Lifting,* NIOSH DHHS Publication No. 81-122, Cincinnati, USA

NIOSH - National Institute for Occupational Safety and Health. (1994). *Applications Manual for the Revised NIOSH Lifting Equation,* NIOSH DHHS Publication No. 94-110, Cincinnati, USA

Owen, B.D. & Garg, A. (1989). Patient handling tasks perceived to be most stressful by nursing assistants, In: *Advances in Industrial Ergonomics and Safety,* A. Mital, (Ed.), 775–781, I. Taylor and Francis, ISBN 978-0850664935, London, United Kingdom

Owen BD. (2000). Preventing injuries using an ergonomic approach. AORN Journal, Vol.72, No.6, (December 2000), pp. 1031-1036, ISSN 0001-2092

Owen, B.D.; Keene, K. & Olson, S. (2002). An ergonomic approach to reducing back/shoulder stress in hospital nursing personnel: a five year follow up. *International Journal of Nursing Studies,* Vol.39, No.3, (March 2002), pp. 295-392, ISSN 0020-7489

Polit, D.F. (January 1996). *Data Analysis and Statistics for Nursing Research,* Prentice-Hall, ISBN 978-0838563298, Upper Saddle River, NJ, USA

Puotiniemi, T.A. & Kyngäs, H. (2004). The coping of an adolescent who has been in psychiatric inpatient care and her mother in every day life. *Journal of Psychiatry and Mental Health Nursing,* Vol.11, No.6, (December 2004), pp. 675-682, ISSN 1351-0126

Rainville, J.; Hartigan, C.; Martinez, E.; Limke, J.; Jouve, C. & Finno, M. (2004). Exercise as a treatment for chronic low back pain. *The Spine Journal,* Vol.4, No.1, (January-February, 2004), pp. 106-115, ISSN 1529-9430

Retsas, A. & Pinikahaba, J. (2000). Manual handling activities and injuries among nurses: an Australian hospital study. *Journal of Advanced Nursing,* Vol.31, No.4, (April 2000), pp. 874-883, ISSN 0309-2402

Rubin, D.I. (2007). Epidemiology and risk factors for spine pain. *Neurologic Clinics,* Vol.25, No.2, (May 2007), pp. 353-371 ISSN 0733-8619

Santaguida, P.L.; Pierrynowski, M.; Goldsmith, C. & Fernie, G. (2005). Comparison of cumulative low back loads of caregivers when transferring patients using overhead and floor mechanical lifting devices. *Clinical Biomechanics,* Vol. 20, No.9, (November 2005), pp. 906-916, ISSN 0268-0033

Shehab, D. & Al-Jarallah, K. (2005). Nonspecific low-back pain in Kuwaiti children and adolescents: Associated factors. *Journal of Adolescent Health,* Vol.36, No.1, (January 2005), pp. 32-35, ISSN 1054-139X

Smedley, J.; Egger, P.; Cooper, C. & Coggon, D. (1995). Manual handling activities and risk of low back pain in nurses. *Occupational and Environmental Medicine,* Vol.52, No.3, (March 1995), pp. 160-163, ISSN 1351-0711

Smedley, J.; Inskip, H.; Trevelyan, F.; Buckle P.; Cooper C. & Coggon D. (2003). Risk factors for incident neck and shoulder pain in hospital nurses. *Occupational and Environmental Medicine,* Vol.60, No.11, (November 2003), pp. 864-869, ISSN 1351-0711

Trinkoff, A.M.; Lipscomb, J.A.; Geiger-Brown, J.; Storr, C.L. & Brady, B.A. (2003). Perceived Physical Demands and Reported Musculoskeletal Problems in Registered Nurses. *American Journal of Preventive Medicine,* Vol.24, No.3, (April 2003), pp. 270-275, ISSN 0749-3797

Turk, Z. (2005). Socialnomedicinski vidiki bolečine v križu. *Rehabilitacija,* Vol.4, No.3-4, (December 2005), pp. 9-12, ISSN 1580-9315

van Tulder, M.W.; Koes, B.W. & Bouter, L.M. (1995). A cost-of-illness study of back pain in The Netherlands. *Pain,* Vol.62, No.2, (August 1995), pp. 233-240, ISSN 0304-3959

Vasiliadou, A.; Karvountzis, G.; Roumeliotis, D.; Soumilas, A.; Plati, C. & Nomikos, I. (1997). Factors associated with back pain in nursing staff: a survey in Athens, Greece, *International Journal of Nursing Practice,* Vol.3, No.1, (March 1997), pp. 15-20, ISSN 1322-7114

Videman, T.; Ojajärvi, A.; Riihimäki, H. & Troup, J.D. (2005). Low back pain among nurses: a follow-up beginning at entry to the nursing school. *Spine,* Vol.30, No.20, (October 2005), pp. 2334-2341, ISSN 0362-2436

Zhuang, Z.; Stobbe, T.J.; Hsiao, H.; Collins, J.W. & Hobbs, G.R. (1999). Biomechanical evaluation of assistive devices for transferring residents. *Applied Ergonomics,* Vol.30, No.4, (August 1999), pp. 285-294, ISSN 0003-6870

Zhuang, Z.; Stobbe T.J.; Collins J.W.; Hsiao, H. & Hobbs, G.R. (2000). Psychophysical assessment of assistive devices for transferring patients/residents. *Applied Ergonomics,* Vol.31, No.1, (February 2000), pp. 35-44, ISSN 0003-6870

Wenig, C.M.; Schmidt, C.O.; Kohlmann, T. & Schweikert, B. (2009). Costs of back pain in Germany, *European Journal of Pain,* Vol.13, No.3, (March 2009), pp. 280-286, ISSN 1090-3801

Whiting, W.C.; Ronald, F. & Zernicke, R.F. (2008). *Biomechanics of Musculoskeletal Injury* (2nd ed), Human Kinetics, ISBN 978-0736054423, Champaign, IL, USA

WHO. (2006). BMI Classification. World Health Organization, Geneva, 17.08.2011, Available from http://apps.who.int/bmi/index.jsp?introPage=intro_3.html

Winkelmolen, G.H.; Landeweerd, J.A. & Drost, M.R. (1994). An evaluation of patient lifting techniques. *Ergonomics,* Vol. 37, No.5, (May 1994), pp. 921-932, ISSN 0014-0139

5

Estimation of Prognosis in Non Specific Low Back Pain from Biopsychosocial Perspectives

J. Nicholas Penney
Centre of National Research on Disability and Rehabilitation Medicine, University of Queensland, Australia

1. Introduction

The significance of low back pain and associated disability across many western nations continues to be an important issue. Pain and disability associated with musculoskeletal conditions represents a significant health and economic burden in Australia, with total direct and indirect costs of musculoskeletal disorders including arthritis being in excess of 15 billion dollars per annum (AAMPG. 2003).

In the USA the data from the 1998 Medical Expenditure Panel Survey, reported that health care expenditure incurred by individuals with back pain reached in excess of 90 billion dollars. Individuals with back pain also incurred 60% more health care costs than those without (Luo, Pietrobon et al. 2003).

There is also a growing literature that supports the contention that low back pain is a complex, multidimensional health issue and should be reviewed within the context of the individual (Young,Waisiak, et al 2011).

Evidence-based clinical practice guidelines, such as those produced in Australia in 2003 emphasise the importance of the biopsychosocial model in the understanding of pain in general and musculoskeletal pain in particular (AAMPG. 2003). The biopsychosocial model focuses on illness, communicating or behaving in a manner that suggests the individual is not well, rather than on disease, the person's experience of illness being influenced by physical, psychological and social factors (Engel. 1980). Engel's model highlighted that in order to respond adequately to an individuals suffering, and give them a sense of being understood, the clinician needed to be able to respond simultaneously to the biological, psychological and social dimensions of illness (Borrell-Carrio,Suchman et al 2004)

The model incorporates the biomedical understanding of nociception as part of the wider holistic biopsychosocial view, rather than treating psychosocial factors as an 'overlay' to the biomedical model.

Philosophically the model is a way of understanding how suffering, disease and illness may be affected by mulitple levels of organisation, from the molecular to societal. Practically, the model provides a way of understanding the patient's subjective experiance as an essential contributor to accurate clinical diagnosis and assessment (Borrell-Carrio et al 2004).

There has been increasing acceptance that psychosocial factors play a significant role in the transition from an acute episode, or episodes, of low back pain to a chronic disorder (Pincus, Burton, et al. 2002). There is also some evidence that these factors may play an aetiological role (Pincus et al. 2002) (Linton. 2000) (Trouchon, and Fillion. L.2000).

The acceptance of the wider biopsychosocial model has been further extended by the World Health Organisation's (WHO) International Classification of Functioning, Disability and Health (ICF) (WHO. 2000).

Many individual psychological factors have been reported over the years as potential obstacles to recovery, with much of the early work centred around fear. Initially the work focussed around the fear avoidance model of exaggerated pain perception in chronic low back develpoed by Lethem and co-workers (Lethem, Slade, Troup, Bentley. 1983). The Fear-Avoidance Belief Questionnaire developed by Waddell and co-workers published in 1993 measured beliefs about physical activity and work (Waddell, Somerville, Henderson, Newton, Main 1993). Workers with low back pain were shown to believe that physical activity including work was feared to increase both spinal pain and damage. These fear avoidant beliefs helped to explain self reported disability in normal daily activities including work(Waddell et al 1993).

Fear of pain together with fear of hurt or harm were further postulated as a fundemental mechanism of disability associated with low back pain were explored by Vlaeyen and Linton. The natural human reaction to pain is an automatic one to try and avoid what is belived to be the cause of the pain, ongoing fear then potentially drives further avoidant behavior(Vlaeyen and Linton 2000).

Contrary to the weight of evidence however, surveys of primary contact practitioners continue to indicate that general practitioners for instance, may only be partially managing low back pain from this evidence-based perspective. This may be due in part to the difficulties reported in changing physician behaviour (Buchbinder, Staples et al. 2009) and then further highlighted by the difficulty reported in integrating the biopsychosocial model into clinical disiplines, such as physiotherapy (Harland and Lavallee. 2003). The potential difficulties in fully incorporating a biopsychosocial approach to patients, appear to transcend professional training and boundaries, as Harding and co-workers reported in 2010. Whilst pain clinic practioners in the UK embrase behavioural based management as part of a biopsychosocial pain management model, little consideration was given to social factors (Harding, Campbell et al 2010).

The estimation of prognosis (identifying those at risk of a poor outcome such as ongoing pain or disability, or failing to return to work) of an episode of low back pain is particularly important to clinicians, patients, employers and third party payers alike. However despite the weight of evidence there remains a tendancy to rely on instruments that quantify prognostic factors from a biomedical perspective alone, rather than the contemporary biopsychosocial model, whilst focusing on return to work as a single outcome. A predictive instrument that may help clinicians fully incorporate the biopsychosocial model into clinical practice clearly has some utility, and whilst it has been suggested that such an instrument needs to capture all the potential biopsychosocial risk factors that may adversely affect functional outcomes (Hilficker, Bachmann, et al. 2007), an initial attempt to produce such a draft questionnaire resulted in a long and unwieldy instrument

The study reported in this chapter tested the hypothesis that it would be feasible to develop a valid and reliable instrument for estimating the prognosis of non specific low back pain from within the biopsychosocial domain, suitable for routine clinical use.

Ethical approval for each step of the instrument's development was obtained from the ethics committee, University of Queensland, Australia.

The components of the resultant instrument (termed the Biopsychosocial Index of Prognosis (BPIP)) were developed from the literature review and perspective of a logical course of clinical enquiry into the current and past episodes of low back pain. The nature and character of the pain together with the severity, spread and duration of the symptoms were also included in the draft questionnaire. Past and present medical and psychological histories were considered together with demographic details including occupation. The items generated were combined into a content map derived from the International Classification of Function (ICF). Initial item generation included items from previously validated instruments identified from the literature where possible. The draft index initially contained 145 items. The large pool of items were initially included in the prototype questionnaire, which was progressively and systematically subjected to item reduction. The necessity for this process of item reduction was established a priori, and driven by the lack of feasibility of carrying a large number of potentially redundant items through to the validation stage of the instruments development (Bellamy, Campbell et al. 2002). The development of the BPIP potentially filled a gap in measurement, estimating prognosis from a variety of biopsychosocial domains and driven by clinical, rather than theoretical perspectives.

Thie chapter describes the development of the BPIP including the steps taken in item reduction and reports on testing the validity of the final instrument, and its reliability against the 'gold standard' measure identified as the Roland and Morris disability questionnaire (RDQ) (Roland and Morris. 1983). The RDQ is one of the most frequently reported instruments used to assess the disability associated with low back pain. The RDQ was also the criterion measure selected for the previous work of Burton and co-workers on psychosocial predictors (Burton, Tillotson, Main and Hollis 1995). A variety of other instruments were considered from the literature including the Orebro Musculoskeletal Pain Questionnaire (Linton and Hallden. 1998) as the potential gold standard. However the focus was on the wider community with low back pain, not just workers with acute low back pain, so the RDQ remained the instrument of choice.

2. Methods

2.1 Development of the BPIP

The initial assessments of the prototype index were undertaken in three distinct phases In phase one, piloting was undertaken with a small group without low back pain, consisting of five health care professionals from a variety of disciplines and from different English spreaking countries including England, Australia and New Zealand. and chosen for their academic and general life experiance. The primary focus of the first pilot trial was to obtain feedback on the pool of items selected for evidence of any ambiguity or repetition, ease of administration and the overall comprehensiveness of the questionnaire.

In phase two, a further pilot study was undertaken with a group of low back pain patients recruited from a variety of primary health care practices on the Sunshine Coast in Australia. Patients were provided with a pack containing the prototype questionnaire, and instruction sheet and two copies of the informed consent form together with two stamped addressed envelopes. Each stage of data collection was subjected to ethical clearance through The University of Queensland's ethics committee.

Phase three was a 24 hour test-retest of the reliability of the amended instrument was completed. BPIP packs containing 2 identical questionniares were distributed with the instruction to complete the first questionniare and then the second one, ideally at the same time of day, 24 hours later without reference to the answers provided the day before. The intention was to establish reliability in a sample of 25% of the total of respondents required for the trial of the main instrument.

No specific exclusion criteria were stated other than children or adolescents, pregnancy or three months post partum. The instrument was designed for use in adults over the age of 18 years with English as a first language.

The overall development process of the BPIP is summarised in Figure 1

BPIP item generation

↓

Draft Index

↓

(Prototype BPIP)

BPIP item reduction

↓

Reliability (test re-test)

↓

BPIP item reduction

↓

Reliability & validity elucidation (Australian) sample

↓

Reliability & validity confirmation (New Zealand) sample

Fig. 1.

A total of one hundred and forty five items were generated from the literature review and clinical perspectives for the draft questionnaire. Redundant and non response items were eliminated following consultation with a panel of five independent healthcare practitioners as the first stage of item reduction. The questionnaire was subsequently reduced to a ninety nine item prototype.

A 24 hour test-retest of the stability of the ninety-nine item questionnaire was undertaken by twenty five respondents who were asked to complete the first questionnaire (A) and then the second (B) at the same time twenty four hours later, without referring back to their previous answers.

2.2 Data collection

Questionnaire packs containing the prototype BPIP, RDQ , an informed consent form and instruction sheet were assembled. The data captured at baseline and twelve weeks, outcomes at twelve weeks having been previously reported as being predictive of outcome at one year and beyond (Burton, McClune, et al .2004)

Recruitment of respondents originally intended to capture a homogeneous cohort drawn from general practice proved impossible despite repeated requests via the faculty of Health Sciences, University of Queensland. Recruitment difficulties therefore resulted in two distinct cohorts, a larger Australian cohort (n = 91) recruited from an osteopathic practice and a diagnostic imaging centre. The smaller New Zealand cohort (n = 27) was recruited from an osteopathic practice and an osteopathic teaching clinic.

The larger Australian group was utilised as an elucidation (or clarification) cohort, and the smaller New Zealand cohort was treated as a small prospective validation of the final version of the BPIP.

2.3 Statistical analysis

The continued process of item reduction, including correlation analysis of baseline BPIP data with the 12 week score on the RDQ resulted in an ordinal scale of initially 24 items, which was further reduced to 12 items for correlation with the RDQ. The BPIP was tested for internal consistency in both the Australian and New Zealand cohorts.

The baseline data from the Australian cohort were assessed for concurrent, predictive and construct validity against the RDQ.

Reliability of the index was evaluated by calculation of Cronbach's Alpha of the baseline BPIP score with the twelve week score on the RDQ in the both cohorts. The mean scores fell within the range of possible scores indicating that the scores were entered into the data set correctly.

The BPIP baseline data from the New Zealand cohort was treated as a small prospective validation of the BPIP scale, with the baseline data from the BPIP correlated with the change score from the baseline to twelve weeks of the RDQ.

The questions retained their original numbers from the draft questionnaire until item reduction was completed, and were then renumbered 1-12 in the final BPIP scale.

Analysis was undertaken using the Statistical Package for Social Sciences (SPSS).

3. Results

The results are reported in the same order as they contributed to the item reduction process, and final assessment of the 12 item BPIP

3.1 Test-re-test of the ninety nine item prototype BPIP

A positive correlation between A and B questionnaires was demonstrated in a one tailed test, df 11-2 = 9. The Pearson product moment correlation coefficient was calculated in Excel: Pearson r = 0.98, $P < 0.0005$.

The calculation of R^2 0.98 x 0.98 = 0.96, demonstrated that 96% of the shared variance between the two test samples was accounted for by the result.

One hundred and eighteen respondents completed the twelve week data collection period. This was comprised of 91 in the Australian cohort and 27 in New Zealand.

The demographics including gender and age, and the percentage make up of the two cohorts are contained in Tables 1 and 2. Table 3 reports on the duration of low back pain measured at baseline in both cohorts.

Gender

	Australian	New Zealand
Male	Aus: 26 (29%)	NZ: 6 (22%)
Female	Aus: 65 (71%)	NZ: 21 (78%)

Table 1.

Age Range

	Australian	New Zealand
20-29	6 (7%)	3 (11%)
30-39	13 (14%)	6 (22%)
40-49	16 (18%)	5 (19%)
50-59	30 (33%)	7 (26%)
60 +	26 (29%)	6 (22%)

Table 2.

Australian Cohort Duration of LBP at Baseline

Weeks duration	0-2 weeks	3-5 weeks	6-8 weeks	9-11 weeks	12 weeks +
Totals	20	15	5	1	50
Percentage	21.9%	16.4%	5.4%	1.0%	54.9%

Table 3.

New Zealand Cohort Duration of LBP at Baseline

Weeks duration	0-2 weeks	3-5 weeks	6-8 weeks	9-11 weeks	12 weeks +
Totals	13	5	2	0	7
Percentage	48.1%	18.5%	7.4%	0.0%	25.9%

Table 4.

3.2 Item reduction and reliability

Correlation analysis (used to describe the strength and direction of the linear relationship between the two variables) of the baseline BPIP Australian data with the twelve week RDQ Australian data resulted in reducing the prototype scale to questions which correlated at or above 0.3. Items which correlated below 0.3 were considered too weak for inclusion, and a total of twenty four questions were retained for further analysis.

Reliability coefficients for internal consistency of the twenty four item BPIP scale were as follows:

The Australian cohort, Cronbach's Alpha = 0.8736.

The New Zealand cohort, Cronbach's Alpha = 0.8628.

A further review of the correlation analysis of the baseline BPIP Australian data with twelve week RDQ Australian data for items that correlated at or above 0.4 resulted in further item reduction of the BPIP to twelve questions. Following this further item reduction, reliability coefficients for internal consistency were calculated and are included in Tables 5 and 6.

	Scale Mean if Item Deleted	Scale Variance if Item Deleted	Corrected Item-Total Correlation	Cronbach's Alpha if Item Deleted
severity	29.97	89.921	.557	.867
Workintrude	30.66	85.438	.741	.857
Socintrude	30.58	81.670	.728	.854
q19	30.50	82.527	.634	.860
q24	29.95	83.289	.606	.862
q25	30.36	80.859	.687	.857
q26	29.86	91.889	.282	.882
Worklimit	30.25	87.524	.553	.866
soclimit	30.21	88.238	.526	.867
q69	30.61	88.213	.517	.868
q73	30.32	84.827	.546	.866
q74	30.84	85.945	.489	.870

Table 5. Inter-item Statistics Baseline BPIP/12 week RDQ; Australian cohort

The Australian cohort, Cronbach's Alpha = 0.875.

The New Zealand cohort, Cronbach's Alpha = 0.776.

Once it was established that the reduced scale reliably measured the underlying construct, regression analysis was undertaken to establish levels of statistical significance.

Regression analysis of the Australian cohort based on the twelve item scale demonstrated that 61.7% of the variance in the RDQ score at twelve weeks was accounted for by the BPIP scale, with $p = 0.0005$.

	Mean	Std. Deviation	N
RDQchange 13	6.4074	7.05069	27
severity	3.59	.970	27
WorkIntrude	3.15	1.199	27
SocIntrude	2.70	1.235	27
q19	2.52	1.553	27
q24	3.30	1.235	27
q25	2.52	1.503	27
q26	3.44	1.502	27
WorkLimit	2.81	.879	27
SOCLIMIT	2.78	.801	27
Q69	3.11	1.311	27
Q73	1.96	1.192	27
Q74	1.70	1.137	27

Table 6. Inter-Item statistics Baseline BPIP/12 week RDQ; New Zealand cohort

Regression analysis of the change score of the RDQ with the twelve item BPIP in the New Zealand cohort demonstrated that 78.2% of the variance in RDQ scores was accounted for by the BPIP scale, with $p = 0.006$.

3.3 Mulitiple regression analysis (Australian cohort)

Standard multiple regression analysis was undertaken as it allows for a more sophisticated examination of the relationship between the dependent and independent variables, in this case how well the BPIP was able to predict outcome of the RDQ.

	Mean	Std. Deviation	N
RDQ12wk aus	5.5843	5.26741	89
severity	3.13	.964	91
WorkIntrude	2.44	1.056	91
SocIntrude	2.52	1.336	91
q19	2.60	1.429	91
q24	3.15	1.421	91
q25	2.74	1.459	91
q26	3.24	1.353	91
WorkLimit	2.85	1.173	91
soclimit	2.89	1.159	91
q69	2.49	1.177	91
q73	2.78	1.413	91
q74	2.26	1.436	91

Table 7. Multiple Regression; Australian cohort: Baseline 12 Item BPIP/12 wk RDQ.

Multiple regression analysis was then performed on the Australian cohort to establish the predictive value of the shortened BPIP scale score at baseline for the 12 week RDQ.

The results of the analysis of the Australian cohort are presented in Table 7, Table 8 contains the ANOVA result which demonstrates levels of significance.

Model		Sum of Squares	df	Mean Square	F	Sig.
1	Regression	1505.555	12	125.463	10.186	.000 a
	Residual	936.063	76	12.317		
	Total	2441.618	88			

a. Predictors: (Constant), q74, q26, q69, severity, soclimit, q73, q24, q19, SocIntrude,q25, WorkIntrude, WorkLimit
b. Dependent Variable: RDQ12wk aus

Table 8.

The variance in the RDQ score (61.7%) at 12 weeks was accounted for by the 12 item BPIP. The null hypothesis that multiple R in this population equals zero was also confirmed by significance in the ANOVA $p = 0.0005$. Multiple R is a measure of how strongly or weakly the criterion variables (BPIP variables) are related to the dependant variable (RDQ)(Stalin. 2003).

3.4 Regression analysis, (New Zealand cohort)

Regression analysis of the 12 item BPIP with the RDQ change scores baseline to 12 weeks was then performed on the New Zealand cohort, as part of the prospective validation of the

	Mean	Std. Deviation	N
RDQchange 13	6.4074	7.05069	27
severity	3.59	.970	27
WorkIntrude	3.15	1.199	27
SocIntrude	2.70	1.235	27
q19	2.52	1.553	27
q24	3.30	1.235	27
q25	2.52	1.503	27
q26	3.44	1.502	27
WorkLimit	2.81	.879	27
SOCLIMIT	2.78	.801	27
Q69	3.11	1.311	27
Q73	1.96	1.192	27
Q74	1.70	1.137	27

Table 9. Multiple Regression of 12 Item BPIP scores with the change score Roland Morris Disability Index, baseline to 12 weeks; New Zealand Cohort

BPIP following the statistical analysis of the Australian data. The change score from baseline to 12 weeks was utilised as the raw baseline to 12 week score in the New Zealand cohort and did not reach statistical significance. The results are summarised in the same order as the Australian results in Tables 9 and 10.

The variance in the change score from baseline to 12 weeks of the Roland Morris Disability Index (78.2%) was accounted for by the 12 item BPIP.

The null hypothesis that multiple R in this New Zealand population equals zero was also confirmed by significance in the ANOVA $p = 0.006$

Model		Sum of Squares	df	Mean Square	F	Sig.
1	Regression	1011.152	12	84.263	4.193	.006 a
	Residual	281.367	14	20.098		
	Total	1292.519	26			

a. Predictors: (Constant), Q74, Q69, WorkLimit, q24, SocIntrude, q26, severity, SOCLIMIT, Q73, q19, WorkIntrude, q25
b. Dependent Variable: RDQchange 13

Table 10.

4. Discussion

The development of the BPIP from the original hypothesis, that it was feasible to develop a biopsychosocial prognostic instrument for eventual use in clinical practice, produced a promising result. The utility of the scale may also enable clinicians to consider the possibility that a slow or poor prognosis may be the result of a number of psychosocial obstacles to recovery being present, rather than assuming that underlying pathophysiologic constraints to recovery are the culprits.

The study built on the seminal study of Burton and co-workers (Burton, Tillotson et al. 1993) which utilised a small number of items from previously validated measures to correlate with the RDQ, to positively demonstrate that psychosocial factors were indeed predictive of outcome. Other biopsychosocial instruments tend to focus on single psychosocial predictors (Hurley, Dusoir. et al 2000) or are designed as screening instruments for identifying those specifically at risk of developing long term incapacity from work such as the Orebro questionnaire (Linton and Hallden. 1997). These instruments also differ from the BPIP in that they primarily focus on screening workers with acute low back pain , rather than the wider patient population often consulted in primary care.

The BPIP was developed from clinical perspectives rather than isolating a single construct such as fear avoidance as a predictive factor of disability. The BPIP's focus is consistant with the current idea of low back pain as a fluctuating and disabling condition (Young, Wasiak,

Phillips and Gross. 2011) that needs to be considered within the context of the indviduals experiance. Recent studies suggest that perceptions of personal control, pain self efficacy, the acute/chronic timeline and illness identity are distinctive psychological obstacles to recovery in primary care patients with low back pain, with depression, catastrophising and fear avoidance being reported as less significant (Foster, Thomas, Bishop, Dunn and Main. 2011). These findings being broadly consistent with the content of the BPIP.

The approach to data collection was to keep exclusion criteria to a minimum and not discriminate against respondents from the arbitrary time dependent classification of 12 weeks between acute and chronic low back pain patients.

4.1 Summary of key findings

A logical sequence of item reduction resulted in the 24 item BPIP scale, which was assessed both for its validity and reliability in separate cohorts, with a similar and strong result in both cases, with alpha value above 0.85.

The Pearson product moment correlation of the total score of the 24 item BPIP scale at baseline with the 12 week RDQ score demonstrated that the New Zealand scores did not reach statistical levels of significance. The small numbers in the cohort (n =27) or the more acute nature of the respondents, (21.9% reported pain of more than twelve weeks duration) may have potentially impacted on the result. However as the two cohorts tested differently, the decision to deal with the two groups as separate cohorts appears to have been justified.

The BPIP was shortened to 12 items following further correlation analysis of the Australian cohort's BPIP scores and questions demonstrating the stronger correlation of 0.4 were retained, reducing the scale to a single sheet of A4 paper, potentially improving the scales clinical utility.

To check that the reduced scale could still be considered reliable, reliability analysis using Cronbach's alpha was again undertaken in the Australian cohort. There was no appreciable difference in the reliability of the 24-item scale over the much shorter 12-item scale.

There was a small decrease in Cronbach's alpha score in the 12 item BPIP in the New Zealand cohort of 0.09 over the 24 item scale although the scale can still be considered as reliable. The correlation analysis of the items was combined with all the other steps of item reduction, to produce the definitive BPIP scale, which proved to be statistically reliable.

The results demonstrate that a high proportion of the variance in the RDQ score at 12 weeks was accounted for by the 12 item BPIP, and statistically significant. The retained questions appear at the end the chapter. The BPIP question which made the strongest unique contribution to the dependent variable was; 'The pain makes me feel that I can't go on with my normal activities'. The individual's perception of their low back pain being the greatest single contributor to their level of functioning, as measured by the RDQ, and interference with work and between episode limitations at work were the next two strongest single contributors.

Interference with work was the strongest single contributor to predicting the dependent variable, which may be expected when the more acute nature of the New Zealand cohort's low back pain is taken into account. Interestingly the next strongest contributor to the prediction of the dependent variable in the New Zealand cohort was the statement that; 'My low back pain is dominating my life', with the statement: 'I have no hope of ever getting back to normal activities' the next strongest predictor. Despite the New Zealand group being a more acute group by duration of low back pain reported at baseline, these perceptions, and mal-adaptive cognitions about the low back pain appear to be evident. This suggests that early on in the duration of an episode of low back pain, perception and mal-adaptive cognitions may well play a part in influencing prognosis, and can be readily quantified by the BPIP.

4.2 Comparison with other studies

The variance in RDQ scores was accounted for by the 12 item BPIP in the New Zealand cohort, (78.2%) which was considerably higher than the result of Burton and co-workers (Burton et al. 1995). This is potentially a reflection on the wider biopsychosocial domains of the BPIP capturing a greater range of influences on function when correlated against the RDQ. The result was also statistically significant.

The variance in RDQ score accounted for by the BPIP is similarly higher than that reported by Foster and co-workers in 2010. The prospective cohort study of Foster and co-workers of 3019 adults in the UK assessed distinctiveness of psychosocial obstacles to recovery and their multivariate model accounted for 47.7% in variance of RDQ score at 6 months.

A poor perception of outcome, high disability levels, and high self rated pain intensity were also identified as indicators of a poor prognosis in a large inception cohort study reported by Costa and co-workers (Costa, Maher et al.2009). The large cohort demonstrated more than 50% of respondents had not recovered fully from pain or disability after 12 months and highlighted the desirability of an early biopsychosocial estimation of prognosis to inform patient management.

The size of the cohort compared favourably with other predictive instrument studies reported in the literature such as Hurley and co-workers (n=118) (Hurley, Dusoir et al 2001) and Stratford and co-workers (n=88) (Stratford, Binkley et al. 1996).

4.3 Limitations

The biopsychosocial model itself is used in a variety of ways within the literature, with any number of interchangeable variables being included from time to time. This makes a definitive statement about the model and which variables to include for statistical analysis somewhat difficult.

There is also some debate about the relative weight that should be attributed to the biomedical or psychosocial dimensions and whether the literature has become too focused on individual aspects of the model, rather than the overall inclusive biopsychosocial concept. However the literature continues to reflect the need for clinicians to be able to consider their patients from a biopsychosocial perspective in order to inform both prognosis and target interventions.

Self-report and perception of the patient's condition has also been identified as being vulnerable to the individual's social experience (Sen.2002).

The sample size also potentially limits the generalisability of the results.

The difficulties in recruitment of respondants may also be considered a limiting factor to the research.

The resulting scale will also require alteration to an entirely ordinal scale to be user friendly for routine clincial use. Scales need to be quick and easy to both administer and score to be a useful clinical resource. These issues will need to be addressed and the results confirmed in other populations in future research.

5. Conclusion

Predicting the outcome from an episode of low back pain has previously been reported and described in terms of the uni-dimensional biomedical perspective, rather than the contemporary biopsychosocial model, although it is evident that psychosocial factors or contextual factors can be a major obstacle to recovery. Clinicians are often encouraged to seek further information such as diagnostic imaging when a patient does not meet their expectation for recovery, rather than considering psychosocial obstacles to recovery. Routine clinical measurement as part of prognostication potentially encourages consideration of all the potential variables that may impact on recovery, and contributes to evidence-based 'best practice'.

When psychosocial obstacles are not identified or duly considered in clinical practice, there is clearly a risk that some patients will go on to develop chronic pain and disability. Early identification of poor prognostic factors may potentially help target specific intervention and improve case management, and an objective measure may potentially contribute to this process. The BPIP potentially fills a gap in measurement, as a valid and reliable prognostic instrument, developed from a clinical perspective and intended for routine clinical use, following further validation in differing groups of low back pain patients.

6. 12-Item BPIP

Q1. Please score the severity of your low back pain as an average over the last 7 days where 0 equals no pain, and 10 equal's worst pain.

0 1 2 3 4 5 6 7 8 9 10

Q2. How much has your low back pain interfered with your normal work (including housework) over the last 7 days?

Please circle one answer

Not at all: A little: Quite a bit: A lot: Totally

Q3. How much has you low back pain interfered with your normal social (inc sport) life over the last 7 days?

Please circle one answer

Not at all: A little: Quite a bit: A lot: Totally

	SD				SA
Q4. I can only walk short distances because of my low back pain	1	2	3	4	5

Q5. Everything I do I consider how it will affect my low back pain	1 2 3 4 5
Q6. My low back pain is dominating my life	1 2 3 4 5
Q7. My low back pain disturbs my sleep	1 2 3 4 5
Q8. The pain makes me feel that I can't go on with my normal activities	1 2 3 4 5
Q9. I believe I will get back to my normal level of activities	1 2 3 4 5
Q10. I have no hope of ever getting back to normal activities	1 2 3 4 5

Q11. In between episodes does your back limit what you can do at work?

Please circle one response

Q12. In between episodes does your back limit what you can do socially (inc sport)?

Please circle one response

Not at all: Occasionally: Often: All the time

7. References

Australian Acute Musculoskeletal Pain Guidelines Group. (AAMPG) Evidenced-Based Management of Acute Musculoskeletal Pain. 2003. Australian Academic Press. Brisbane

Bellamy, N., Campbell, J., Haraouit, B., Buchbinder, R., Hobby, K., Roth, J.H., and MacDermid, J.C. Dimensionality and clinical importance of pain and disability in hand osteoarthritis: Development of the Australian/Canadian (AUSCAN) osteoarthritis hand index. Osteoarthritis and Cartilage. 2002.10:855-862

Borrell-Carrio, F., Suchman, A.L., Epstien, R.M. The Biopsychosocial model 25 years later:principals, practice and scientific enquiry. Annals of family medicine. 2004.2:6:576-582.

Buchbinder, R., Staples, M., and Jolley, D. Doctors with a special interest in back pain have poorer knowledge about how to treat back pain. Spine. 2009. 34:11:1218-1226.

Burton, A.K., Tillotson, K.M., Main, C. J., and Hollis, S. Psychosocial predictors of outcome in acute and subchronic low back trouble. Spine.1995. 20:6: 722-728.

Burton, A.K., McClune, T.D., Clark, R.D., and Main C.J. Long term follow-up of patients with low back pain attending for manipulative care: outcomes and predictors. Manual Therapy. 2004.9:30-35

Costa, L, C, .Menezes.Maher, C.G., McAuley, J.H., Hancock, M.J., Herbert, R.D., Refshauge, K.M., and Henschke, N. Prognosis for patients with chronic low back pain: inception cohort trial. BMJ. 2009 doi:10.1136/bmj/b3829

Engel, G.L. The clinical application of the Biopsychosocial model. American Journal of Psychiatry.1980. 137:5: 535-44.

Foster, N.E., Thomas, E., Bishop, A., Dunn, K.M., Main, C.J. Distictiveness of psychological obstacles to recovery in low back pain patients in primary care .Pain.2010.148:398-406

Harding, G., Campbell, J., Parsons, S., Rachman, A., Underwood, M. British pain clinic practitioners'recognition and use of the biopsychosocial pain management model for patients when physical interventions and ineffective or inappropriate. BMC musculoskeletal disordersdoi:1471-2474/11/51.

Harland, N., and Lavallee, D. Biopsychosocial management of chronic low back pain patients with psychological assessment and management tools. Physiotherapy. 2003. 89;5:305-312.

Hilficker, R., Bachmann, L.M., Heitz, C., Lorenz, T., Joronen, H., and Klipstein, A. Value of predictive instruments to determine persisting restriction of function in patients with subacute non specific low back pain. Systematic review. Eur Spine Journal. 2007. DOI 10.1007/s00586-007-0433-8

Hurley, D.A., Dusoir, T.E., McDonough, S.M., Moore, A.P., Linton, S.J., Baxter, D. Biopsychosocial screening questionnaire for patients with low back pain: Preliminary report of utility in physiotherapy practice in Northern Ireland. Clinical Journal of Pain.2000.16:3:214-228

Hurley, D.A., Dusoir, T.E., McDonough, S.M., Moore, A.P., and Baxter, D. How effective is the acute low back pain screening questionnaire for predicting 1 year follow-up in patients with low back pain? The Clinical Journal of Pain.2001.17:256-263Linton, S.J. A review of psychological risk factors in back and neck pain. Spine. 2000. 25:9: 1148-1156.

Lethem, J., Slade, P.D., Troup, J.D.G., and Bentley, G. Outline of a fearavoidance model of exaggerated pain perception.Behavioral Research and Therapy.1983.21:401-408.

Linton, S.J and Hallden, K. Risk factors and the natural course of acute and recurrent musculoskeletal pain: Developing a screening instrument. Progress in Pain Research and Management Vol 8.1997 Eds: Jensen, T.S., Turner, J.A., and Wiesenfield-Hallin. IASP press. Seattle.

Luo, X., Pietrobon, R., Sun, S.X., Liu, G.G., and Hey, L. Estimates and Patterns of Direct Health Care Expenditures among Individuals with Back Pain in the United States. Spine.2003. 29:1:: 79-86.

Pincus, T., Burton, A.K., Vogel, S., and Field, A.P. A systematic review of psychological factors as predictors of chronicity/disability in prospective cohorts of low back pain. Spine.2002 27:5:: E109-E120.

Roland, M., and Morris, R. A study of the natural history of back pain. Part 1: Development of a reliable and sensitive measure of disability and low back pain. Spine.1983.8: 141-144.

Sen, A. Health: Perception versus Observation.BMJ.2002.324:860-861

Stalin, L.J. Multidimensional scaling. In: Grimm, L.G., and Yarnold P.R. (Eds) Reading and understanding multivariate statistics. 2003. Page 167. American Psychological Association . Washington DC.

Stratford, P.W., Binkley, J., Solomon, P., Finch, E., Gill, C., and Morland, J. Assessing change over time in patients with low back pain.1994 Physical Therapy74:528-533.

Trouchon, M., and Fillion, L. Biopsychosocial determinants of chronic disability and low back pain: A review. Journal of Occupational Rehabilitation.2000 10:2: 117-141.

Vlaeyen, J.W.S.and Linton, S.J.Fear avoidnace and its consequences in chronic musculoskeletal pain: a state of the art. 2000. Pain.85:115-125

Waddell, G., Sommerville, D., Henderson, L., Newton, M., and Main C.J. A Fear avoidance beliefs questionnaire(FABQ) and the role of fear avoidance beliefs in chronic low back pain and disability.Pain.52:157-168.

World health organisation. (WHO). International classification of functioning, disability and health. 2003. World Health Organisation. Geneva.

Young, A.E., Wasiak, R., Phillips, L., and Gross D.P.Workers persepctives on low back pain recurrence: „It comes and it goes and comes and goes, but it's always there' 2011.Pain:152:204-211

6

The Use of Event-Related Potentials in Chronic Back Pain Patients

Carine Vossen, Helen Vossen, Wiesje van de Wetering,
Marco Marcus, Jim van Os and Richel Lousberg
*Maastricht University Medical Centre,
The Netherlands*

1. Introduction

Chronic back pain is one of the most common pain syndromes, with a lifetime incidence of 60% to 90%. An important question in the field of chronic pain is how acute pain transits to a chronic pain state: why do some persons develop chronic pain while others do not? Approximately 10% to 20% of patients with chronic low back pain (CLBP) still have persisting complaints after 6 weeks (Bekkering et al., 2003). If more insight is gained into chronification mechanisms and, as a consequence, the ability to predict which individual with acute pain develops chronic pain, it may become possible to intervene in the process at an early stage.

In acute pain states, pain is often causally related to physical damage, whereas this relationship is less pronounced in chronic pain states. With increasing duration of pain complaints, other factors, such as psychological, cognitive, and environmental factors, are likely to become more involved (Gamsa, 1994). As a result, pain is conceptualized as a multidimensional phenomenon, making pain measurement complex. However, due to the subjective nature of the pain experience, it can not be measured directly. In fact, only derivatives of pain can be measured. The most frequently measured aspect of pain is its intensity. Two often used measures are the Visual Analog Scale (VAS) and Numeric Rating Scale (NRS). Despite some limitations, their psychometric properties have been demonstrated to be adequate (Jensen et al., 1986; Seymour, 1982). To evaluate several other components of pain, pain-related aspects, and risk factors for chronic back pain (such as fear avoidance, inadequate coping strategies, etc.), clinicians use questionnaires. Although many of these instruments provide reliable and valid results (for an overview, see the Handbook of Pain Assessment, edited by Turk & Melzack, 2011), all subjective measures have the potential for several forms of bias (Magnusson et al., 1995). In an attempt to measure relatively unbiased pain responses, a large number of studies in the 70s and 80s investigated the usefulness of psychophysiological recordings. The results of these studies showed that small but significant correlations could be demonstrated between the subjective pain experience on the one hand and skin conductance, heart rate, electromyography, and finger pulse volume on the other (Flor & Meyer, 2011). The most promising results, however, were obtained from experiments studying event (pain)-related potentials (ERPs), a measure that is derived from electroencephalography (EEG). This technique has been used to study cerebral responses to (non-)noxious stimuli and to gain more insight into the cortical processing of pain. Pain-ERP studies are typically performed in a laboratory setting under strict experimental control. In contrast to the other aforementioned psychophysiological measures, specific ERP components correlate relatively highly with subjective pain estimates (Bromm et al., 1984; Chen et al., 1979; Miltner et al., 1989). In addition, ERPs have been shown to contain information not only on pain intensity but also on many other important (pain-related) factors, such as habituation, personality, and coping strategies. In other words, making use of ERPs, a large number of aspects of the pain construct, interrelations, and mechanisms can be quantified and studied (see Loesers "onion" model in Fig. 1).

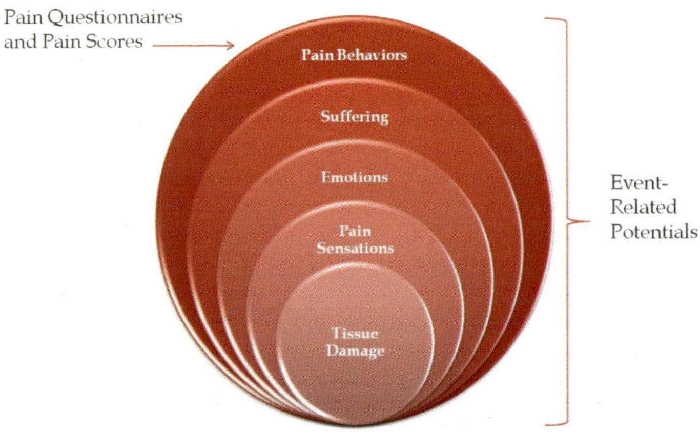

Fig. 1. Loesers "onion" model, modified with the addition of the position of questionnaires and event-related potentials.

This chapter starts with a general description of event-related potentials and their components. Second, factors related to the pain-ERP, such as personality and genetics, are discussed. Special attention will be paid to methods of analyzing the ERP signal. After some discussion of methodological considerations, we will propose an alternative ERP analysis. In addition, we will present preliminary data to illustrate the usefulness of this alternative method. In the last section, some future directions of ERP will be discussed.

2. ERP structure

The ERP represents a cortical response to a specific stimulus—for instance, a sound, a light signal, or a pain stimulus. Event-related potentials are regarded as manifestations of specific (psycho)physiological, stimulus-related processes. An ERP is derived from EEG. Electrodes are attached to specific locations on the scalp (Jasper, 1958). Potential differences between the scalp electrodes and a reference electrode are sampled at a certain frequency, most commonly between 500 and 5000 Hz (cycles per second). The essence of an ERP is that the signal (the cortical reaction to the stimulus) has to be discriminated from background EEG noise. The procedure to achieve this goal is to compute an average of a number of time-locked EEG samples, called epochs or segments. As a general rule, it can be stated that the larger the number of epochs, the better the signal-to-noise ratio. Within each person or condition, the averaging procedure results in a voltage-by-time graph. When averaging ERPs from different persons or conditions, the result is called a grand average.

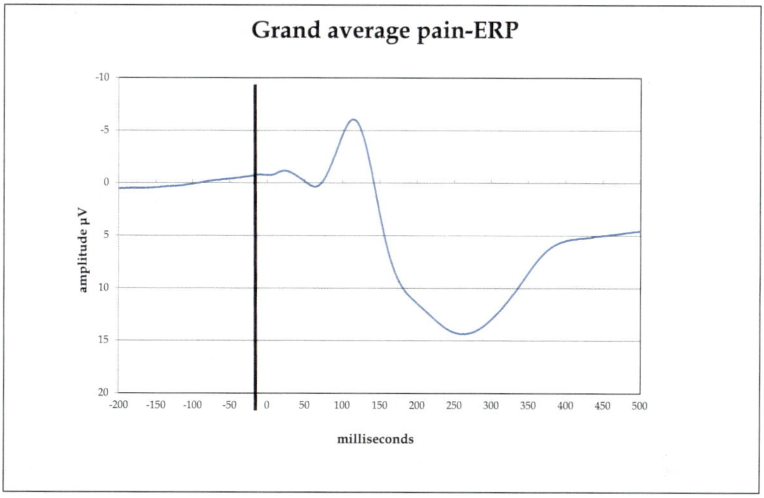

Fig. 2. Example of a grand average pain-ERP on Cz.

In Figure 2, a grand average pain-ERP (Cz location) is shown. This ERP was obtained from a paradigm in which subjects received a series of 150 painful and non-painful shocks of 10 ms in duration (Vossen, 2010c). As can be seen from Figure 2, three peaks can be clearly distinguished. The most common way to describe these peaks is by polarity and latency (time in ms after stimulus onset). For instance, the large positive peak between 250 and 300 ms is called P300. There is also a system that numbers the sequence of the peaks; e.g., the second positive peak is called P2. In this ERP, P300 is the second positive peak, and thus, P2 and P300 are abbreviations pointing to the same peak. In ERP experiments, researchers try to explain the meaning of the peaks. Which (stimulus) characteristics or processes are 'responsible' for the amplitude and latency of the peaks? Early peaks, also called 'exogenous' components, are believed to represent stimulus parameters, such as the intensity and other properties of the stimulus. Later components are thought to be representations of 'endogenous' processes, such as attention (Luck, 2005). Further, it is known that (slight) differences in the paradigm that is used (not only with respect to the stimulus but also to instructions, environmental characteristics, time of the day, etc.) result in changes in the ERP. These changes pertain to latency and amplitude effects and even profound morphological changes. It should be noted that an ERP has a high temporal but low spatial resolution. The latter means that it is difficult to draw valid conclusions on the underlying cerebral source that is generating the electrical activity (Makeig, 2004).

3. Influences on the pain-evoked potentials

In this section, we will discuss the influence of a variety of stimulus-related and person-related factors on the pain-ERP. Special attention will be paid to the predictive relationship of pain-ERPs to the clinical experience of low back pain.

3.1 Stimulus intensity and subjective pain experience

Intensity is an essential property of a stimulus. Is there a relationship between the intensity of a stimulus and peaks of the ERP? Accumulating evidence confirms the relationship between stimulus intensity and increased peak values of N200 and P300 (Becker et al., 1993; Bromm & Meier, 1984; Stowell, 1977). Does an increase in certain peak amplitudes relate to the amount of pain that a subject experiences? One of the first studies that investigated this association demonstrated that an increase in the N200 and P300 peak amplitudes was accompanied by an increase in VAS scores (r = 0.67-0.77) (Harkins & Chapman, 1978). These results were replicated by Chen (1979) and Garcia-Larrea (1997). These authors also found a strong linear association (r = 0.67 and r = 0.41, respectively) between the N200/P300 peak-to-peak amplitude and subjective pain ratings. Miltner and colleagues (1987), however, could not find such a relationship when investigating habituation of noxious stimuli. They observed a significant decrease in peak-to-peak amplitudes of the N150-P360 across trials, but without a corresponding effect on VAS ratings. They suggested that the association between ERP amplitudes and subjective ratings might not be as strong as was claimed previously.

The subjective pain experience seems to be limited not only to these peak amplitude effects. Kanda and colleagues (2002) discovered a late positive component around 600 ms that was associated with pain report, which they called the 'intensity assessment-related potential' (IAP). The IAP was not influenced by intensity, suggesting that this component solely reflects the psychological processes of pain. A recent study, again investigating the relationship between stimulus intensity, peak amplitudes, and subjective pain experience, was performed by Vossen and colleagues (2011). Their methodological comments on common pain-ERP analyses relate to the problems inherent in the averaging technique (see also paragraph 4). The authors argued that averaging eliminates any unwanted 'noise' in the ERP, but in doing so, it assumes no difference between repeated trials. This assumption can not hold, since single trials likely differ from one another because of processes, such as habituation. Moreover, averaging across trials eliminates all information about possible within-subject correlations between ERP and subjective pain. As an alternative, they introduced multilevel random regression analysis, applied on pain-ERP, making it possible to model time (habituation), stimulus intensity, and their random within-person effects. The findings of this study show that the relationships between these three variables are confounded and moderated by several other variables, such as the intensity of the previous stimulus. This means that a certain pain rating after a stimulus also depends on the intensity of the previous stimulus, which makes clinical sense. A pain patient who is asked to evaluate his/her perceived pain is highly likely to base this evaluation on previous pain experiences. In sum, the relationship between stimulus intensity, ERP peaks, and pain experience is probably far more complex than previously thought.

3.2 Habituation and pain-evoked potentials

Habituation is the process that refers to a decrease in a behavioral response to a repeatedly presented stimulus (Thompson & Spencer, 1966). It could be hypothesized that altered habituation might be an explanation for the chronification of pain. It is thought that chronic pain patients may have a deficit in habituation or even an inability to habituate to painful experiences, resulting in persistent pain. Older studies, using pain rating as an outcome measure, reported mixed results. One study investigated the habituation difference between CLBP patients and controls, using eight successive trials of the cold pressure test (Brandt & Schmidt, 1987). Healthy controls could be divided into a subgroup that habituated over trials and a subgroup that sensitized. The CLBP group did not habituate or sensitize over time. Additionally, they found a lower pain tolerance in CLBP patients while reporting higher pain ratings. It was hypothesized that CLBP patients had already undergone a learning process in which sensitization had taken place. Arntz and colleagues (1991) also studied habituation in CLBP patients and controls. They did not observe a difference in habituation between the groups, measured by pain intensity ratings, EMG, and heart rate. A third study (Peters et al., 1989) confirmed the results of Brandt & Schmidt (1987) but did not find differences in physiological measures, such as heart rate and skin conductance. More recently, Smith and colleagues (2008) reported differences in habituation of subjective pain ratings between women with fibromyalgia and pain-free controls. They found that women with fibromyalgia habituated at a lower rate to repeated heat stimuli.

In addition, there are some recent studies that have used ERP as a measure to study habituation. They are suggestive of a deficit in habituation in chronic pain patients, although different chronic pain populations were used. Valeriani and colleagues (2003) studied habituation in response to painful CO_2 laser stimulation in migraine patients. They found reduced habituation of ERP amplitudes in migraine sufferers compared to pain-free controls. In disconfirmation, another study found that patients with migraine did not show any habituation, whereas healthy controls did (De Tommaso, 2005). Vossen et al. (2010c) studied habituation in a group of chronic low back pain patients compared to pain-free controls, measuring ERP in response to 20 painful stimuli. They found a significant interaction between group and trial number on the P300 component at C4 and T4. This means that chronic low back pain patients appeared to habituate to a lesser degree than pain-free controls. They also examined the influence of state-depression on habituation, using the BDI score. The results revealed a significant three-way interaction between BDI, group, and $trial_{inverse}$, suggesting that the difference in habituation between groups depends on the level of depression. Only in the presence of depression did CLBP patients show a deficit in habituation. Interestingly, a recent study in fibromyalgia patients also found evidence for reduced habituation of the N200 vertex component, facilitated by the presence of symptoms of depression (De Tommaso, 2011). In conclusion, habituation seems to be different in chronic back pain patients compared to controls but is probably also influenced by factors, such as depression.

3.3 Influence of neuroticism on pain-evoked potentials

"Personality" can be defined as a dynamic and organized set of characteristics possessed by a person that uniquely influence his or her cognitions, motivations, and behaviors in various situations (Ryckman, 2008). Individuals with different personalities will differ in reaction to a specific situation. Likewise, it is conceivable that persons with diverse personality structures will react differently to a pain stimulus. This theoretical claim is frequently being confirmed in clinical practice. There is a large variety in 'pain behaviors' when patients are confronted with painful medical procedures (injections, stitches, etc.). One of the most important personality factors that are known to influence the experience of pain is neuroticism (Wade et al., 1992). Neuroticism is defined as a tendency to experience negative emotions in stressful situations (Costa & McCrae, 1980). One of the most commonly used questionnaire measuring neuroticism, is the NEO-Big 5 (Costa & McCrae, 1985), which also gives information on six neuroticism facets—namely anxiety, impulsivity, depression, self-consciousness, irritability, and vulnerability.

There are several mechanisms that explain the hypothesized relationship between neuroticism and pain. In the first explanation, the relationship between neuroticism and pain is thought to arise from over-reporting of pain-related complaints, an exaggerated expression of disturbance, and a more focussed view on bodily states. Persons with high levels of neuroticism tend to be more aware of their bodily states than others and thus report more physical complaints (Groth-Marnat & Fletcher, 2000). Costa and McCrae (1980) suggest that in patients with high levels of neuroticism, physical complaints can be viewed as exaggerations of bodily concerns, linking neuroticism to hypochondria. In yet another explanation, neuroticism can be seen as a vulnerability factor. When a patient is confronted with a stressor, such as low back pain, patients with high neuroticism levels already might perceive pain as threatening at lower thresholds, which consequently may evoke catastrophic thoughts (Goubert et al., 2004). In a study on a large sample (n = 1441) of CLBP patients, Bendebba found a correlation between the severity of perceived pain and psychological distress. A correlation between psychological distress and the duration of the complaint, however, could not be demonstrated (Bendebba, 1997).

Note that the aforementioned studies are based on data derived from questionnaires. ERP can be used as an additional tool to get more insight into the mechanism(s) of pain and neuroticism. Vossen et al. performed a study in 75 healthy subjects in which they studied the influence of neuroticism and two NEO-big 5 facets (depression and anxiety) on the pain-ERP. They found that subjects with relatively high neuroticism scores showed more positive ERP amplitudes. These amplitude effects were observed frontally in a broad latency range, from 250 to 1500 ms, with significant effects between 340-400 ms, 730-860 ms, and 1240-1450 ms, suggesting stronger pain processing. Comparing the effects of the neuroticism facets anxiety and depression, opposite effects were found. Anxiety was associated with a negative effect (enlarging negative amplitudes) early in the ERP (100-200 ms), whereas depression exerted an opposite effect in the same latency range. Another study of 14 healthy participants also found anxiety to be related with a larger N140 component (Warbrick, 2006). In addition, the authors also observed no effect of anxiety in the P300 range. It is known that the N140 increases when attention to a stimulus is heightened (Kida et al., 2004). It is plausible that participants focus their attention more when they are more anxious, thus increasing the amplitude of N140. This would support the idea of a greater focus on bodily states in anxious patients. In conclusion, the number of pain-ERP studies investigating the relationship between personality factors (especially neuroticism) is relatively small. More experimental data are needed to unravel mechanisms involving pain report, personality, and cortical pain processing.

3.4 The influence of gene polymorphisms on pain-evoked potentials

There is a rising interest in genetic factors in pain research, as they likely explain a substantial portion of the interindividual differences in pain perception and response to pain treatment (Fillingim et al., 2008). Twin studies give the opportunity to determine the proportion of variability in pain response that is accounted for by genes (heritability).

Heritability for migraine has been estimated at 35% (Stam et al., 2010), 55% for menstrual pain (Treloar et al., 1998), and 33% to 50% for low back pain (Bengtsson & Thorson, 1991 Battié et al., 2007). The main aim in pain genetics, however, is to identify the actual genes and gene polymorphisms that influence the pain pathways. Linkage and association studies have attempted to identify specific genes that affect the peripheral nervous system through the voltage-gated sodium channels on the one hand and genes that affect the central nervous system and modulate sensory-discriminatory and affective-evaluative elements of pain perception that affects the central nervous system on the other (for an extensive overview, see Foulkes & Wood, 2008). Many candidate genes have been proposed, but the effects of these genes are small and even together, if true, explain only a fraction of the heritability involved. A possible explanation for this is the complexity of pain as a phenotype. Measurement of the pain experience plays an important part in this. In human studies, three single-nucleotide polymorphisms (SNPs) have been proposed to impact pain perception: COMT Val158Met (rs4680), BDNF Val66Met (rs6265), and OPRM A118G (rs1799971). COMT Val158Met is a gene polymorphism that alters the activity of the COMT enzyme, which degrades catecholamines, such as dopamine, epinephrine, and norepinephrine (Nackley et al., 2006). It has been demonstrated that Met/Met homozygotes have decreased mu-opioid system activation in response to pain (Zubieta et al., 2001, 2003); however, further replication is required. Brain-derived neurotrophic factor (BDNF) is a neurotrophin that supports the growth, differentiation, and survival of neurons in both the peripheral and the central nervous system. BDNF is released when nociceptors are activated and is involved in the activity-dependent pathogenesis of nociceptive pathways, which may lead to chronification of pain (Merighi et al., 2008; Sen et al., 2008). One piece of genetic variation within the BDNF gene is a valine-to-metionine substitution at codon 66 (Val66Met), resulting in reduced secretion of the BDNF protein and impaired BDNF signaling. The Met carriers are believed to be more sensitive to pain; however, here, replication in large and systematic studies is also required.

Experimental designs represent a particularly powerful approach to study genetic effects on psychological phenotypes, as they allow for controlled conditions and investigation of underlying mechanisms (van Os et al., 2008).

Lötsch and colleagues (2006) studied the influence of the G allele of the OPRM1 A118G polymorphism on ERP pain processing of experimental pain stimuli. This polymorphism replaces adenine with guanine, increasing the receptor affinity of b-endorphin 3-fold, resulting in decreased pain responses (Bond et al., 1998; Filligim et al., 2005). Lötsch and colleagues concluded that ERP amplitudes (N1 component) of carriers of the G allele were, on average, half as high as the amplitude of the non-carriers, suggesting lower pain processing for the G allele carriers.

In a more recent study, we investigated the influence of the COMT Val158Met, BDNF Val66Met, and BDNF Val66Met polymorphisms on pain using ERPs (Vossen et al., 2010a). The sample of this study consisted of chronic low back pain patients, as well as healthy controls. The results suggest that the COMT Val158Met and the BDNF Val66Met polymorphisms influence the cortical processing of experimental electrical pain stimuli. However, no main gene effects were observed. Rather, genetic effects appeared to be moderated by the concurrent presence of chronic pain complaints. In the presence of chronic pain, the COMT Met allele and the BDNF Met allele augmented cortical pain processing at the N2 and P1 components, respectively, whilst reducing pain processing in pain-free controls. The findings of Lötsch and colleagues (2006) concerning the OPRM1 A118G polymorphism could not be replicated in our study. The influence of chronic pain complaints on gene effects may indicate a gene-environment interaction and may even implicate epigenetic modification. It is clear that genetic findings remain preliminary, and well-conducted systematic studies with larger samples sizes are required.

Up to now, limited attention has gone out to gene-environment interplay in pain research, especially with event-related potentials as pain measure. In future studies investigating gene-environment interplay, the complexity of the phenotype and the overall small direct effect of genes (Manolio et al., 2009) should be considered. Longitudinal designs using event-related potentials can contribute to the study of genetic influences in causal pathways of the chronification of pain.

3.5 The predictive relationship of pain-ERPs to clinical experience of pain

Since chronic low back pain is a very common problem and accompanied by high costs in health care, it is important to be able to predict the likelihood of developing chronic disabling back pain. In 2010, Chou & Chelleke performed a systematic review of 20 studies to investigate the usefulness of individual risk factors for chronification in low back pain. Identified risk factors, although individually relatively weak, were maladaptive pain coping behaviors, nonorganic signs, functional impairment, a poor general health status, and presence of psychiatric comorbidities. They also reviewed risk-predicting instruments, which are usually based on self-reported questionnaires. To date, no instrument has been used routinely and no recommendations exist, since evidence is insufficient (Chou & Chelleke, 2010). Could the pain-ERP serve as a predictor for chronic low back pain? The experimentally induced pain-ERP has been demonstrated to be a relatively objective measure of experimental pain compared to subjective pain ratings (Becker et al., 2000; Bromm, 1984; Stowell, 1977). An important issue, however, concerns the relevance and translation of the experimentally induced pain-ERP to pain in daily life. Stated in another way, can the pain-ERP serve as a predictor for clinical pain? There are two fundamental problems, which are related to the meaning of experimentally induced pain and its generalizability to pain in daily life. First, the characteristics of experimentally induced pain stimuli are typically not comparable with those of clinical pain (e.g., the intensity and duration). Second, in an experimental environment, the subject has at least partial control of the experimentally induced pain (escape is possible by stopping the participation), a controllability that cannot be exerted in a clinical setting. Consequently, a straightforward translation of experimentally induced pain to clinical pain is simply not possible. Nevertheless, event-related potentials have already been used to predict depression (Kemp et al., 2006), awakening from a coma (Daltrozzo et al., 2006), and in the discrimination of Alzheimer's disease from controls (Benvenuto et al., 2002). The prediction of pain, using ERPs, has not been studied intensively. To our knowledge, only one study investigated the prediction of chronic low back pain complaints (Vossen et al., 2010b). Even-related potentials in response to experimental pain were measured in 75 CLBP patients. The ERP mean amplitudes of the peaks (N1, P1, N2, P3) served as predictors for the mean pain ratings, registered during a 2-week period after the experiment. The N2 component of Cz and C4 appeared to be significantly related to the daily pain ratings, collected over 2 consecutive weeks. Surprisingly, the ERP variables related more strongly to the clinical pain ratings than the accompanying subjective ratings of the experimental pain stimuli. Although care must be taken in the interpretation of these results, the findings suggest that it might be possible to make inferences on clinical pain, based on experimentally derived pain-ERPs. More studies are needed to confirm these results and to investigate the usefulness of predicting long-term complaints in patients with acute or chronic back pain.

4. Analyzing event-related potentials

In the last 2 decades, the methods of analyzing ERPs have not been changed essentially. In the first paragraph, we will describe the most commonly used method. In the second paragraph, we will discuss several issues concerning the methodology. Additionally, we will introduce an alternative method and present preliminary results.

4.1 Common methods in analyzing pain-ERPs

In an experimental ERP paradigm, stimuli are repeated to allow averaging of the epochs and to compare different experimentally induced conditions. Although many variants are possible, the most common procedure of ERP analysis is as follows (Luck, 2005; Mouraux & Iannetti, 2008) : The first step is to filter the raw EEG data. The second step is the creation of segments or epochs, based on markers of the stimuli in the EEG. The duration of these epochs varies but is usually between 500 and 1500 ms. The third step concerns identification of invalid epochs. Epochs are qualified as valid or not, depending on whether an epoch is likely to be confounded by an artifact: electrical activity that does not arise from the brain—for example, an eyelid movement, tension of the muscles in the head and neck, or electrical activity from the heart. Basically, there are two procedures for dealing with invalid epochs. The first method is a rejection of invalid epochs in the computation of the averaged ERP. This simply reduces the maximum number of analyzable segments, and as a result, information is lost. The second option is a correction for confounding effects by commonly accepted statistical algorithms, such as the so-called Gratton and Coles ocular correction (Gratton, 1983). To date, it is not clear which of these two methods is preferable. After the averaging of all epochs per individual (step 4), a grand average of ERP segments across subjects (per experimental condition) is calculated (step 5). The next action is to carefully identify peaks with their corresponding latency windows: a time range surrounding a specific peak. The seventh step is to apply these 'peak latency windows' at the within-subject epoch level: within the defined latency window, the maximum (or minimum) amplitude is determined. These maximum amplitudes form the input for the computation of the peak average for each individual. The final action is to use these maximum or minimum amplitudes as a dependent variable in statistical analyses, such as ANOVA (Hoormann et al., 1998).

4.2 Methodological considerations

Although this procedure of ERP analysis is plausible, functional, and generally accepted, there are some critical issues that need to be considered, particularly given recent developments in statistics that may provide superior analytical approaches. First, each time-locked EEG segment consists of the aimed signal and a noise element (all background ongoing EEG activity). Averaging of the trials will separate the signal from the noise, because the signal element is thought to be constant in every trial, while the noise element is considered to be random. However, one can dispute the fact that a signal is constant over trials in pain experiments, since processes, such as habituation, play an important role (Woestenburg et al., 1983; Vossen et al., 2006). In addition, within-subject variance (trial-to-trial variance) is lost by averaging, which may contain clinically important information on cortical processes. Second, it is known that in consecutive trials, the latency of maximum peak values is likely to differ. Although it is possible to take the variability of latency into account in the analysis (as a covariate), this solution is not ideal, since the trial-to-trial latency information is lost. A third unsolved problem is how to deal with peak values located on the borders of the latency window. A final critical point regards the fact that peaks contain information on many processes: it is generally known that P300 is sensitive for attention, evaluation, stimulus intensity, and many other stimulus-related and person-related factors (Zaslansky et al., 1996). Multilevel random regression analysis, as already discussed in paragraph 3.2, tackles the problems associated with averaging and habituation. Nonetheless, the methodological problems concerning peak definition and peak measurement can not be solved with multilevel analysis.

Without a doubt, averaged maximized peak values carry important information. However, theoretically spoken, each (!) latency point contains meaningful information. To be able to analyze amplitude information that is not related to peaks, area under the curve (AUC) can be computed for specific latency ranges. Usually, AUC is applied to quantify peaks as well as to calculate averaged group differences located on the flanks/limbs of a peak (Luck, 2005). AUC is not often applied in pain-ERPs, since it has been postulated that more noise is introduced when averaging trials (Picton, 2000). However, when using AUCs of single-trial data, the problem of introducing noise is substantially reduced.

5. Introducing an alternative method

In this section, we will discuss an alternative method for analyzing ERP data. We will present preliminary results using this method in a previously used dataset of CLBP patients and pain-free controls.

5.1 Fixed-interval AUC segment analysis

From a statistical point of view, the main goal of ERP analysis is to explain variance in the pain-ERP as much as possible, using a series of predictors. It seems reasonable to focus not only on the explanation of maximum peak amplitudes but also on effects in other latencies. This assertion is supported by the fact that several above-cited publications (e.g., Kanda et al., 2002; Vossen et al., 2006) report stimulus- and person-related effects in non-peak latencies. We felt that the concept of AUC is valuable but should be applied to small fixed intervals, independent of peaks. This implicates a partitioning of the whole epoch in small event-related fixed interval areas (ERFIAs). To illustrate this line of reasoning, three averaged pain-ERPs are presented. In the first picture, three ERPs are depicted, each representing another level of stimulus intensity. As can be observed, there are intensity effects on P1 and N2 and a large effect on P2: the larger the intensity, the larger the peak amplitude. However, the intensity effects are not limited to these peaks. The effect on the P2 already starts at approximately 200 ms and lasts at least until 500 ms. Also, the intensity effect between P1 and N2 can not be ignored. The second graph illustrates the effects on habituation. The three ERPs represent three blocks of trials delivered in the experiment. Again, habituation is not restricted visually to the peaks. Also, habituation seems to reduce the amplitude. In the third graph, two grand averages are shown of ERPs on Cz: one from a pain-free control group (n = 76) and the other from a group of chronic low back patients (n = 75). There seem to be small amplitude group effects on the P1 and N2 but not on the P2. In addition, there seem to be non-peak-related group effects. Care must be taken in the interpretation of differences observed in these grand averages, since they represent a reduced, oversimplified representation of the pain experience. In the intensity ERPs, the information on habituation is averaged out and vice versa.

Based on these observations, we performed a number of (unpublished) pilot analyses on ERP datasets of previous studies to determine a pragmatic width of AUC segments (ERFIAs). This led to our choice of segments of 20 ms. In our view, this seems to be a reasonable compromise between specific AUC segments that are too large on the one hand and segments that are too small, resulting in multiple testing problems on the other.

We decided to reanalyze part of the data pertaining to the PhD thesis, defended by H. Vossen. We focused the preliminary analysis on three electrodes, namely C3, C4, and Cz, because these locations represent the sensomotoric cortex and are of anatomical importance in pain processing (Kupers & Kehlet, 2006). Also, we restricted the range to 0-500 ms post-stimulus. The reanalysis took place in an explorative, hypothesis-generating fashion. Basically, we were interested in to what degree the proposed ERFIA method would yield significant relationships between stimulus intensity and habituation and to what degree these findings would correspond to known results, based on peak analyses. In addition, there was one special point of interest: Do the ERPs of chronic pain patients differ from pain-free controls, analyzed with fixed-interval AUCs?

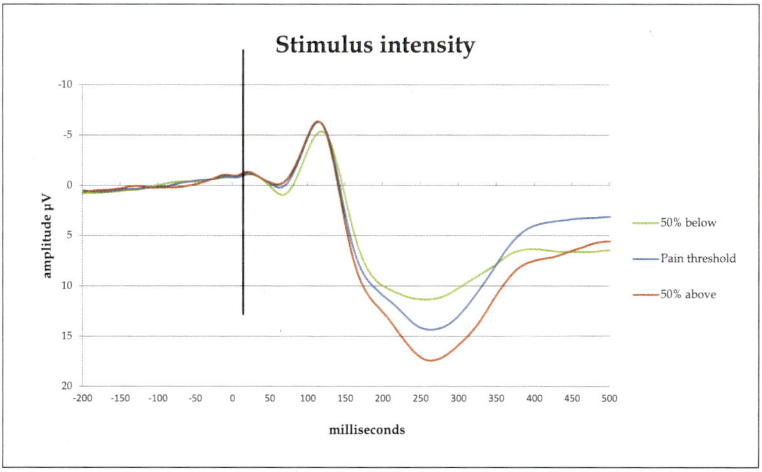

Fig. 3. Grand ERPs of stimulus intensity on Cz.

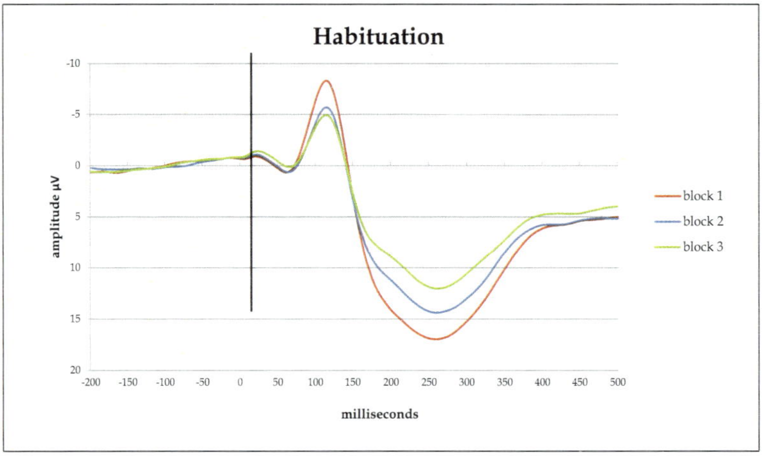

Fig. 4. Grand ERPs of the three consecutive blocks of stimuli on Cz.

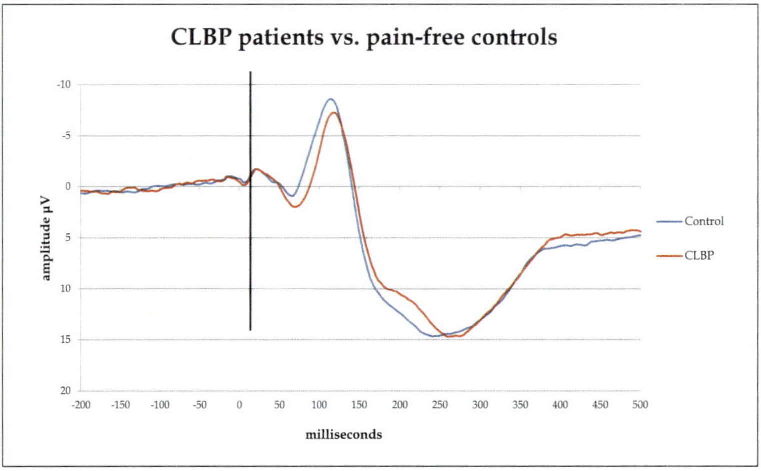

Fig. 5. Grand ERPs of CLBP patients and a pain-free control group on Cz.

5.2 Study design

The dataset we are using is based on previously collected raw EEG data. For a detailed description of the protocol, we refer to Vossen et al., 2010a & 2011. Here, a summary of the design is given. Seventy-six pain-free subjects and 75 patients with chronic low back pain participated in the study. All CLBP subjects suffered from low back pain for at least 6 months and were recruited from the general population. All subjects underwent a rating paradigm of 150 semi-randomly presented electrical stimuli. The used stimuli, administered intracutaneously on the top of the left middle finger, consisted of electrical pulses, each with a duration of 10 ms, and an inter-stimulus interval (ISI) ranging from 9 to 11 seconds. Before starting the experiment, the sensory and pain threshold were determined. In the experiment, five different intensities, based on the participant's pain threshold, were administered. The five used intensities were -50% and -25% below the pain threshold, the pain threshold itself (0%), and 25% and 50% above the pain threshold. After each stimulus, subjects were asked to rate the intensity on a numeric rating scale (NRS) ranging from 0 to 100. During the entire experiment, EEG was recorded with a 1000-Hz sampling rate. The ERP epochs were selected from the continuous EEG and segmented at 200 ms prior to the stimulus to 500 ms post-stimulus. For each stimulus, we calculated 20-ms ERFIAs in the range of 0 to 500 ms. ERFIA segments with EOG activity exceeding +25 mA or -25 mA were excluded from the analysis. The calculated ERFIAs were used as dependent variables in a multilevel random regression model (see equations 1 and 2). This resulted in 25 separate multilevel regression analyses per electrode. All analyses were performed with SPSS 18.0.

Mulilevel regression model with main effects:

$$\begin{gathered} Y_{ti} = \beta_0 + \beta_1\text{*intensity}_{\text{linear}} + \beta_2\text{*trial}_{\text{linear}} + \beta_3\text{*trial}_{\text{quadratic}} + \beta_4\text{*trial}_{\text{inverse}} + \\ \beta_5\text{*group} + \beta_6\text{*age} + \beta_7\text{*gender} + \beta_8\text{*sensation threshold} + \beta_9\text{*pain threshold} + \\ \beta_{10}\text{*intensity}_{\text{linear}} \text{ of previous trial} + e_{ti} + u_{1*}\text{*intensity}_{\text{linear}} + \\ u_2\text{ *trial}_{\text{linear}} + u_3\text{* trial}_{\text{inverse}} + u_4\text{* trial}_{\text{quadratic}} \end{gathered} \quad (1)$$

Mulilevel regression model with three group-interaction effects:

$$\begin{gathered} Y_{ti} = \beta_0 + \beta_1\text{*intensity}_{\text{linear}} + \beta_2\text{*trial}_{\text{linear}} + \beta_3\text{*trial}_{\text{quadratic}} + \beta_4\text{*trial}_{\text{inverse}} + \beta_5\text{*group} + \\ \beta_6\text{*age} + \beta_7\text{*gender} + \beta_8\text{*sensation threshold} + \beta_9\text{*pain threshold} + \beta_{10}\text{*intensity}_{\text{linear}} \\ \text{of previous trial} + \beta_{11}\text{*group*intensity}_{\text{linear}} + \beta_{12}\text{*group*trial}_{\text{linear}} + \\ \beta_{13}\text{*group*trial}_{\text{quadratic +}} + \beta_{14}\text{*group*trial}_{\text{inverse}} + \beta_{15}\text{*group*intensity}_{\text{linear}} \text{ of previous} \\ \text{trial} + \beta_{16}\text{*group*pain threshold} + \beta_{17}\text{*group*sensory threshold} + e_{ti} + \\ u_{1*}\text{*intensity}_{\text{linear}} + u_2\text{ *trial}_{\text{linear}} + u_3\text{* trial}_{\text{inverse}} + u_4\text{* trial}_{\text{quadratic}} \end{gathered} \quad (2)$$

5.3 Preliminary results

First, some general group characteristics are presented in Table 1. The CLBP patients report much more pain and pain interference. In addition, as might be expected, their mood is negatively affected, which is expressed in a higher depression score.

	Pain-free control (N = 76)	CLBP patients (N = 75)	*T*-value/χ^2	*p*-value
Age	34.68	42.11	3.15	0.002
Gender male	26	34	2.26	0.09
Gender female	50	41		
Pain magnitude (SF-36)	1.65	3.51	13.73	0.000
Pain interference (SF-36)	1.18	2.23	9.84	0.000
Depression (BDI)	3.35	7.09	5.8	0.000

Table 1. Characteristics of the two experimental groups.

Because of the preliminary aspect of the analyses, a full description of all results is beyond the scope of this chapter. Therefore, the focus will be on the robust and salient results of the analyses.

We present the results of four independent variables, applied in the first multilevel model (see equation 1): intensity, the intensity of the previous trial, habituation (analyzed with a linear contrast), and group (CLBP patients versus pain-free controls). The results for the 20-ms periods between 0 and 500 ms are shown in Figures 6-9.

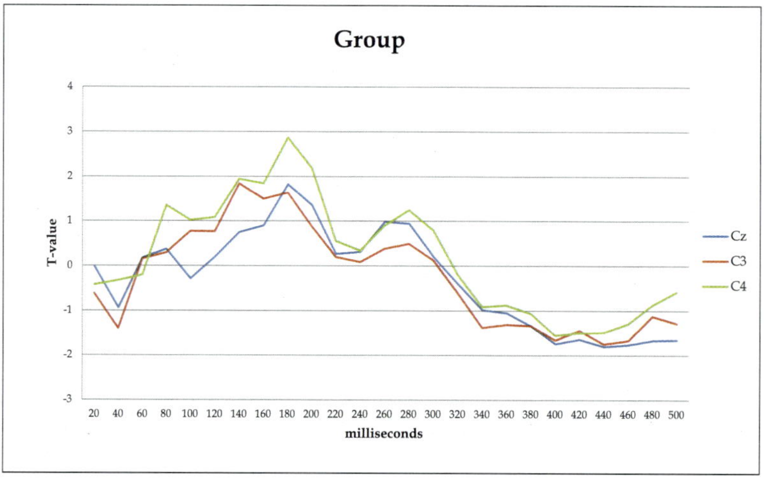

Fig. 6.

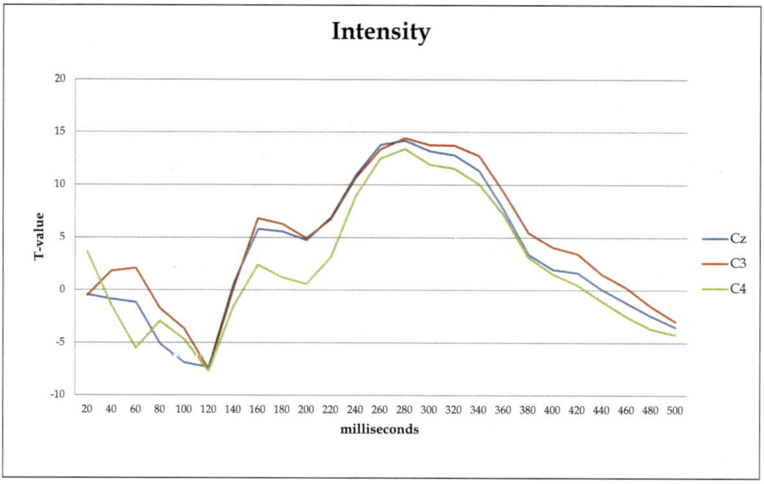

Fig. 7.

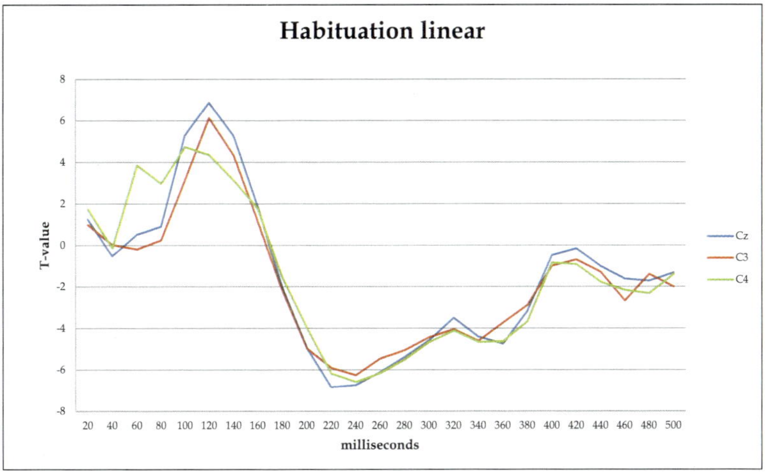

Fig. 8.

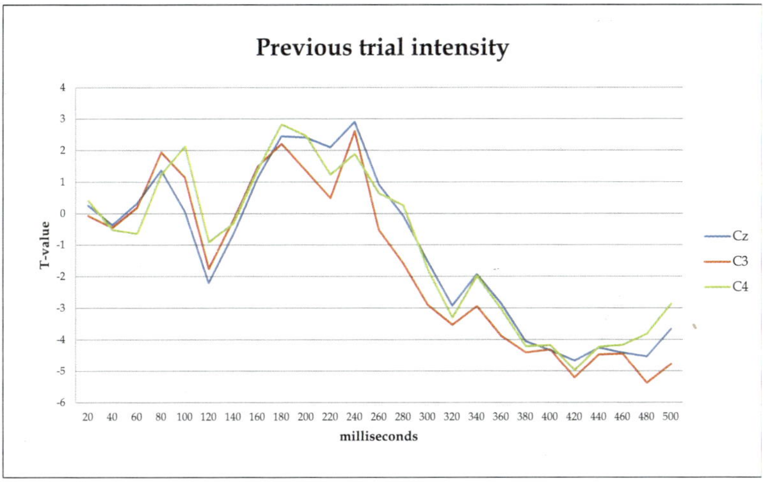

Fig. 9.

Fig. 6-9. T-values per 20-ms AUC of four separate independent variables.

On the vertical axis, the T-value of the variable is depicted, and the horizontal axis represents latency (i.e., the 25 consecutive 20-ms ERFIAs). The variable intensity, habituation (linear), and previous trial intensity show profound and long-lasting, significant effects, as shown in the figure. Note a significant negative effect of stimulus intensity on all three electrodes from 60 to 120 ms and a very strong positive effect from 160 to 400 ms. Remarkably, two positive intensity processes in the latency range between 100 and 400 ms are apparent (from 140-200 ms and from 200-400 ms). In addition, an asymmetry can be observed between C4 and C3/Cz in the 140-to-200-ms range, where C4 demonstrates no clear significance. In contrast to the results presented by Vossen and colleagues (2011), where no main effects of the previous trial intensity variable were found in peak amplitude analyses, the ERFIAs show a large and consistent negative effect from 320 to 500 ms at all three electrodes. There are some small, significant, positive effects in 180-to-260-ms latency. With respect to linear habituation, large and long-lasting significant t-values can also be identified. The linear habituation emerges from the 100-140-ms range as a significant positive effect and becomes significantly negative in the range from 200-380 ms. Although less pronounced, the linear habituation t-curve appears to be opposite compared to the intensity t-curve; whereas intensity has an amplitude-inflating effect in the range from 140 to 400 ms, linear habituation has the opposite effect. Although not displayed, significant effects were observed for the inverse variables habituation (1/trial) and quadratic habituation. Inverse habituation had a clear, significant (T-values between -2 and -4) amplitude-reducing effect during a latency period of 360-500 ms, and quadratic habituation showed strong, significant amplitude-inflating effects (T-values up to 4) in the range of 200-300 ms. No convincing main effect of group, independent of the effect of all other variables in the model, could be demonstrated. The only area of interest appears to be located on C4 and is situated between 140 and 200 ms, but taking the number of tests into account (3x25=75), this effect is questionable.

Finally, we investigated whether there were significant interaction effects with the group variable (see equation 2). A priori (see Vossen et al., 2011), we expected a group*habituation interaction showing CLBP patients to have a reduced habituation. We were also interested in whether the intensity effect was modified by group. In order to limit the number of figures, we present the results on the group by intensity and group by linear habituation interactions (note that group was coded "1" for CLBP patients and "0" for pain-free controls). As can be seen from Figures 10 and 11, the group effect may depend on stimulus intensity (especially in the 200-300-ms range) as well as linear habituation (320-440 ms, especially on Cz). There were also clear significant effects (T-values between 2 and 3 between 320 and 440 ms) for the group by quadratic habituation (no graphs included).

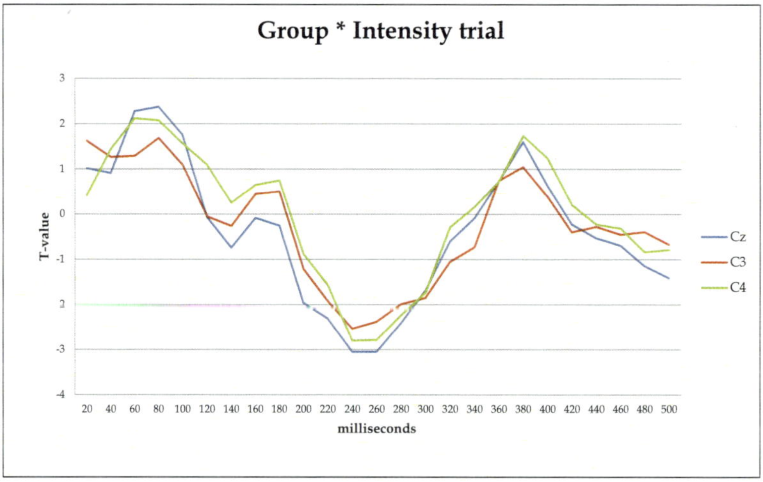

Fig. 10.

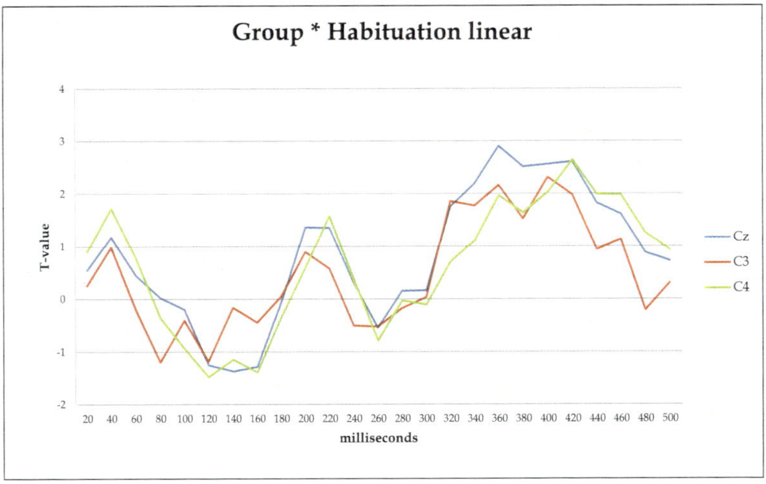

Fig. 11.

Fig. 10,11. T-values per 20-ms ERFIAs of two interaction effects.

5.4 Discussion of the preliminary findings

In paragraph 4.2, several critical points were discussed in relation to ERP peak measures, followed by the proposal of an alternative approach based on AUC, analyzed with multilevel random regression techniques. A number of explorative analyses were performed. We are aware of the fact that the results are merely explorative, since we only analyzed three cranial locations and restricted the analyses to a 500-ms post-stimulus time range. However, given these limitations, we think the analyses show promising results and illustrate proof of concept.

As a first step, we investigated whether the 'new' method would yield comparable results, with respect to already established relationships between peak-ERP, stimulus intensity, and habituation. Reviewing our results, the answer seems to be affirmative. Consistent results were found for all three central electrodes. A large number of the 20-ms ERFIA segments were significantly related to stimulus intensity and habituation. When examining the areas in which we would expect significant results for the intensity and habituation variables *a priori*, the alternative method produced results comparable to other studies (e.g., Bromm & Meier, 1984; Stowell, 1977). For example, the main effect of the variable intensity was very significant in the N2 range and the P3 range. A similar observation could be made for linear habituation in the N2 range (De Tommaso, 2011).

In addition to these basic 'validating' analyses, we were also interested in whether ERP-pain processing of CLBP patients differs from pain-free controls. No clear main group effect could be observed. However, the results strongly suggest that the effects on intensity and linear and quadratic habituation depend on being a CLBP patient or not. An interesting observation was that the group*intensity interaction took place at an earlier latency range compared to the group*habituation interaction in the ERP. The group*intensity interaction effect is situated in the latency range of the P3 and probably can be replicated using peak amplitudes. The group*habituation effect, however, is situated after the P3 and, as a consequence, most likely can not be found in peak analyses. These off-peak effects may be valuable in the search for chronification mechanisms.

All group interaction effects are based on a contrast of a subclinical CLBP population to pain free-controls. The choice of this CLBP group may be disputed, since this subclinical group is likely to be heterogeneous with respect to underlying pathology. Nonetheless, the CLBP group clearly differs from the control group with regard to the key variable pain (see Table 1). The analyses of the ERFIA segments seem to produce more pronounced and significant results, compared to the peak results published by Vossen (2010c). This can be concluded not only from the very large T-values (up to 14) but also from the prolonged latency effects. A typical example is the very broad latency window (from 160-420 ms) of the main effect on intensity. Also, effects of linear habituation are significantly embedded in a large range of consecutive ERFIA segments. Interestingly, intensity of a previous stimulus, indicative for a 'memory' of painful events, showed a significant long-lasting influence (see Figure 5). Since no apparent peaks emerge after 300 ms in the averaged pain-ERP (see Figure 1), The ERFIA method seems to be more useful to detect such late effects than the peak method. This is demonstrated by the fact that we could not find a main effect of the previous stimulus intensity in earlier analyses (Vossen et al., 2011). By plotting the T-values of consecutive ERFIAs, we observed another advantage in the interpretation of the results. In time, variables become more significant and reach a 'peak significance,' followed by a decrease. This information gives insight into the start and end of an influential effect of a variable. To illustrate, intensity seems to have two main effects in the latency range of 140-400 ms. One could speculate that this T-value graph (Figure 3) is indicative for two 'intensity' processes.

Some critical aspects need to be considered in the application of the proposed ERFIA method. First, a large number of consecutive ERFIA segments may result in an unacceptable number of statistical tests. In our view, a rigid correction method for multiple testing, such as the Bonferroni correction, would increase the risk of rejecting 'real' effects in this early, explorative phase of the study. However, an appropriate correction for multiple testing is required. Another critical point concerns the optimal width of ERFIAs. In the present study, we used fixed segments of 20 ms. In order to get a general impression of effects within a relatively large window (500 ms or more), we judge the 20-ms criterion to be appropriate. When investigating small effects, one could argue for the use of smaller areas. Enlargement of the width would reduce the number of tests but may introduce more noise. A third note is related to EOG rejection. In the present analyses, we used a ±25-μV criterion to reject AUCs. It remains to be investigated whether this criterion is optimal. In handling confounded EOG segments, the use of multilevel analyses is especially worthwhile, since all valid, analyzable segments are included, whereas in analysis of variance, a whole subject would have been excluded in the case of too many invalid segments. Finally, one major disadvantage of both peak and AUC measures is the poor spatial resolution. Other techniques in analyzing ERP have been developed to overcome this problem. As an example, probabilistic independent component analysis (PICA) has been applied to gain more insight in the source of underlying multimodal and modality-specific neural activities (Jung et al., 2001; Makeigh et al., 1997; Mouraux et al., 2009). Also, many fMRI studies and magnetoencephalography studies are emerging, with high spatial resolution (Bromm, 2001; Makeig, 004; Stancak et al., 2011; Peyron et al., 2000). Combining ERP methods with fMRI will allow investigation of pain processing in a temporal as well as a spatial superior fashion.

6. Conclusion

In conclusion, without doubting the importance of maximized data derived from peak analyses, one could express doubt whether this approach represents too large a reduction and oversimplification of the post-stimulus cortical processing. In this respect, the present alternative method seems to be more appropriate. A direct comparison of the methods is difficult, if not impossible, since the ERFIA method is based on fixed latency intervals for all trials, whereas in the peak method, the latency of the maximum amplitude differs per trial. Future research has to clarify when to use peak amplitude analysis and in which situations a fixed-AUC method is more suitable.

Using ERP measures, many interesting insights in cortical processing of pain are emerging, such as habituation processes, genetic influences, and influences of personality. These phenomena may contribute to finding explanations for the transition of acute pain to chronic (low back) pain states. Nevertheless, longitudinal research designs are necessary to study this process in detail, as well as a combination of ERP with other methods, such as fMRI, and magnetoencephalography. Furthermore, the application of mixed regression will enable a better understanding of the variance in the pain-ERP. Once the pain-ERP and its underlying cortical processes are understood more completely, the path to remediation in clinical practice is open. Then, development of diagnostic tools could be in reach.

7. Acknowledgments

We are grateful to Jacco Ronner and his colleagues, Department of Instrumentation, Faculty of Psychology and Neuroscience, Maastricht University, for their technical assistance and programming.

8. References

Arntz, A. Merckelbach, H. Peters, M. & Schmidt, A. (1991). Chronic Low back pain, response specificity and habituation to painful stimuli, *Joural of Psychosomatic Research*, Vol. 5, pp. 15-28.

Battié, MC. Videman, T. Levalahti, E. Gill, K. & Kaprio, J. (2007). Heritability of low back pain and the role of disc degeneration. *Pain*, Vol.13, pp.272-280

Becker, DE. Yingling, CD. & Fein G. (1993). Identification of pain, intensity and P300 components in the pain evoked potential. *Electroencephology and clinical Neuropsychology*, Vol.88, pp. 290-301.

Becker, DE. Haly, DW. Urena, WM. & Yingling, CD. (2000). Pain measurement with evoked potentials: combination of subjective ratings, randomized intensities, and long intertimulus intervals procedures a P300-like confound. *Pain*, Vol.84, pp. 257-290.

Bekkering, GE. Hendriks, HJM, Koes, BW. Oostendorp, RAB, Ostelo, RWJG. Thomassen, JMC. & Tulder van, MW. (2003). KNGF-guidelines for physical therapy in patients with low back pain. Nederlands Tijdschrift voor Fysiotheraptie, Vol.111, https://www.cebo.nl/media/m162.pdf.

BenDebba, M. Torgerson, WS. & Long, DM. (1997). Personality traits, pain duration and severity, functional impairment, and psychological distress in patients with persistent low back pain. Pain, Vol. 72, pp. 115-125.

Bengtsson, B. & Thorson, S. (1991). Back pain: a study of Twins. *Acta Genet Med Gemellol (Roma)*, Vol.40. pp. 83-90.

Benvenuto, J. Jin, Y. Casale, M. Lynch, G. & Granger, R. (2002). Identification of diagnostic evoked response potentials segments in Alzheimer's disease. *Experimental Neurology*. Vol. 176, pp. 269-276.

Bond, C. LaForge, KS. Tian, M. Melia, D. Zhang, S. et al. (1998). Single-Nucleotide Polymorphism in the human m-opioid receptor gene alters b-endorphin binding and activity: Possible implications for opiate addiction. *Proc Natl Acad Sci USA* Vol.95, pp. 9608–9613.

Bromm, B. & Meier, W. (1984). The intracutaneous stimulus: a new pain model for algesimetric studies. *Methods and Findings in Experimental Clinical Pharmacology*, Vol.6, pp. 405-410.

Bromm, B. (2001). Brain images of pain. *News in Physiological Sciences*. Vol.16, pp. 244-249.

Chatrian, GE. Canfield, RC. Knauss, TA. & Lettich, E. (1975). Cerebral responses to electrical tooth pulp stimulation in man. Neurology, Vol. 25, pp. 745-757.

Chen, ACN. Chapman, CR. & Harkins, SW. (1979). Brain potentials are functional correlates of induced pain in man. *Pain*, Vol.6, pp. 365-374.

Chou, R & Schelleke P. (2010). Will this patient develop chronic persisting low back pain? *JAMA*. Vol.303, pp. 1295-1302.

Costa, PT. & McCrae, RR. (1980). Somatic complaints in males as a function of age and neuroticism: A longitudinal analysis. *Journal of Behavioural Medicine*, Vol.3, pp. 245-257.

Costa, PT. & McCrae, RR. (1985). *The NEO Personality Inventory Manual*, Psychological Assessment Resources Inc, Odessa, Florida.

Daltrozzo, J. Wioland, L. Mutschler, V. & Kotchoubey, B. (2007). Predicting coma and other low responsive patients's outcome using event-related potentials: a meta-analysis. *Clinical Neurophysiology*. Vol.118, pp. 606-614.

De Tommaso, M. Libro, G. Guido, M. Losito, L. & Lamberti, P. et al. (2005). Habituation of single CO2 laser evoked responses during interictal phase of migraine. *Journal of Headache Pain*, Vol.6, pp. 195-198.

De Tommaso, M. Federici, A. Santostasi, R. Calabrese, R. Vecchio, E. Lapadula, G. Iannone, F. Lamberti, P. Livrea, P. (2011). Laser-evoked potentials habituation in fibromyalgia. J Pain. Vol. 12, pp. 116-24.

Fillingim, RB. Kaplan, L. Staud, R. Ness, TJ. Glover, TL. et al. (2005). The A118G single nucleotide polymorphism of the mu-opioid receptor gene (OPRM1) is associated with pressure pain sensitivity in humans. *J Pain* Vol.6, pp. 159–167.

Fillingim, RB. Wallace, MR. Herbstman, DM. Ribeiro-Dasilva, M. Staud, R. (2008). Genetic contributions to pain: a review of findings in humans. *Oral Diseases* Vol.14, pp. 673-682.

Flor, H. & Meyer, P. (2011). Chapter 8: Psychophysiological and Neuroimaging measures in the assessment of patients with chronic pain. In: *Handbook of Pain Assessment* (3rd revised edition), Turk, D. & Melzack, R., pp.(151-175). Guilford Publications, ISBN 978-1606239766, New York.

Foulkes, T. & Wood JS. (2008). Pain genes. *PLoSONE genetics*, Vol. 25. pp. e1000086.

Gamsa, A. (1994). The role of psychological factors in chronic pain. I. A half century of study. *Pain*. Vol. 57, pp. 5-15.

Garcia-Larrea, L. Peyron, R. Laurent, B. Mauguiere, F. (1997). Association and dissociation between laser-evoked potentials and pain perception. *Neuroreport*, Vol. 8, pp. 3785-3789.

Goubert, L. Crombez, G. & Van Damme, S. (2004). The role of neuroticism, pain catastrophizing and pain-related fear in vigilance to pain: a structural equations approach, *Pain*. Vol.107, pp. 234-241.

Gratton, G. Coles, M. & Donchin, E. (1983). A new method for off-line removal of ocular artifact. *Electroencephalography and Clinical Neurophysiology*, Vol.55, pp. 468-484.

Groth-Marnat, G. & Fletcher, A. (2000). Influence of neuroticism, catastrophizing, pain duration, and the receipt of compensation on short-term response to nerve block treatment for chronic back pain. *Journal of Behavioural Medicine*. Vol.23, pp. 173-182.

Harkins, SW. & Chapman, CR. (1979). Cerebral evoked responses to noxious dental stimulation: relationship to subjective pain report. Psychophysiology, Vol.15, pp. 248-252.

Hoormann, J. Falkenstein, M. Schwarzenau, P. & Hohnsbein, J. (1998). Methods for the quantification and statistical testing of ERP differences across conditions. *Behavioural Research Methods Instruments & Computers*, Vol.30, pp. 371-375.

Jasper, HH. (1958). The ten-twenty electrode system of the International Federation. *Journal of Electroencephalopgraphy Clinical Neurophysiology*, Vol. 20. pp. 371-375.

Jensen, MP. Karoly, P. & Braver, S. (1986). The measurement of clinical pain intensity: a comparison of six methods. *Pain*. Vol.27, pp. 117-126.

Jung, TP. Makeig, S. Westerfield, JT. Courchesne, E. & Seijnowski, T. (2001). Analysis and Vizualisation of Single-Trial event-Related Potentials. *Human Brain Mapping*, Vol. 14, pp. 166-185.

Kanda, M. Matsuhashi, M. Sawamoto, N. Oga, T. Mima, T. Nagamine, T. & Shibasaki, H. (2002). Cortical potentials related to assessment of pain intensity with visual analogue scale (VAS). Clinical Neurophysiology, Vol.113, pp. 1013-1024.

Kemp, AH. Hopkinson, PJ. Stephan, BC. Clark, R. Gordon, E. Bryant, RA. & Willems, LM. (2006). Predicting severity of non-clinical depression: preliminary findings using an integrated approach. Journal of Integrated Neuroscience, Vol.5, pp. 89-110.

Kida, T. Nishihira, Y. Wasaka, T. Nakata, H. & Sakamoto, M. (2004). Differential modulation of temporal and frontal components of the somatosensory N140 and the effect of interstimulus interval in a selective attention task. *Cognitive Brain Research*, Vol.19, pp. 33–39.

Kupers, R. & Kehlet, H. (2006). Brain imaging of clinical pain states: a critical review and strategies for future research. *Lancet Neurology*, Vol.5, pp. 1033-1044.

Lötsch, J. Stuck, B. & Hummel, T. (2006). The Human m-Opioid Receptor Gene Polymorphism 118A.G Decreases Cortical Activation in Response to Specific Nociceptive Stimulation. *Behavioral Neuroscience* Vol.120, pp. 1218–1224

Luck, SJ. (2005). An introduction to the event-related potential technique. ISBN 0262621967 MIT press, Masachusetts.

Makeig, S. Debener, S. Onton, J. Delorme, A. (2004). Mining event-related brain dynamics. Vol.8, pp. 204-210.

Magnusson, T. List, T. & Helkomo, M. (1995). Self-assessment of pain and discomfort in patients with temporomandibular disorders: a comparison of five different scales with respect to their precision in sensitivity as well as their capacity to register memory of pain and discomfort. *Journal of Oral Rehabilitation*. Vol.22, pp. 549-556.

Manolio, TA. Collins, FS. Cox, NJ. Goldstein, DB. Hindorff, LA. et al. (2009). Finding the missing heritability of complex diseases. *Nature* Vol.461, pp. 747–753.

Merighi, A. Salio, C. Ghirri, A. Lossi, L. Ferrini, F. et al. (2008). BDNF as a pain modulator. *Prog Neurobiol*. Vol.85, pp. 297–317.

Mouraux, A. & Iannetti, GD. (2008). Across-trial averaging of event-related EEG responses and beyond. *Magnetic Resonance Imaging*. Vol. 26, pp. 1041-1054.

Mouraux, A. & Iannetti, GD. (2009). Nociceptive Laser-Evoked Brain Potentials do not reflect Nociceptive-Specific Neural Activity. *Journal of Neurophysiology*. Vol.101, pp. 3258-3269.

Miltner, W. Johnson, R. & Braun, C. (1989). Somatosensory event-related potentials to painful and non-painful stimuli: effects of attention. *Pain*. Vol.38, pp. 303-312.

Nackley, AG. Shabalina, SA. Tchivileva, IE. Satterfield, K. Korchynskyi, O. et al. (2006). Human Catechol-O-Methyltransferase Haplotypes Modulate Protein Expression by Altering mRNA Secondary Structure. *Science*, Vol. 314, pp. 1930–1933.

Os van, J. Rutten, BP & Poulton, R. (2008). Gene-environment interactions in schizophrenia: Review of epidemiological findings and future directions. *Schizophrenic Bulletin* Vol.34, pp. 1066-82.

Peyron, R. Laurent, B. &. García-Larrea, L. (2000). Functional imaging of brain responses to pain. A review and meta-analysis. *Neurophysiol Clin*. Vol.30, pp. 263-88.

Picton, TW. Bentin, S. Berg, Donchin, PE. Hillyard, SA. Johnson, R. Miller, GA. Ritter, W. Ruchkin, DS. Rugg, MD. & Taylor, MJ. (2000). Guidelines for using human even-related potentials to study cognition: recording standards and publication criteria. *Psychophysiology*. Vol.37, pp. 127-152.

Ryckman, RM. (2008). *Theories of Personality* (9th ed.). Cengage Learning/Wadsworth, Belmont.

Sen, S. Duman, R. Sanacora, G. (2008). Serum brain-derived neurotrophic factor,depression and antidepressant medications: meta-analyses and implications. *Biol Psychiatry* Vol.15, pp. 527–532.

Seymour, RA. (1982). The use of pain scales in assessing the efficacy of analgesics in post-operative dental pain. *European Journal of Clinical Pharmacology*. Vol.23, pp. 441-444.

Smith, BW. Tooley, EM. Montague, EQ. Robinson, AE. Cosper, CJ. & Mullins, PG. (2008). Habituation and sensitization to heat and cold pain in women with fibromyalgia and healthy controls. *Pain*. Vol.140, pp. 420-428.

Stam, AH. de Vries, B. Janssens, AC. Vanmolkot, KR. Aulchenko, YS. Henneman, P. Oostra, BA. Frants, RR. van den Maagdenberg, AM. Ferrari, MD. van Duijn, CM. & Terwindt, GM. (2010). Shared genetic factors for migraine and depression. *Neurology*, Vol.74, pp. 288-294.

Stancak, A. Alghamidi, J. Nurmikko, TJ. (2011). Cortical activation changes during repeated laser stimulation: a magnetoencephalographic study. *PloS One*. Vol.10; e319744.

Stowell, H. (1977). Cerebral slow waves related to the perception of pain in man. Brain Research Bulletin, Vol. 2, pp. 23-30.

Thompson, RF. & Spencer, WA. (1966). Habituation: A model phenomenon for the study of neuronal substrates of behavior. *Psychological Review*, Vol. 73. pp. 513-519.

Treloar, SA. Martin, NG. & Heath, AC. (1998). Longitudinal genetic analysis of menstrual flow, pain and limitation in a sample of Australian twins. *Behavioural Genetics*, Vol. 28, pp. 107-116.

Turk, DC. & Melzack, R. (Ed(s).). *Handbook of Pain Assessment* (3rd revised edition), Guilford Publications, ISBN 978-1606239766, New York.

Valeriani, M. de Tommaso, M. Restuccia D. le Pera, D. & Giudo, M. et al. (2003). Reduced habituation to experimental pain in migraine patients: a CO2 laser evoked potential study. *Pain*. Vol.105, pp. 57-64.

Vossen, HGM. Van Os, J. Hermens, & H. Lousberg, R. (2006). Evidence that Trait-Anxiety and Trait-Depression Differentially Moderate Cortical Processing of Pain. *Clinical Journal of pain*, Vol.22, pp. 725-729.

Vossen, HGM. Kenis, G. Rutten, B. van Os, J. & Hermens, H. et al. (2010a). The genetic influence on the cortical processing of experimental pain and the moderating effect of pain status. *PLoS ONE* 5(10): e13641.doi:10.1371/journal.pone.0013641.

Vossen, HGM. Van Os, J. Hermens, H. & Lousberg, R. (2010b). The predictive value of pain event-related potentials for the clinical experience of pain. *Journal of Integrative Neuroscience*, Vol.9 pp. 1-10.

Vossen, HGM. (2010c). Thesis Cortical Processing of Pain: a bridge between experimental findings and clinical implications. ISBN 9789090251486.

Vossen, HGM. Van Breukelen, GJP. Hermens, H. Van Os, J. & Lousberg, R. (2011). More Potential in Statistical Analyses of event-Related Potentials: A Mixed Regression Approach. *International Journal of Methods in Psychiatric Research*. DOI: 10.1002/mpr.

Wade, JB. Dougherty, LM, Hart, RP. & Rafii, A. et al. (1992) A canonical correlation analysis of the influence of neuroticism and extraversion on chronic pain, suffering and pain behavior. *Pain*, Vol. 1, pp. 67-73.

Warbrick, T. Sheffield, D. & Nouwen A. (2006). Effects of pain-related anxiety on components of the pain event-related potential. *Psychophysiology*. Vol.43, pp. 481-485.

Woestenberg, JC. Verbaten, MN. Hees van, HH. & Slangen, JL. (1983). Single trial ERP estimation in the frequency domain using orthogonal polynomial trend analyses (OPTA): estimation of individual habituation. *Biological Psychology*, Vol.17, pp. 39-49.

Zaslansky, R. Sprecher, E. Tenke, CE. Hemli, JA. Yarnitsky, G. (1996). The P300 in evoked potentials. *Pain*, Vol.66, pp. 39-49.

Zubieta, JK. Smith, YR. Bueller, JA. Xu, K. Kilbourn, MR. et al. (2001). Regional mu-opioid receptor regulation of sensory and affective Dimensions of Pain. *Science* Vol.293, pp. 311–315.

Zubieta, JK. Heitzeg, MM. Smith, YR. Bueller, JA. Xu, K. et al. (2003). COMT val158met Genotype Affects m-Opioid neurotransmitter Responses to a Pain Stressor. *Science* Vol.299, pp. 1240–1243.

7

Muscular Performance Assessment of Trunk Extensors: A Critical Appraisal of the Literature

Christophe Demoulin** et al.*
Department of Motricity Sciences, Liege University and Liege University Hospital Centre (CHU), Belgium

1. Introduction

Despite growing research efforts, non-specific low back pain (LBP) remains a major public health burden throughout the industrialized world. Epidemiological data indicate a point prevalence ranging from 19% (Hillman et al., 1996) to 27% (Picavet & Schouten, 2003) and a lifetime prevalence of about 60% (Hillman et al., 1996). Costs to society stem mainly from chronic forms, which account for only 5–10% of cases (Nachemson et al., 2000).

Some literature suggests that muscle dysfunction or increased fatigability might jeopardize the function of the spine and be a risk factor in the development, persistence or recurrence of LBP (Biering-Sorensen, 1984; Parnianpour et al., 1988; Alaranta et al., 1995; Hides et al., 1996). Besides, several studies suggest that patients with chronic low back pain (CLBP) may benefit from an active multidisciplinary approach involving an individually tailored reconditioning program (Bendix et al., 1998; Smeets et al., 2008; Demoulin et al., 2010); some authors even reported benefits of programs based mainly on trunk muscles training (Manniche et al., 1988; Mooney et al., 1995; Nelson et al., 1995; Carpenter & Nelson, 1999; Mannion et al., 1999b). As a result, tests of trunk muscle performance are essential to get insight in the muscle strength/endurance. Furthermore, accurate evaluation of patients' deficiencies is essential for the planning of a successful rehabilitation program, for documenting program efficacy and for providing the patients with information on their physical potential and ability to make progress, thereby leading to favourable behavioural changes. Therefore, several reviews have been published targeting performance of trunk muscles (Beimborn & Morrissey, 1988; Newton & Waddell, 1993; Moreau et al., 2001; Malliou et al., 2006). Currently, assessments are performed by means of various methods and no consensus has been reached regarding the optimal test to be used. Most of the time, assessment of trunk extensors has been performed by means of maximum effort tests;

* Stéphanie Grosdent[1,**], Rob Smeets[2], Jeanine Verbunt[2], Boris Jidovtseff[1], Geneviève Mahieu[3,**], Jean-Michel Crielaard[1,**], Marc Vanderthommen[1,**]
[1] *Department of Motricity Sciences, Liege University and Liege University Hospital Centre (CHU), Belgium*
[2] *Department of Rehabilitation Medicine, School of Caphri, Maastricht University and Maastricht University Medical Centre, Adelante, Centre of Expertise in Rehabilitation and Audiology, The Netherlands*
[3] *Back Unit, Dinant Hospital Centre, Belgium*
** *Member of the Belgian Back Society*

however, alternatives to maximum effort tests have also been developed. Therefore the aim of the current review is to present a critical appraisal of the literature on this topic.

2. Assessment of trunk extensors by means of maximum effort tests

2.1 Non-dynamometric tests

Trunk extensor performance has been measured with clinical tests for more than 50 years (Hansen, 1964). These tests, which usually assess endurance of trunk extensors, have the main advantages that they don't require specific equipment, are inexpensive, quick and easy to perform. However, they are not adapted to assess muscle strength and they do not provide a stabilization system to limit hip extensors activation (making them unable to assess spinal muscles specifically). These tests have most often been used in healthy subjects and in patients with CLBP, but they have also been used in other populations (e.g. patients after back surgery (Hakkinen et al., 2003), in schoolchildren (Salminen et al., 1992), etc.).

2.1.1 Static tests

The **Sorensen test** is by far the most widely used and studied test for assessing trunk extensor muscles (Demoulin et al., 2006b). In this test, the subject lies on an examining table in the prone position with the pelvis aligned with the edge of the table. Calves, thighs, and buttocks are secured and upon command, the subject is asked to maintain the horizontal position as long as possible with the arms folded across the chest (Fig 1a). This test was first described by Hansen in 1964 (Hansen, 1964), but it became known as the "Sorensen test" following a study by Biering-Sorensen in 1984, according to which good isometric endurance might prevent first-time LBP occurrence (Biering-Sorensen, 1984). Although some authors have reported similar findings (Alaranta et al., 1995; Adams et al., 1999; Sjolie & Ljunggren, 2001), such association was not confirmed in other studies (Salminen et al., 1995; Gibbons et al., 1997b; Hamberg-van Reenen et al., 2006).

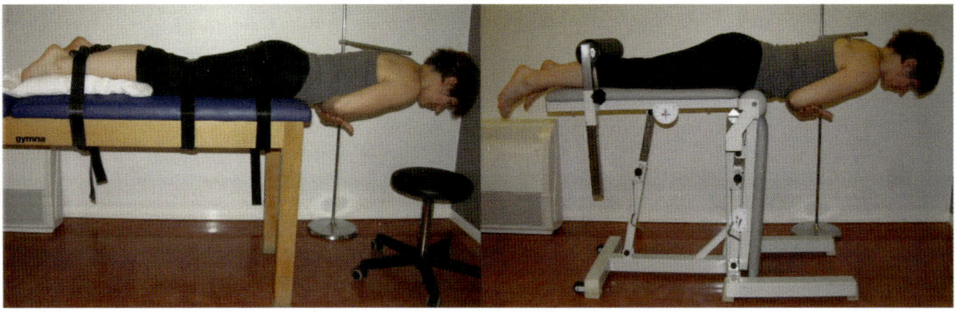

a) b)

Fig. 1a. Original Sorensen test

Fig. 1b. Sorensen test with a Roman chair

Since 1984, the Sorensen test has been used in several studies, either in its original or in adapted versions: the differences concerned the arm position, number of straps, criteria for stopping the test, etc. (Demoulin et al., 2006b); the test has also been performed on a roman chair (Fig 1b) in a few studies (Hultman et al., 1993; Mayer et al., 1995; Keller et al., 2001), sometimes with 45 degrees of hip flexion (Champagne et al., 2008). These numerous methodological variations can affect muscle activity considerably (Mayer et al., 1999; Champagne et al., 2008) and result in considerable discrepancies in study findings. However, concordance was found between some studies regarding the mean holding time in healthy subjects: whereas Latimer et al. measured a holding time of 133s in mixed males and females (Latimer et al., 1999), Mannion et al. reported a holding time reaching 142s and 116s in females and males, respectively (Mannion & Dolan, 1994). Such a gender-related difference was reported in most other studies (Biering-Sorensen, 1984; Mannion et al., 1997a; Kankaanpaa et al., 1998a; McGill et al., 1999; Muller et al., 2010). Differences between genders regarding the weight of the upper body, the degree of lumbar lordosis, the muscles composition (Demoulin et al., 2006b) and the neuromuscular activation patterns (Lariviere et al., 2006) are all hypotheses mentioned.

The Sorensen test has sometimes been considered as a specific tool for evaluating the back muscles (Alaranta et al., 1995). Although spinal muscles are really solicited, most notably the multifidus muscle (Ng et al., 1997; Coorevits et al., 2008; Muller et al., 2010), the test solicits also the other muscles involved in extension of the trunk i.e. the hip extensor muscles (Kankaanpaa et al., 1998a; Plamondon et al., 2002; Plamondon et al., 2004; Champagne et al., 2008; Coorevits et al., 2008; Muller et al., 2010). However muscle fatigue of the hip extensor muscles (reflected by electromyographic parameters) is less correlated to the test holding time than back muscle fatigue (Coorevits et al., 2008).

Although some authors call it a "strength test" (Salminen et al., 1992; Tekin et al., 2009), it rather assesses muscle static endurance (Crowther et al., 2007). Indeed, the elicited contractions were found to be no greater than 40-52% of the maximal voluntary contraction (MVC) (Mannion & Dolan, 1994; Ng et al., 1997; Plamondon et al., 1999; Muller et al., 2010) and the electromyographic (EMG) activity of the spinal erector muscles rarely exceeded 40% of its maximal value (Plamondon et al., 1999; Plamondon et al., 2002).

Although the reproducibility of the Sorensen test has been evaluated in several studies, most of these suffered from methodological weakness (Essendrop et al., 2002; Demoulin et al., 2006b). In general, investigations reported a moderate or high† intra-session, inter-session and inter-tester reproducibility (Simmonds et al., 1998; Latimer et al., 1999; Demoulin et al., 2008b; Gruther et al., 2009), except in case a Roman chair was used (Mayer et al., 1995; Keller et al., 2001). Although the reproducibility is satisfactory in patients with LBP (Simmonds et al., 1998; Latimer et al., 1999) it might be relevant to repeat the test twice (with a 15-minute rest in between) to avoid a learning effect which has been found in some patients (Demoulin et al., 2008b).

Most studies have reported a good discriminative validity of the Sorensen test reflected by a holding-time being significantly lower in patients with LBP compared to healthy subjects (Biering-Sorensen, 1984; Hultman et al., 1993; Simmonds et al., 1998; Latimer et al., 1999; Ljungquist et al., 1999; Arab et al., 2007; Gruther et al., 2009). The safety of the test has also been investigated. A small number of subjects reported back pain during the test (Demoulin et al., 2008b; Demoulin et al., 2009), sometimes resulting in the interruption of the test (Biering-Sorensen, 1984; Latikka et al., 1995; Latimer et al., 1999); however, no persistent adverse effects have been reported following the test (Simmonds et al., 1998; Demoulin et

† based on the classification of Wind et al. (J Occup Rehabil, 2005, 15(2):253-272) which will also be used in the rest of the chapter.

al., 2008b) and it could even be applied in elderly people (Champagne et al., 2009). In view of the stress induced on the cardiovascular system, the Sorensen test might better be avoided in patients suffering from cardiovascular disease because of a pressure overload of the cardiovascular system (Suni et al., 1998; Demoulin et al., 2009).

The **Ito test,** sometimes called "prone isometric chest raise test", has been described in a couple of studies (Shirado et al., 1995b; Ito et al., 1996; Arab et al., 2007; Durmus et al., 2009; Muller et al., 2010); it consists of lifting the upper body while lying prone with a pad under the abdomen, the arms along the sides, the neck flexed as much as possible and the gluteus maximus muscles contracted for stabilizing the pelvis (Fig. 2a) (Shirado et al., 1995b); this position has to be held as long as possible (Ito et al., 1996). Its discriminative power and high reproducibility were reported in the original study (Ito et al., 1996); furthermore, fatigue of the iliocostalis and the multifidi has clearly been linked to the holding time (Muller et al., 2010). Although this test is attractive because it is easy to perform and because it seems to induce less spine loading and limit the risk of lumbar hyperlordosis as compared to the Sorensen test (Ito et al., 1996), no study really confirmed this assumption. Furthermore, a study suggested that this test was less comfortable and more difficult to standardize (with regard to the extent of the upper body lift) than the Sorensen test (Demoulin et al., 2008b). These differences might explain the controversial correlations found when comparing holding times of both tests (Demoulin et al., 2008b; Muller et al., 2010).

The **prone double straight-leg raise test** has been described for evaluating the isometric endurance of the lower spinal extensor muscles (McIntosh et al., 1998; Moreau et al., 2001). In this test, the subject lies prone with hips extended and the hands underneath the forehead (Fig. 2b). The subject is asked to raise both legs until knee clearance as long as possible. According to Arab et al., this test is as reproducible as the other static endurance tests and has good sensitivity, specificity and predictive values in LBP (Arab et al., 2007). However, information about its validity, safety and responsiveness is lacking.

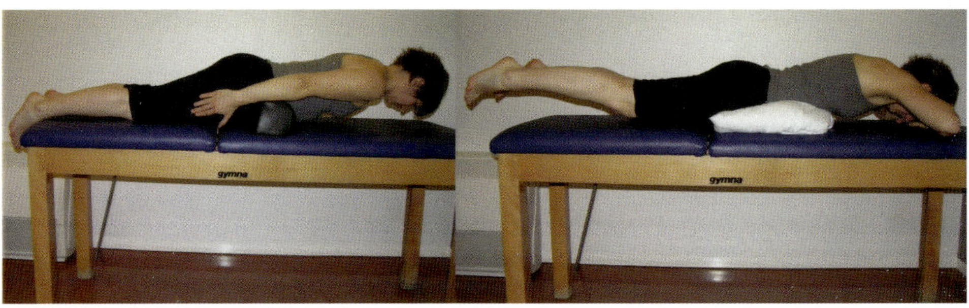

a) b)

Fig. 2. a) Ito test, b) Prone double straight leg raise test

2.1.2 Dynamic tests ("arch-up tests")

The "arch-up tests", sometimes considered as dynamic variants of the Sorensen test, are usually used to assess dynamic endurance of trunk extensors. These tests, performed with the subject prone with the torso cantilevered over the edge of a table, consist in flexing the trunk to a specific position (e.g. 30° trunk flexion), then returning to the initial position as many times as possible at a determined rate of arch-ups per minute (Fig. 3) (Alaranta et al., 1994; Gronblad et al., 1997; Moreland et al., 1997; Udermann et al., 2003). Whereas the static tests have been widely studied, the dynamic tests have received less attention and have been performed in various ways regarding the support (examination table, roman chair, etc.), the range of motion, the rate per minute, etc. As the original Sorensen test, the dynamic tests are not specifically testing the back muscles (Konrad et al., 2001). Although moderate reliability is suggested (Alaranta et al., 1994; Moreland et al., 1997), little is known about the other clinimetric properties of such tests. Furthermore, a recent study, which compared the static Sorensen test with its dynamic variant, revealed that the latter was less comfortable and more difficult to standardize (Demoulin et al., 2008b). In a few studies, the subjects were asked to perform as many repetitions as possible in 30 seconds (Viljanen et al., 1991; Kujala et al., 1996).

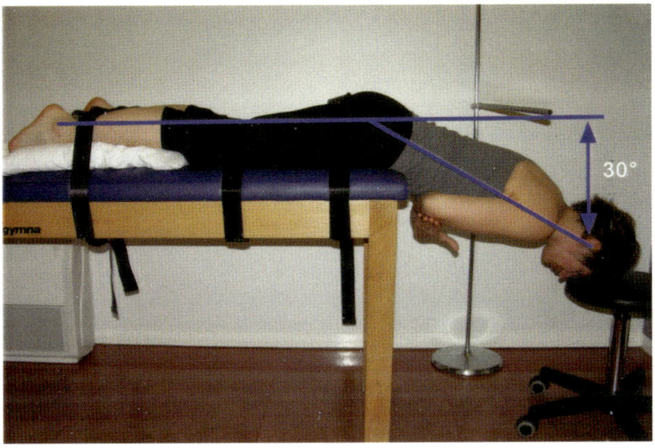

Fig. 3. Arch-up test

2.2 Dynamometric tests

Today, various dynamometric testing machines have been developed to assess trunk muscle performance: these tests allow more complete, precise and specific assessments than the non-dynamometric tests. These measurement systems, also designed to train muscles, differ in terms of contraction mode (static, isotonic, isokinetic), subject position (standing, sitting, lying prone) etc., and generally enable the assessment of several muscular qualities.

2.2.1 Muscle strength tests

MVC tests of trunk extensor muscles have been used in several studies to assess maximal strength in healthy subjects and patients with LBP but also in other populations (e.g. patients following back surgery (Hakkinen et al., 2003), elderly subjects (Rantanen et al., 1997), etc.). Patients with CLBP had reduced values compared to healthy controls in most studies (Reid et al., 1991; Hultman et al., 1993; Kankaanpaa et al., 1998b; Handa et al., 2000; Bayramoglu et al., 2001; Kramer et al., 2005; Gruther et al., 2009), but not all studies (Shirado et al., 1992; Cassisi et al., 1993; Takemasa et al., 1995; da Silva et al., 2005). Several methods (see below) have been used for testing maximal strength.

2.2.1.1 Static strength test

Usually, after a muscular warming-up and sometimes a familiarization period, the subject is instructed to build up the force with increasing intensity. In most studies, about three MVC are measured at short periods intervals; sometimes additional trials are permitted and the best result of the contractions is selected (Demoulin et al., 2006a; Schenk et al., 2006).

Trunk extensors strength can be assessed by means of a **hand-held dynamometer** that is held by the investigator in the interscapular area; the subject, lying prone, has to perform a maximal static effort against it (Fig. 4a). This test which has been confidentially described (Moreland et al., 1997; Swezey et al., 2000; Durmus et al., 2009) appears to be difficult to perform in a standardized manner (Moreland et al., 1997; Swezey et al., 2000) and has a low reproducibility (Moreland et al., 1997).

MVC of trunk extensors has also been assessed by means of a **strain gauge** (Fig. 4b) attached to a wall and connected to a strap around the shoulders; a pelvic fixation is provided so that the rotation axis is set at the hip joint level. The subject, in standing position, has to perform an isometric backward extension ("pulling test") (Biering-Sorensen, 1984; Nicolaisen & Jorgensen, 1985; Kumar et al., 1995; Kujala et al., 1996). In some studies, a more sophisticated apparatus (e.g. with a frame) has been developed (da Silva et al., 2005). Tests in sitting (Kumar et al., 1995) or in prone positions (Plamondon et al., 2004; da Silva et al., 2005) have also been described. Reliability of the pulling tests seems high to moderate (Jorgensen, 1997; Lariviere et al., 2001); however, little is known about the other clinimetric qualities.

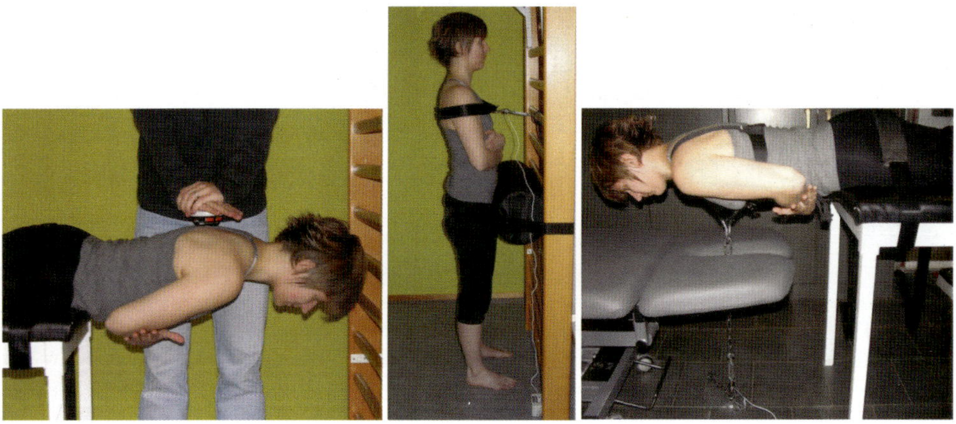

a) b) c)

Fig. 4. a) Hand-held dynamometer, b) "Pulling test" in standing position, c) "Pulling test" in prone position

Specialized and commercialized equipments have also been developed to assess and train trunk muscles. The subject is seated in the equipment and a control of the pelvis is provided by means of a stabilization system designed to limit the activation of hip extensors (Graves et al., 1994; San Juan et al., 2005; Smith et al., 2008); however relevance of such stabilization systems which differ from one device to another remains controversial (Udermann et al., 1999; Walsworth, 2004).

Most studies concerned the MedX™ (MedX Corp. Ocala, FL, USA) which is a dynamometer developed to assess and train spinal muscles (Graves et al., 1990) (Fig. 5). MedX™ assessment consists of measuring the extensor isometric MVC at 7 angles of trunk flexion within the patient's range of motion (i.e. 0-12-24-36-48-60-72°) (Graves et al., 1990). This device is unique in the fact that it uses a gravity correction system (Pollock et al., 1991; Graves et al., 1994). Literature suggests a moderate to high reproducibility of peak torque values in healthy individuals (Graves et al., 1990) and patients with CLBP (Robinson et al., 1992).

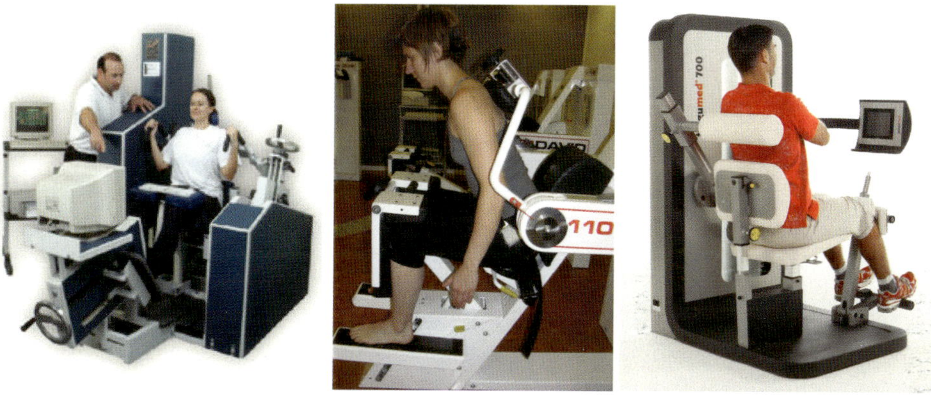

Fig. 5. MedX™, David® and Tergumed® dynamometers, respectively

Other companies (David®, Tergumed®, Schnell®, DBC®) propose a complete set of four individual units for training (Taimela & Harkapaa, 1996; Daniels & Denner, 1999; Mannion et al., 1999b; Giemza et al., 2006) and assessing the trunk extensor, flexor, rotator and lateral-flexor muscles, respectively (Demoulin et al., 2006a; Roussel et al., 2008). The extension device (Fig. 5) differs between the various systems of the companies regarding the hip stabilization system, position of the thighs, legs and feet, etc. Although these protocol differences might concur meaningful inter-system comparison, significant correlations were observed between the MVCs measured by the David®, Tergumed® and Schnell® systems as well when considering the absolute values ($r \geq 0.8$) as when considering the relative values expressed in percentage of specific normative data ($r \geq 0.69$) (Demoulin et al., 2008a). Although spinal muscles seem to be well activated (≥80% maximal EMG activity) during an isometric extension MVC on such dynamometers (Denner, 1997; Vanderthommen et al., 2007), a significant activation of hip extensor muscles has also been observed (about 50% of maximal EMG activity) (Vanderthommen et al., 2007). Several authors reported a high inter-session (Elfving et al., 1999; Demoulin et al., 2006a) and inter-tester (Demoulin et al., 2006a) reproducibility of MVC measurements in healthy subjects and in patients with CLBP (Elfving et al., 2003; Roussel et al., 2008); however, the inter-site reproducibility (in healthy subjects) revealed small but significant differences in measurements between identical devices (Demoulin et al., 2006a). The cardiovascular stress of such maximal isometric effort seems to be limited in healthy middle-aged individuals (maximal systolic and diastolic blood pressure monitored at the end of the MVC test: 165 and 105 mmHg, respectively) (Demoulin et al., 2009); however these results need to be confirmed with instantaneous blood pressure measurement.

A positive relationship between lifting and LBP has been reported (Cole & Grimshaw, 2003); as a result some **functional assessments (lifting test)** have been developed to measure the strength of the functional chain (upper limbs-trunk-lower limbs) during static lifting tasks (Newton et al., 1993; Mannion et al., 1997a; da Silva et al., 2005; Ropponen, 2006). While standing and bending forward, the subject is asked to pull upward a handlebar which is fixed by a chain to a floor-mounted load cell. Methods of testing described in the literature differ regarding materials, knee flexion, the bar height, etc. Though it is a lifting task, the real functional aspect of such test remains questionable because it involves no movement; the safety of such lifting maximal isometric task remains also controversial (Hansson et al., 1984). Limited evidence is available about the clinimetric qualities of such tests.

2.2.1.2 Isokinetic test

Isokinetic dynamometry has been one of the most widely used approaches to train and measure strength of trunk muscles (Newton et al., 1993) for more than 30 years (Hasue et al., 1980). Such dynamometers can measure **trunk flexion and extension strength** (allowing to calculate agonist/antagonist ratios (Newton et al., 1993))(Fig. 6a), at various angular speeds and contraction modes (concentric most often but also eccentric (Shirado et al., 1992) and isometric (Bayramoglu et al., 2001; McGregor et al., 2004; Gruther et al., 2009)). Another advantage of isokinetic dynamometry is that it provides a variable resistance accommodating to a painful arc during the movement. Test-retest reliability of isokinetic measurements appears high in healthy subjects in most studies (Delitto et al., 1991; Newton et al., 1993; Keller et al., 2001; Karatas et al., 2002). In patients with LBP, an increase in performance between test and retest, interpreted as "learning effect", has often been reported (Grabiner et al., 1990; Newton et al., 1993; Keller et al., 2001; Gruther et al., 2009). Inter-site reliability, tested in healthy volunteers, also seems to be high (Byl & Sadowski, 1993).

However, use of isokinetic dynamometry to perform trunk muscle assessment suffers from several limitations: although some authors tried to propose a standard method of testing (Dvir & Keating, 2001), no consensus has been established yet regarding the optimal parameters for testing i.e. movement speed (which can affect testing accuracy (Keller et al., 2001)), range of motion, number of repetitions (Genty & Schmidt, 2001), etc. Differences between the existing isokinetic trunk testing machines in terms of subject position (sitting vs standing)(Morini et al., 2008), ways to reduce the artefacts, stabilization system, gravity correction system (Hupli et al., 1997; Findley et al., 2000) limit meaningful inter-system comparison (Hupli et al., 1997). Besides, the stabilization systems might be inefficient to avoid involvement of hip muscles, especially in the standing position (Morini et al., 2008). Finally, according to some authors (Ayers & Pollock, 1999), the validity of the isokinetic tests of trunk extensors remain controversial due to the impact forces at the end of the movements which can induce artefacts (overshoot). Furthermore, these tests could induce vagal disturbances (Genty & Schmidt, 2001) and pain during testing (Shirado et al., 1995a; Genty & Schmidt, 2001).

Isokinetic dynamometer has also been used to measure the **strength of the functional chain (liftask)** (Newton et al., 1993; Latikka et al., 1995; Gibbons et al., 1997b; Ropponen, 2006). As for the static lifting tests, various methods of testing have been described in the literature; besides, though it is a lifting task, the real functional aspect of such test remains questionable because it involves a movement in a constant speed. Limited evidence is available about the clinimetric qualities of such tests except for reliability which is high in LBP patients and healthy subjects (Newton et al., 1993; Latikka et al., 1995). The high correlations found between the isokinetic flexion-extension and lifting tests suggest that performing both tests is not necessary in clinical practice (Newton et al., 1993).

2.2.1.3 Isoinertial measurements

The Isostation B-200® (Fig. 6b) has been used in a huge number of studies to assess trunk muscle performance but is less used nowadays. In addition to mobility and isometric MVC measurements, this triaxial lumbar dynamometer allows for isoinertial tests (i.e. use of a constant load throughout the range of motion) (Parnianpour et al., 1989b; Gomez et al., 1991; Balague et al., 2010). For the isoinertial flexion-repetition test, the resistance (free weights) is set at a determined percentage of the MVC of flexion (e.g. 25% or 50% (Hutten & Hermens, 1997)) for the sagittal axis and the subject is asked to bend and then return backward as fast as possible (maximum effort) about five times while functional indices (maximal or average velocity, power index and work index) can be simultaneously assessed (Gomez et al., 1991; Rytokoski et al., 1994). This assessment appears to be safe (Newton & Waddell, 1993) and reliable (Rytokoski et al., 1994) as well in healthy persons (Parnianpour et al., 1989a) as in patients with CLBP (Szpalski et al., 1992; Hutten & Hermens, 1997) except for mobility assessments. Unfortunately, axis of rotation of the device is behind the estimated axis for lumbar spine for flexion and extension (Dillard et al., 1991). Furthermore, the device might be inefficient to fully stabilize the pelvis and its relevance to improve functional physical capacity remains controversial (Sachs et al., 1994).

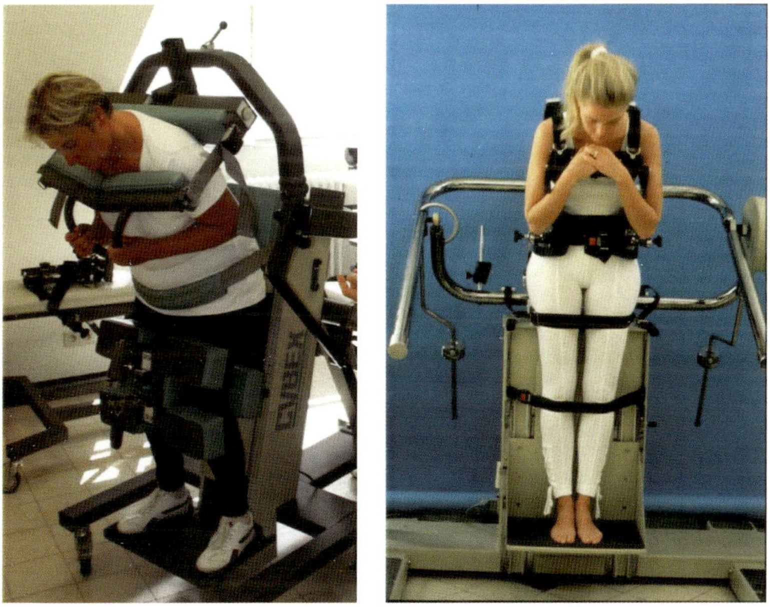

a) b)

Fig. 6. a) Isokinetic dynamometer, b) Isostation B-200®

2.2.2 Endurance tests

2.2.2.1 Static endurance

Muscle static endurance can be assessed with several dynamometers by measuring the time during which a subject is able to maintain a specific torque level corresponding at a preset relative percentage (often 40-60%) of the MVC previously determined (Jorgensen, 1997; Kankaanpaa et al., 1998b; Udermann et al., 2003; Demoulin et al., 2009). A visual feedback system, displaying the torque in real time, is generally positioned in front of the subject in order to keep a constant torque. This test performed in standing position, used for more than 25 years (Nicolaisen & Jorgensen, 1985), is sometimes considered to be more appropriate than the Sorensen test because it is less sensitive to heterogeneous physiques (Jorgensen, 1997; Kankaanpaa et al., 1998a; da Silva et al., 2005). Demoulin et al. compared a seated endurance test performed on a specific dynamometer (David®) (Fig. 7a) to the Sorensen test in healthy subjects; they reported limited pain in the back during performance of both tests and similar subjective level of exertion and cardiovascular stress (Demoulin et al., 2009). As for the MVC test performed on this device, this seated endurance test induces hip extensors activation in spite of the hip stabilization system (Kankaanpaa et al., 1998b); unfortunately, this endurance test has a low test-retest reliability as well in healthy subjects as in patients with CLBP (Demoulin, 2008). Static endurance of trunk extensors have also been measured while the subject performs a lifting test (Mannion et al., 1997a; da Silva et al., 2005); however, such tests produce less fatigue in the back muscles than the Sorensen or the pulling tests (da Silva et al., 2005).

2.2.2.2 Dynamic endurance

Muscle dynamic endurance can be assessed with dynamometers by measuring the maximal number of repetitions performed with a specific load, with a preset speed and range of motion. The literature reports only few studies using such tests: on the David® device (Fig. 7b), the load used corresponded to [0.4 x height (meter)] x [0.6 x Weight (kg)] x 0.82 (Kankaanpaa et al., 1997). This test seems to be less reproducible and well tolerated than the MVC strength and static endurance tests (Demoulin, 2008). Similar tests have been described with the Isostation B-200® (Morlock et al., 1997) and the MedX™ (Udermann et al., 2003).

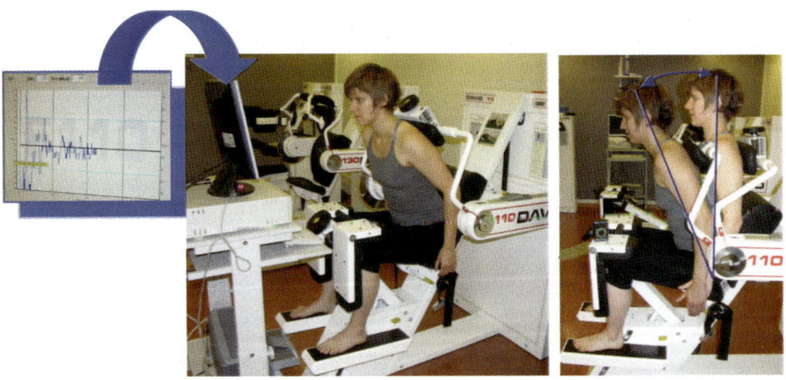

a) b)

Fig. 7. a) Static endurance test, b) Dynamic endurance test

2.2.3 Muscle fatigue tests

Muscle fatigue can be defined as "an exercise-induced reduction in the ability of muscle to produce force or power whether or not the task can be sustained" (Enoka & Duchateau, 2008). Fatigue can be calculated by comparing the maximal strength (MVCs) prior and after an exhaustion task; in the study of Al-Obaidi et al., the task consisted in performing as many extension movements as possible against a predefined individual resistance (corresponding at 50% of the pre-MVC) (Al-Obaidi et al., 2003). Plamondon et al. submitted healthy students to an intermittent prone back extension exercise (100 dynamic repetitions) and reported fatigue of trunk extensors according to the decrease of MVC values (14-20%) measured with a strain gauge in a prone position (Plamondon et al., 2004). Corin et al. compared several ways to test muscle fatigue (Corin et al., 2005) but according to our knowledge, no study has really investigated the clinimetric properties of such assessments.

The isokinetic dynamometers enable to assess fatigue resistance of trunk extensors by requiring more than 15 repetitions at maximal intensity; the torque decrease (fatigue index) throughout the test is generally considered as a good indicator of fatigue resistance (Cale-Benzoor et al., 1992; Genty & Schmidt, 2001; McGregor et al., 2004). The high cardiovascular stress induced by such tests, which can be an important factor-limiting performance (Rantanen et al., 1995), might explain why they have been poorly investigated; furthermore, dizziness has been reported after such exercise (Peel & Alland, 1990) and a huge increase in heart rate (HR), which could reach 90% of maximal theoretical HR at the end of 20 repetitions, was reported (Rantanen et al., 1995). Therefore, caution is needed when testing patients with suspected heart problems (Rantanen et al., 1995).

Nowadays, for fatigue assessment, the surface electromyography (S-EMG) technique is often used and coupled to the endurance tests previously described, which are most of the time limited in time; thus S-EMG is used as an alternative to maximum effort tests to assess trunk muscle performance (see below).

2.3 Interpretation of results

Maximum effort tests have generally pointed out decreased trunk muscle performance in patients with CLBP. Most authors having observed such changes suggested that they could result from physical deconditioning and the associated alterations in the size (decrease in cross-sectional surface area of spinal muscles), density (fatty infiltration) and structure (fibers size reduction) of the trunk muscles (Hultman et al., 1993; Gibbons et al., 1997b; Raty et al., 1999; Danneels et al., 2000; Barker et al., 2004; Demoulin et al., 2007). However, several more recent papers consider that there is minimal research evidence that patients with CLBP really suffer from disuse, physical deconditioning (Smeets & Wittink, 2007; Verbunt et al., 2010) and morphologic alterations (Crossman et al., 2004; Smeets & Wittink, 2007; Verbunt et al., 2010).

The decrease in performance found in patients could partly result from of a lack of validity of such assessments which require maximal collaboration of subjects to produce a maximal effort in terms of intensity or duration (Newton & Waddell, 1993). Therefore, results can be influenced by several individual confounding factors such as motivation, pain tolerance, competitiveness (Mannion & Dolan, 1994); furthermore pain on exertion, anticipation or fear of pain and reflex inhibition of motor activation can be additional factors resulting in inability or unwillingness to produce a truly maximal effort in patients with LBP (Menard et al., 1994; Vlaeyen et al., 1995; Crombez et al., 1996; Keller et al., 1999; Rashiq et al., 2003; Rainville et al., 2004; Al-Obaidi et al., 2005; Ropponen et al., 2005; Verbunt et al., 2005; Thomas et al., 2008; Huijnen et al., 2010). These individual factors might explain the absence or low correlations found in some studies between morphologic variables and performance (Parkkola et al., 1993; Gibbons et al., 1997a). They might also explain the significant learning effect observed in some patients, reflected by performance higher at the second trial than at the first one (Grabiner et al., 1990; Newton & Waddell, 1993; Lariviere et al., 2003b; Gruther et al., 2009). Such learning effect might explain partly the increase in trunk extensor performance sometimes observed after only a few training sessions (Mannion et al., 2001; Demoulin et al., 2010). Therefore, such increase in performance should always be interpreted with caution.

Therefore, although several studies reported no or low correlations between pain or disability and trunk extensor performance (Newton et al., 1993; Gronblad et al., 1997; Bayramoglu et al., 2001; da Silva et al., 2005), these maximum effort tests could also be considered as psychophysical test, reflecting in some cases more the fears and pain tolerance than the muscle function. Consequently, the relevance of using such tests in very painful patients is doubtful. Besides, a period of familiarization with the test appears absolutely necessary in order to eliminate the learning effect and the risk to underestimate real performance.

The technique of twitch interpolation seems a research method able to identify the role of non-physiological factors during strength testing (Verbunt et al., 2003). It is based on the registration of a twitch contraction elicited by a supramaximal electrical stimulus delivered to the muscle or nerve during a MVC. The force increment in response to this stimulus reflects the muscle force reserve or the difference between the maximum force that can be generated by the muscle and the maximum voluntary contraction force, in which nonphysiological factors play a role (Verbunt et al., 2003). This technique was used to compare healthy subjects with patients with LBP regarding knee extensor inhibition in a few studies (Suter & Lindsay, 2001; Verbunt et al., 2005); a lower central activation ratio was reported in patients experiencing increased psychological distress and with higher pain intensity (Verbunt et al., 2005).

3. Alternative to maximum effort tests to assess trunk muscle performance

A few studies examined whether trunk extensor strength could be predicted by anthropometric variables (Mannion et al., 1999a; Wang et al., 2005); indeed, such a prediction is of particular interest in patients who cannot perform maximal tests in order to determine appropriate loads for rehabilitation training (Mannion et al., 1999a). If these variables seem to influence muscle performance, their ability to predict accurately muscle capacity remains limited (Lariviere et al., 2003b).

Taimela et al. developed a submaximal dynamic back extension endurance test utilising subjective perception of low back fatigue (Taimela et al., 1998). They reported that the perceived fatigue (assessed by means of a Borg scale every 15 seconds) increased faster in patients with LBP disorders than in healthy subjects and suggested that this test might be a low-risk, low-cost evaluation method for assessing LBP patient when combined with other clinical data (Taimela et al., 1998). However, according to our knowledge, no other study has used this test.

Mannion et al. conducted a very interesting study to determine whether the twitch superimposition technique could be used to predict maximum force (isometric lifting test) of the spinal muscles from submaximal efforts (Mannion et al., 1997b). Although they reported an excellent curvilinear relationship between twitch force and submaximal force being sustained, they observed that the predicted MVC (extrapolated from the relationship) underestimated the true strength by about 18%. Such difference might result partly from the difficulty in stimulating the spinal muscle mass as a whole. The authors concluded that another testing apparatus and/or subject's posture might result in a more accurate prediction of maximal force (Mannion et al., 1997b). However, no other studies have used the twitch superimposition technique to predict back muscle maximal force since then.

Surface electromyography (S-EMG) technique is sometimes considered as the best tool to assess objectively trunk extensors muscle function because it enables to investigate and compare simultaneously and specifically several back muscles. Furthermore, this technique can be used during a submaximal and time-limited effort in order to limit the influence of individual factors (motivation, fears, etc.). Therefore S-EMG coupled to the endurance field (Sorensen, etc.) and dynamometric (static or dynamic) tests previously described have been frequently used in the literature (Mannion et al., 1997a; Elfving et al., 2000; Koumantakis et al., 2001, Ng et al., 1997; Kankaanpaa et al., 2005; Demoulin et al., 2007). Some devices such as the Back Analysis System (NeuroMuscular Research Center, Boston University, Boston, USA) were even developed to standardize assessments of back muscle dysfunction (i.e. repeated isometric extensions at a given percentage of the MVC associated to S-EMG monitoring) (De Luca, 1993; Roy et al., 1995). The EMG power spectrum has been widely used to calculate the median frequency (MF), mean power frequency (MPF), as well as their rates of decline during prolonged exercise in order to reflect muscle fatigue (Vollestad, 1997). Several studies observed that EMG fatigue parameters recorded after a prespecified period (often 45-60 seconds) of a fatiguing task were significantly correlated to the parameters monitored at the end of the endurance test (van Dieen et al., 1998; Suter & Lindsay, 2001) as well as to the maximal holding time (Kankaanpaa et al., 1997; Mannion et al., 1997a; van Dieen et al., 1998; Dedering et al., 1999). Furthermore, EMG fatigue parameters could be a better predictor of low back disorder than the maximal holding time (Mannion et al., 1997a).

Though submaximal tests coupled to S-EMG have become very popular, the validity of the EMG submaximal endurance tests performed at a given percentage of the MVC can be questioned. Indeed, the intensity of effort during such tests depends on the factors (motivation, pain, fears, etc.) influencing the MVC test previously performed; the absence of difference in EMG parameters between healthy and patients with CLBP and the smaller decrease in power frequency (reflecting lower fatigue) found in the latter group in some studies could be explained by the underestimation of the patients MVC resulting in a lower load level (Elfving et al., 2003; Lariviere et al., 2003a; Kramer et al., 2005). In order to avoid such a bias and to limit the influence of the anthropometric variables, Larivière et al. recently proposed a promising assessment based on S-EMG monitoring during intermittent submaximal static contractions (6,5 seconds contraction / 1,5 second rest) performed in a non-commercial trunk dynamometer at a specific intensity (90 N.m) during 5 to 10 minutes

(Lariviere et al., 2008a; Lariviere et al., 2009). Their results based on healthy subjects suggest that the EMG indices used in the study could predict absolute endurance as well as strength with the use of a single intermittent and time-limited endurance test (Lariviere et al., 2008b).

Although S-EMG technique appears attractive, it presents some drawbacks. Indeed, EMG results are influenced by many factors including the type, size, and location of the electrodes, the impedance of the source and amplifier, the location of the motor points, the type of contraction, the temperature of the muscle and skin, the force produced by the contraction, the fiber composition, the blood flow and the fat layer thickness (De Luca, 1993). Whereas intra-session reproducibility of EMG parameters seems generally satisfactory (Ng & Richardson, 1996), inter-session and inter-operator reproducibility remains controversial (Peach et al., 1998; Elfving et al., 1999; Danneels et al., 2001). Furthermore, S-EMG might not reliably isolate the activity of the different back muscles (Stokes et al., 2003) and the interpretation of EMG measurements at an individual level remains impossible at the moment because of the considerable inter-individual variability (Elfving et al., 2000; Arnall et al., 2002), thereby limiting its diagnostic usefulness (Pullman et al., 2000; Lariviere et al., 2002). Finally, the absence of standardized EMG protocols prevents from performing several comparative studies.

4. Conclusions

As shown in this review, several methods have been used to assess trunk extensor muscle performance. Unfortunately there is not yet a consensus regarding the optimal test to be used and the present literature review does not enable such a test to be determined. Further studies about the clinimetric properties of the maximal effort tests as well as comparison studies between the various existing tests and tools are needed. Anyway, when using such tests, several methodological cautions are necessary in clinical practice (e.g. a familiarization period to the device and to the test, several trials authorized, etc.) in order to avoid a learning effect; furthermore, results interpretation should always be careful, especially in painful or fearful subjects considering the risk of underestimating the true muscle performance. Additional effort to develop a submaximal test remains essential. Although the S-EMG technique appears to be a key investigation tool for research because individual factors do not influence the outcomes, further investigations are necessary to make the measurement interpretation possible at an individual level.

5. Acknowledgements

The authors thank Prof M. Szpalsky and F. Balagué for providing some pictures as well as A. Depaifve and S. Wolfs for their help, cooperation and valuable assistance.

6. References

Adams, M.A.; Mannion, A.F. & Dolan, P. (1999). Personal risk factors for first-time low back pain. *Spine,* Vol.24, No.23, pp. 2497-2505.

Al-Obaidi, S.; Al-Zoabi, B.; Chowdhury, R. & Al-Shuwai, N. (2003). Fatigue susceptibility of the lumbar extensor muscles among smokers. *Physiotherapy,* Vol.89, No.4, pp. 238-248.

Al-Obaidi, S.M.; Beattie, P.; Al-Zoabi, B. & Al-Wekeel, S. (2005). The relationship of anticipated pain and fear avoidance beliefs to outcome in patients with chronic low back pain who are not receiving workers' compensation. *Spine*, Vol.30, No.9, pp. 1051-1057.

Alaranta, H.; Hurri, H.; Heliovaara, M.; Soukka, A. & Harju, R. (1994). Non-dynamometric trunk performance tests: reliability and normative data. *Scandinavian Journal of Rehabilitation Medicine*, Vol.26, No.4, pp. 211-215.

Alaranta, H.; Luoto, S.; Heliovaara, M. & Hurri, H. (1995). Static back endurance and the risk of low-back pain. *Clinical Biomechanics*, Vol.10, No.6, pp. 323-324.

Arab, A.M.; Salavati, M.; Ebrahimi, I. & Ebrahim Mousavi, M. (2007). Sensitivity, specificity and predictive value of the clinical trunk muscle endurance tests in low back pain. *Clinical Rehabilitation*, Vol.21, No.7, pp. 640-647.

Arnall, F.A.; Koumantakis, G.A.; Oldham, J.A. & Cooper, R.G. (2002). Between-days reliability of electromyographic measures of paraspinal muscle fatigue at 40, 50 and 60% levels of maximal voluntary contractile force. *Clinical Rehabilitation*, Vol.16, No.7, pp. 761-771.

Ayers, S. & Pollock, M. (1999). Isometric dynamometry, In: *Spinal rehabilitation*, D.E. Stude, (Ed.), 339-367, Appleton & Lange, Stamford Connecticut.

Balague, F.; Bibbo, E.; Melot, C.; Szpalski, M.; Gunzburg, R. & Keller, T.S. (2010). The association between isoinertial trunk muscle performance and low back pain in male adolescents. *European Spine Journal*, Vol.19, No.4, pp. 624-632.

Barker, K.L.; Shamley, D.R. & Jackson, D. (2004). Changes in the cross-sectional area of multifidus and psoas in patients with unilateral back pain: the relationship to pain and disability. *Spine*, Vol.29, No.22, pp. E515-519.

Bayramoglu, M.; Akman, M.N.; Kilinc, S.; Cetin, N.; Yavuz, N. & Ozker, R. (2001). Isokinetic measurement of trunk muscle strength in women with chronic low-back pain. *American Journal of Physical Medicine and Rehabilitation*, Vol.80, No.9, pp. 650-655.

Beimborn, D.S. & Morrissey, M.C. (1988). A review of the literature related to trunk muscle performance. *Spine*, Vol.13, No.6, pp. 655-660.

Bendix, A.E.; Bendix, T.; Haestrup, C. & Busch, E. (1998). A prospective, randomized 5-year follow-up study of functional restoration in chronic low back pain patients. *European Spine Journal*, Vol.7, No.2, pp. 111-119.

Biering-Sorensen, F. (1984). Physical measurements as risk indicators for low-back trouble over a one-year period. *Spine*, Vol.9, No.2, pp. 106-119.

Byl, N. & Sadowski, S. (1993). Inter-site reliability of repeated isokinetic measurements: Cybex back systems including trunk rotation, trunk extension flexion and lift task. *Isokinetics and Exercise Science*, Vol.3, pp. 139-147.

Cale-Benzoor, M.; Albert, M.S.; Grodin, A. & Woodruff, L.D. (1992). Isokinetic trunk muscle performance characteristics of classical ballet dancers. *Journal of Orthopaedic and Sports Physical Therapy*, Vol.15, No.2, pp. 99-106.

Carpenter, D.M. & Nelson, B.W. (1999). Low back strengthening for the prevention and treatment of low back pain. *Medicine and Science in Sports and Exercise*, Vol.31, No.1, pp. 18-24.

Cassisi, J.E.; Robinson, M.E.; O'conner, P. & Macmillan, M. (1993). Trunk strength and lumbar paraspinal muscle activity during isometric exercise in chronic low-back pain patients and controls. *Spine*, Vol.18, No.2, pp. 245-251.

Champagne, A.; Descarreaux, M. & Lafond, D. (2008). Back and hip extensor muscles fatigue in healthy subjects: task-dependency effect of two variants of the Sorensen test. *European Spine Journal,* Vol.17, No.12, pp. 1721-1726.

Champagne, A.; Descarreaux, M. & Lafond, D. (2009). Comparison between elderly and young males' lumbopelvic extensor muscle endurance assessed during a clinical isometric back extension test. *Journal of Manipulative and Physiological Therapeutics,* Vol.32, No.7, pp. 521-526.

Cole, M.H. & Grimshaw, P.N. (2003). Low back pain and lifting: a review of epidemiology and aetiology. *Work,* Vol.21, No.2, pp. 173-184.

Coorevits, P.; Danneels, L.; Cambier, D.; Ramon, H. & Vanderstraeten, G. (2008). Assessment of the validity of the Biering-Sorensen test for measuring back muscle fatigue based on EMG median frequency characteristics of back and hip muscles. *Journal of Electromyography and Kinesiology,* Vol.18, No.6, pp. 997-1005.

Corin, G.; Strutton, P.H. & Mcgregor, A.H. (2005). Establishment of a protocol to test fatigue of the trunk muscles. *British Journal of Sports Medicine,* Vol.39, No.10, pp. 731-735.

Crombez, G.; Vervaet, L.; Baeyens, F.; Lysens, R. & Eelen, P. (1996). Do pain expectancies cause pain in chronic low back patients? A clinical investigation. *Behaviour Research and Therapy,* Vol.34, No.11-12, pp. 919-925.

Crossman, K.; Mahon, M.; Watson, P.J.; Oldham, J.A. & Cooper, R.G. (2004). Chronic low back pain-associated paraspinal muscle dysfunction is not the result of a constitutionally determined "adverse" fiber-type composition. *Spine,* Vol.29, No.6, pp. 628-634.

Crowther, A.; Mcgregor, A. & Strutton, P. (2007). Testing isometric fatigue in the trunk muscles. *Isokinetics and Exercise Science,* Vol.15, pp. 91-97.

Da Silva, R.A.; Arsenault, A.B.; Gravel, D.; Lariviere, C. & De Oliveira, E. (2005). Back muscle strength and fatigue in healthy and chronic low back pain subjects: a comparative study of 3 assessment protocols. *Archives of Physical Medicine and Rehabilitation,* Vol.86, No.4, pp. 722-729.

Daniels, K. & Denner, A. (1999). Analysis based medical training therapy for the spine (FPZ concept): quality assurance in the scope of evidence-based medicine. *Zeitschrift für Arztliche Fortbildung und Qualitatssicherung,* Vol.93, No.5, pp. IV-V.

Danneels, L.A.; Vanderstraeten, G.G.; Cambier, D.C.; Witvrouw, E.E. & De Cuyper, H.J. (2000). CT imaging of trunk muscles in chronic low back pain patients and healthy control subjects. *European Spine Journal,* Vol.9, No.4, pp. 266-272.

Danneels, L.A.; Cagnie, B.J.; Cools, A.M.; Vanderstraeten, G.G.; Cambier, D.C.; Witvrouw, E.E. & De Cuyper, H.J. (2001). Intra-operator and inter-operator reliability of surface electromyography in the clinical evaluation of back muscles. *Manual Therapy,* Vol.6, No.3, pp. 145-153.

De Luca, C.J. (1993). Use of the surface EMG signal for performance evaluation of back muscles. *Muscle Nerve,* Vol.16, No.2, pp. 210-216.

Dedering, A.; Nemeth, G. & Harms-Ringdahl, K. (1999). Correlation between electromyographic spectral changes and subjective assessment of lumbar muscle fatigue in subjects without pain from the lower back. *Clinical Biomechanics,* Vol.14, No.2, pp. 103-111.

Delitto, A.; Rose, S.J.; Crandell, C.E. & Strube, M.J. (1991). Reliability of isokinetic measurements of trunk muscle performance. *Spine,* Vol.16, No.7, pp. 800-803.

Demoulin, C.; Grosdent, S.; Debois, I.; Mahieu, G.; Maquet, D.; Jidovsteff, B.; Croisier, J.; Crielaard, J. & Vanderthommen, M. (2006a). Inter-session, inter-rater and inter-site reproducibility of isometric trunk muscle strength measurements. *Isokinetics and Exercise Science,* Vol.14, pp. 317-325.

Demoulin, C.; Vanderthommen, M.; Duysens, C. & Crielaard, J.M. (2006b). Spinal muscle evaluation using the Sorensen test: a critical appraisal of the literature. *Joint Bone Spine,* Vol.73, No.1, pp. 43-50.

Demoulin, C.; Crielaard, J.M. & Vanderthommen, M. (2007). Spinal muscle evaluation in healthy individuals and low-back-pain patients: a literature review. *Joint Bone Spine,* Vol.74, No.1, pp. 9-13.

Demoulin, C. (2008). Contribution à l'évaluation et à la rééducation de la fonction musculaire du sujet lombalgique chronique. PhD Thesis, 192 pages. Département des Sciences de la Motricité, Université de Liège (ULg), Liège, Belgique.

Demoulin, C.; Koninckx, S.; Mahieu, G.; Feiereisen, P.; Koch, D.; Crielaard, J.-M. & Vanderthommen, M. (2008a). Analyse corrélative des résultats de différents dynamomètres spécifiques pour l'évaluation des muscles du tronc *Revue du Rhumatisme,* Vol.75, No.10-11, pp. 1180.

Demoulin, C.; Sac, D.; Serre, L.; Maquet, D.; Crielaard, J. & Vanderthommen, M. (2008b). Reproducibility and suitability of clinical assessments of trunk flexor and extensor muscles. *Journal of Musculoskeletal Pain,* Vol.16, pp. 301-311.

Demoulin, C.; Grosdent, S.; Bury, T.; Croisier, J.-L.; Maquet, D.; Lehance, C.; Crielaard, J.M. & Vanderthommen, M. (2009). Cardiovascular responses to static assessments of trunk muscles. *Journal of Musculoskeletal Pain,* Vol.17, No.4, pp. 378-389.

Demoulin, C.; Grosdent, S.; Capron, L.; Tomasella, M.; Somville, P.R.; Crielaard, J.M. & Vanderthommen, M. (2010). Effectiveness of a semi-intensive multidisciplinary outpatient rehabilitation program in chronic low back pain. *Joint Bone Spine,* Vol.77, No.1, pp. 58-63.

Denner, A. (1997). *Muskuläre Profile der Wirbelsäule,* Springer, Berlin.

Dillard; J., Trafimow, J.; Andersson, G.B. & Cronin, K. (1991). Motion of the lumbar spine. Reliability of two measurement techniques. *Spine,* Vol.16, No.3, pp. 321-324.

Durmus, D.; Akyol, Y.; Alayli, G.; Tander, B.; Zahiroglu, Y. & Canturk, F. (2009). Effects of electrical stimulation program on trunk muscle strength, functional capacity, quality of life, and depression in the patients with low back pain: a randomized controlled trial. *Rheumatology International,* Vol.29, No.8, pp. 947-954.

Dvir, Z. & Keating, J. (2001). Reproducibility and validity of a new test protocol for measuring isokinetic trunk extension strength. *Clinical Biomechanics,* Vol.16, No.7, pp. 627-630.

Elfving, B.; Nemeth, G.; Arvidsson, I. & Lamontagne, M. (1999). Reliability of EMG spectral parameters in repeated measurements of back muscle fatigue. *Journal of Electromyography and Kinesiology,* Vol.9, No.4, pp. 235-243.

Elfving, B.; Nemeth, G. & Arvidsson, I. (2000). Back muscle fatigue in healthy men and women studied by electromyography spectral parameters and subjective ratings. *Scandinavian Journal of Rehabilitation Medicine,* Vol.32, No.3, pp. 117-123.

Elfving, B.; Dedering, A. & Nemeth, G. (2003). Lumbar muscle fatigue and recovery in patients with long-term low-back trouble--electromyography and health-related factors. *Clinical Biomechanics,* Vol.18, No.7, pp. 619-630.

Enoka, R.M. & Duchateau, J. (2008). Muscle fatigue: what, why and how it influences muscle function. *Journal of Physiology,* Vol.586, No.1, pp. 11-23.

Essendrop, M.; Maul, I.; Laubli, T.; Riihimaki, H. & Schibye, B. (2002). Measures of low back function: a review of reproducibility studies. *Clinical Biomechanics,* Vol.17, No.4, pp. 235-249.

Findley, B.; Brown, L.; Whitehurst, M.; Gilbert, R.; Groo, D. & O'neal, J. (2000). Sitting versus standing isokinetic trunk extension and flexion performance differences. *Journal of Strength and Conditioning Research,* Vol.14, No.3, pp. 310-315.

Genty, M. & Schmidt, D. (2001). Utilisation de l'isocinétisme dans les programmes de rééducation du rachis (modalités pratiques, protocoles proposés), In: *Isocinétisme et rachis,* P. Codine, C. Hérisson, B. Denat, (Eds), 99-106, Masson, Paris.

Gibbons, L.E.; Latikka, P.; Videman, T.; Manninen, H. & Battie, M.C. (1997a). The association of trunk muscle cross-sectional area and magnetic resonance image parameters with isokinetic and psychophysical lifting strength and static back muscle endurance in men. *Journal of Spinal Disorders,* Vol.10, No.5, pp. 398-403.

Gibbons, L.E.; Videman, T. & Battie, M.C. (1997b). Isokinetic and psychophysical lifting strength, static back muscle endurance, and magnetic resonance imaging of the paraspinal muscles as predictors of low back pain in men. *Scandinavian Journal of Rehabilitation Medicine,* Vol.29, No.3, pp. 187-191.

Giemza, C.; Bodnar, A.; Kabala, T.; Gruszecka, D.; Lipnicki, W.; Magiera, P. & Kowalski, J. (2006). The efficiency assessment of rehabilitation with DBC method in low back pain patients. *Ortopedia Traumatologia Rehabilitacja,* Vol.8, No.6, pp. 650-657.

Gomez, T.; Beach, G.; Cooke, C.; Hrudey, W. & Goyert, P. (1991). Normative database for trunk range of motion, strength, velocity, and endurance with the Isostation B-200 Lumbar Dynamometer. *Spine,* Vol.16, No.1, pp. 15-21.

Grabiner, M.D.; Jeziorowski, J.J. & Divekar, A.D. (1990). Isokinetic measurements of trunk extension and flexion performance collected with the biodex clinical data station. *Journal of Orthopaedic and Sports Physical Therapy,* Vol.11, No.12, pp. 590-598.

Graves, J.E.; Pollock, M.L.; Carpenter, D.M.; Leggett, S.H.; Jones, A.; Macmillan, M. & Fulton, M. (1990). Quantitative assessment of full range-of-motion isometric lumbar extension strength. *Spine,* Vol.15, No.4, pp. 289-294.

Graves, J.E.; Webb, D.C.; Pollock, M.L.; Matkozich, J.; Leggett, S.H.; Carpenter, D.M.; Foster, D.N. & Cirulli, J. (1994). Pelvic stabilization during resistance training: its effect on the development of lumbar extension strength. *Archives of Physical Medicine and Rehabilitation,* Vol.75, No.2, pp. 210-215.

Gronblad, M.; Hurri, H. & Kouri, J.P. (1997). Relationships between spinal mobility, physical performance tests, pain intensity and disability assessments in chronic low back pain patients. *Scandinavian Journal of Rehabilitation Medicine,* Vol.29, No.1, pp. 17-24.

Gruther, W.; Wick, F.; Paul, B.; Leitner, C.; Posch, M.; Matzner, M.; Crevenna, R. & Ebenbichler, G. (2009). Diagnostic accuracy and reliability of muscle strength and endurance measurements in patients with chronic low back pain. *J Rehabil Med,* Vol.41, No.8, pp. 613-619.

Hakkinen, A.; Kuukkanen, T.; Tarvainen, U. & Ylinen, J. (2003). Trunk muscle strength in flexion, extension, and axial rotation in patients managed with lumbar disc herniation surgery and in healthy control subjects. *Spine,* Vol.28, No.10, pp. 1068-1073.

Hamberg-Van Reenen, H.H.; Ariens, G.A.; Blatter, B.M.; Twisk, J.W.; Van Mechelen, W. & Bongers, P.M. (2006). Physical capacity in relation to low back, neck, or shoulder pain in a working population. *Occupational and Environmental Medicine,* Vol.63, No.6, pp. 371-377.

Handa, N.; Yamamoto, H.; Tani, T.; Kawakami, T. & Takemasa, R. (2000). The effect of trunk muscle exercises in patients over 40 years of age with chronic low back pain. *Journal of Orthopaedic Science*, Vol.5, No.3, pp. 210-216.

Hansen, J.W. (1964). Postoperative Management in Lumbar Disc Protrusions. I. Indications, Method and Results. II. Follow-up on a Trained and an Untrained Group of Patients. *Acta Orthopaedica Scandinavica (Suppl)*, Vol.71, pp. 1-47.

Hansson, T.H.; Bigos, S.J.; Wortley, M.K. & Spengler, D.M. (1984). The load on the lumbar spine during isometric strength testing. *Spine*, Vol.9, No.7, pp. 720-724.

Hasue, M.; Fujiwara, M. & Kikuchi, S. (1980). A new method of quantitative measurement of abdominal and back muscle strength. *Spine*, Vol.5, No.2, pp. 143-148.

Hides, J.A.; Richardson, C.A. & Jull, G.A. (1996). Multifidus muscle recovery is not automatic after resolution of acute, first-episode low back pain. *Spine*, Vol.21, No.23, pp. 2763-2769.

Hillman, M.; Wright, A.; Rajaratnam, G.; Tennant, A. & Chamberlain, M.A. (1996). Prevalence of low back pain in the community: implications for service provision in Bradford, UK. *Journal of Epidemiology and Community Health*, Vol.50, No.3, pp. 347-352.

Huijnen, I.P.; Verbunt, J.A.; Peters, M.L. & Seelen, H.A. (2010). Is physical functioning influenced by activity-related pain prediction and fear of movement in patients with subacute low back pain? *European Journal of Pain*, Vol.14, No.6, pp. 661-666.

Hultman, G.; Nordin, M.; Saraste, H. & Ohlsen, H. (1993). Body composition, endurance, strength, cross-sectional area, and density of MM erector spinae in men with and without low back pain. *Journal of Spinal Disorders*, Vol.6, No.2, pp. 114-123.

Hupli, M.; Sainio, P.; Hurri, H. & Alaranta, H. (1997). Comparison of trunk strength measurements between two different isokinetic devices used at clinical settings. *Journal of Spinal Disorders*, Vol.10, No.5, pp. 391-397.

Hutten, M.M. & Hermens, H.J. (1997). Reliability of lumbar dynamometry measurements in patients with chronic low back pain with test-retest measurements on different days. *European Spine Journal*, Vol.6, No.1, pp. 54-62.

Ito, T.; Shirado, O.; Suzuki, H.; Takahashi, M.; Kaneda, K. & Strax, T.E. (1996). Lumbar trunk muscle endurance testing: an inexpensive alternative to a machine for evaluation. *Archives of Physical Medicine and Rehabilitation*, Vol.77, No.1, pp. 75-79.

Jorgensen, K. (1997). Human trunk extensor muscles physiology and ergonomics. *Acta Physiologica Scandinavica (Suppl)*, Vol.637, pp. 1-58.

Kankaanpaa, M.; Taimela, S.; Webber, C.L., Jr.; Airaksinen, O. & Hanninen, O. (1997). Lumbar paraspinal muscle fatigability in repetitive isoinertial loading: EMG spectral indices, Borg scale and endurance time. *European Journal of Applied Physiology and Occupational Physiology*, Vol.76, No.3, pp. 236-242.

Kankaanpaa, M.; Laaksonen, D.; Taimela, S.; Kokko, S.M.; Airaksinen, O. & Hanninen, O. (1998a). Age, sex, and body mass index as determinants of back and hip extensor fatigue in the isometric Sorensen back endurance test. *Archives of Physical Medicine and Rehabilitation*, Vol.79, No.9, pp. 1069-1075.

Kankaanpaa, M.; Taimela, S.; Laaksonen, D.; Hanninen, O. & Airaksinen, O. (1998b). Back and hip extensor fatigability in chronic low back pain patients and controls. *Archives of Physical Medicine and Rehabilitation*, Vol.79, No.4, pp. 412-417.

Kankaanpaa, M.; Colier, W.N.; Taimela, S.; Anders, C.; Airaksinen, O.; Kokko-Aro, S.M. & Hanninen, O. (2005). Back extensor muscle oxygenation and fatigability in healthy subjects and low back pain patients during dynamic back extension exertion. *Pathophysiology,* Vol.12, No.4, pp. 267-273.

Karatas, G.K.; Gogus, F. & Meray, J. (2002). Reliability of isokinetic trunk muscle strength measurement. *American Journal of Physical Medicine and Rehabilitation,* Vol.81, No.2, pp. 79-85.

Keller, A.; Johansen, J.G.; Hellesnes, J. & Brox, J.I. (1999). Predictors of isokinetic back muscle strength in patients with low back pain. *Spine,* Vol.24, No.3, pp. 275-280.

Keller, A.; Hellesnes, J. & Brox, J.I. (2001). Reliability of the isokinetic trunk extensor test, Biering-Sorensen test, and Astrand bicycle test: assessment of intraclass correlation coefficient and critical difference in patients with chronic low back pain and healthy individuals. *Spine,* Vol.26, No.7, pp. 771-777.

Konrad, P.; Schmitz, K. & Denner, A. (2001). Neuromuscular Evaluation of Trunk-Training Exercises. *Journal of Athletic Training,* Vol.36, No.2, pp. 109-118.

Koumantakis, G.A.; Arnall, F.; Cooper, R.G. & Oldham, J.A. (2001). Paraspinal muscle EMG fatigue testing with two methods in healthy volunteers. Reliability in the context of clinical applications. *Clinical Biomechanics,* Vol.16, No.3, pp. 263-266.

Kramer, M.; Ebert, V.; Kinzl, L.; Dehner, C.; Elbel, M. & Hartwig, E. (2005). Surface electromyography of the paravertebral muscles in patients with chronic low back pain. *Archives of Physical Medicine and Rehabilitation,* Vol.86, No.1, pp. 31-36.

Kujala, U.M.; Taimela, S.; Viljanen, T. ; Jutila, H. ; Viitasalo, J.T. ; Videman, T. & Battie, M.C. (1996). Physical loading and performance as predictors of back pain in healthy adults. A 5-year prospective study. *European Journal of Applied Physiology and Occupational Physiology,* Vol.73, No.5, pp. 452-458.

Kumar, S.; Dufresne, R.M. & Van Schoor, T. (1995). Human trunk strength profile in flexion and extension. *Spine,* Vol.20, No.2, pp. 160-168.

Lariviere, C.; Gagnon, D.; Gravel, D.; Arsenault, A.B.; Dumas, J.; Goyette, M. & Loisel, P. (2001). A triaxial dynamometer to monitor lateral bending and axial rotation moments during static trunk extension efforts. *Clinical Biomechanics,* Vol.16, No.1, pp. 80-83.

Lariviere, C.; Arsenault, A.B.; Gravel, D. ; Gagnon, D. & Loisel, P. (2002). Evaluation of measurement strategies to increase the reliability of EMG indices to assess back muscle fatigue and recovery. *Journal of Electromyography and Kinesiology,* Vol.12, No.2, pp. 91-102.

Lariviere, C.; Arsenault, A.B.; Gravel, D. ; Gagnon, D. & Loisel, P. (2003a). Surface electromyography assessment of back muscle intrinsic properties. *Journal of Electromyography and Kinesiology,* Vol.13, No.4, pp. 305-318.

Lariviere, C.; Gravel, D.; Gagnon, D. ; Arsenault, A.B. ; Loisel, P. & Lepage, Y. (2003b). Back strength cannot be predicted accurately from anthropometric measures in subjects with and without chronic low back pain. *Clinical Biomechanics,* Vol.18, No.6, pp. 473-479.

Lariviere, C.; Gravel, D.; Gagnon, D.; Gardiner, P.; Arsenault, A.B. & Gaudreault, N. (2006). Gender influence on fatigability of back muscles during intermittent isometric contractions: a study of neuromuscular activation patterns. *Clinical Biomechanics,* Vol.21, No.9, pp. 893-904.

Lariviere, C.; Gagnon, D.; Gravel, D. & Arsenault, A.B. (2008a). The assessment of back muscle capacity using intermittent static contractions. Part I - Validity and reliability of electromyographic indices of fatigue. *Journal of Electromyography and Kinesiology,* Vol.18, No.6, pp. 1006-1019.

Lariviere, C.; Gravel, D.; Gagnon, D. & Arsenault, A.B. (2008b). The assessment of back muscle capacity using intermittent static contractions. Part II: validity and reliability of biomechanical correlates of muscle fatigue. *Journal of Electromyography and Kinesiology*, Vol.18, No.6, pp. 1020-1031.

Lariviere, C.; Gravel, D.; Gagnon, D. & Arsenault, A.B. (2009). Toward the development of predictive equations of back muscle capacity based on frequency- and temporal-domain electromyographic indices computed from intermittent static contractions. *Spine Journal*, Vol.9, No.1, pp. 87-95.

Latikka, P.; Battie, M.C.; Videman, T. & Gibbons, L.E. (1995). Correlations of isokinetic and psychophysical back lift and static back extensor endurance tests in men. *Clinical Biomechanics*, Vol.10, No.6, pp. 325-330.

Latimer, J.; Maher, C.G.; Refshauge, K. & Colaco, I. (1999). The reliability and validity of the Biering-Sorensen test in asymptomatic subjects and subjects reporting current or previous nonspecific low back pain. *Spine*, Vol.24, No.20, pp. 2085-2090.

Ljungquist, T.; Fransson, B.; Harms-Ringdahl, K.; Bjornham, A. & Nygren, A. (1999). A physiotherapy test package for assessing back and neck dysfunction--discriminative ability for patients versus healthy control subjects. *Physiotherapy Research International*, Vol.4, No.2, pp. 123-140.

Malliou, P.; Gioftsidou, A.; Beneka, A. & Godolias, G. (2006). Measurements and evaluations in low back pain patients. *Scandinavian Journal of Medicine and Science in Sports*, Vol.16, No.4, pp. 219-230.

Manniche, C.; Hesselsoe, G.; Bentzen, L.; Christensen, I. & Lundberg, E. (1988). Clinical trial of intensive muscle training for chronic low back pain. *Lancet*, Vol.2, No.8626-8627, pp. 1473-1476.

Mannion, A.F. & Dolan, P. (1994). Electromyographic median frequency changes during isometric contraction of the back extensors to fatigue. *Spine*, Vol.19, No.11, pp. 1223-1229.

Mannion, A.F.; Connolly, B.; Wood, K. & Dolan, P. (1997a). The use of surface EMG power spectral analysis in the evaluation of back muscle function. *Journal of Rehabilitation Research and Development*, Vol.34, No.4, pp. 427-439.

Mannion, A.F.; Dolan, P.; Adam, G.G.; Adams, M.A. & Cooper, R.G. (1997b). Can maximal back muscle strength be predicted from submaximal efforts ? *Journal of Back and Musculoskeletal Rehabilitation*, Vol.9, No.1, pp. 49-51.

Mannion, A.F.; Adams, M.A.; Cooper, R.G. & Dolan, P. (1999a). Prediction of maximal back muscle strength from indices of body mass and fat-free body mass. *Rheumatology*, Vol.38, No.7, pp. 652-655.

Mannion, A.F.; Muntener, M.; Taimela, S. & Dvorak, J. (1999b). A randomized clinical trial of three active therapies for chronic low back pain. *Spine*, Vol.24, No.23, pp. 2435-2448.

Mannion, A.F.; Dvorak, J.; Taimela, S. & Muntener, M. (2001). Increase in strength after active therapy in chronic low back pain (CLBP) patients: muscular adaptations and clinical relevance. *Schmerz*, Vol.15, No.6, pp. 468-473.

Mayer, J.M.; Graves, J.E.; Robertson, V.L.; Pierra, E.A.; Verna, J.L. & Ploutz-Snyder, L.L. (1999). Electromyographic activity of the lumbar extensor muscles: effect of angle and hand position during Roman chair exercise. *Archives of Physical Medicine and Rehabilitation*, Vol.80, No.7, pp. 751-755.

Mayer, T.; Gatchel, R.; Betancur, J. & Bovasso, E. (1995). Trunk muscle endurance measurement. Isometric contrasted to isokinetic testing in normal subjects. *Spine*, Vol.20, No.8, pp. 920-927.

McGill, S.M.; Childs, A. & Liebenson, C. (1999). Endurance times for low back stabilization exercises: clinical targets for testing and training from a normal database. *Archives of Physical Medicine and Rehabilitation,* Vol.80, No.8, pp. 941-944.

McGregor, A.; Hill, A. & Grewar, J. (2004). Trunk strength patterns in elite rowers. *Isokinetics and Exercise Science,* Vol.12, pp. 253-261.

McIntosh, G.; Wilson, L.; Affieck, M. & Hall, H. (1998). Trunk and lower extremity muscle endurance: normative data for adults. *Journal of Rehabilitation Outcome Measurement,* Vol.2, pp. 20-39.

Menard, M.R.; Cooke, C.; Locke, S.R.; Beach, G.N. & Butler, T.B. (1994). Pattern of performance in workers with low back pain during a comprehensive motor performance evaluation. *Spine,* Vol.19, No.12, pp. 1359-1366.

Mooney, V.; Kron, M.; Rummerfield, P. & Holmes, B. (1995). The effect of workplace based strengthening on low back injury rates: a case study in the strip mining industry. *Journal of Occupational Rehabilitation,* Vol.5, No.3, pp. 157-167.

Moreau, C.E.; Green, B.N.; Johnson, C.D. & Moreau, S.R. (2001). Isometric back extension endurance tests: a review of the literature. *Journal of Manipulative and Physiological Therapeutics,* Vol.24, No.2, pp. 110-122.

Moreland, J.; Finch, E.; Stratford, P.; Balsor, B. & Gill, C. (1997). Interrater reliability of six tests of trunk muscle function and endurance. *Journal of Orthopaedic and Sports Physical Therapy,* Vol.26, No.4, pp. 200-208.

Morini, S.; Ciccarelli, A.; Cerulli, C.; Giombini, A.; Di Cesare, A. & Ripani, M. (2008). Functional anatomy of trunk flexion-extension in isokinetic exercise: muscle activity in standing and seated positions. *Journal of Sports Medicine and Physical Fitness,* Vol.48, No.1, pp. 17-23.

Morlock, M.M.; Bonin, V.; Muller, G. & Schneider, E. (1997). Trunk muscle fatigue and associated EMG changes during a dynamic iso-inertial test. *European Journal of Applied Physiology and Occupational Physiology,* Vol.76, No.1, pp. 75-80.

Muller, R.; Strassle, K. & Wirth, B. (2010). Isometric back muscle endurance: an EMG study on the criterion validity of the Ito test. *Journal of Electromyography and Kinesiology,* Vol.20, No.5, pp. 845-850.

Nachemson, A.; Waddell, G. & Norlund, A. (2000). Epidemiology of neck and low back pain, In: *Neck and back pain: The scientific evidence of causes, diagnosis and treatment,* A. Nachemson, (Ed), 165-188, Lippincott Williams & Wilkins, Philadelphia.

Nelson, B.W.; O'reilly, E.; Miller, M.; Hogan, M.; Wegner, J.A. & Kelly, C. (1995). The clinical effects of intensive, specific exercise on chronic low back pain: a controlled study of 895 consecutive patients with 1-year follow up. *Orthopedics,* Vol.18, No.10, pp. 971-981.

Newton, M.; Thow, M.; Somerville, D.; Henderson, I. & Waddell, G. (1993). Trunk strength testing with iso-machines. Part 2: Experimental evaluation of the Cybex II Back Testing System in normal subjects and patients with chronic low back pain. *Spine,* Vol.18, No.7, pp. 812-824.

Newton, M. & Waddell, G. (1993). Trunk strength testing with iso machines. Part 1: Review of a decade of scientific evidence. *Spine,* Vol.18, No.7, pp. 801-811.

Ng, J.K. & Richardson, C.A. (1996). Reliability of electromyographic power spectral analysis of back muscle endurance in healthy subjects. *Archives of Physical Medicine and Rehabilitation,* Vol.77, No.3, pp. 259-264.

Ng, J.K.; Richardson, C.A. & Jull, G.A. (1997). Electromyographic amplitude and frequency changes in the iliocostalis lumborum and multifidus muscles during a trunk holding test. *Physical Therapy*, Vol.77, No.9, pp. 954-961.

Nicolaisen, T. & Jorgensen, K. (1985). Trunk strength, back muscle endurance and low-back trouble. *Scandinavian Journal of Rehabilitation Medicine*, Vol.17, No.3, pp. 121-127.

Parkkola, R.; Rytokoski, U. & Kormano, M. (1993). Magnetic resonance imaging of the discs and trunk muscles in patients with chronic low back pain and healthy control subjects. *Spine*, Vol.18, No.7, pp. 830-836.

Parnianpour, M.; Nordin, M.; Kahanovitz, N. & Frankel, V. (1988). 1988 Volvo award in biomechanics. The triaxial coupling of torque generation of trunk muscles during isometric exertions and the effect of fatiguing isoinertial movements on the motor output and movement patterns. *Spine*, Vol.13, No.9, pp. 982-992.

Parnianpour, M.; Li, F.; Nordin, M. & Frankel, V.H. (1989a). Reproducibility of trunk isoinertial performances in the sagittal, coronal, and transverse planes. *Bulletin of the Hospital for Joint Diseases Orthopaedic Institute*, Vol.49, No.2, pp. 148-154.

Parnianpour, M.; Li, F.; Nordin, M. & Kahanovitz, N. (1989b). A database of isoinertial trunk strength tests against three resistance levels in sagittal, frontal, and transverse planes in normal male subjects. *Spine*, Vol.14, No.4, pp. 409-411.

Peach, J.P.; Gunning, J. & Mcgill, S.M. (1998). Reliability of spectral EMG parameters of healthy back extensors during submaximum isometric fatiguing contractions and recovery. *Journal of Electromyography and Kinesiology*, Vol.8, No.6, pp. 403-410.

Peel, C. & Alland, M.J. (1990). Cardiovascular responses to isokinetic trunk exercise. *Physical Therapy*, Vol.70, No.8, pp. 503-510.

Picavet, H.S. & Schouten, J.S. (2003). Musculoskeletal pain in the Netherlands: prevalences, consequences and risk groups, the DMC(3)-study. *Pain*, Vol.102, No.1-2, pp. 167-178.

Plamondon, A. ; Marceau, C.; Stainton, S. & Desjardins, P. (1999). Toward a better prescription of the prone back extension exercise to strengthen the back muscles. *Scandinavian Journal of Medicine and Science in Sports*, Vol.9, No.4, pp. 226-232.

Plamondon, A.; Serresse, O. ; Boyd, K. ; Ladouceur, D. & Desjardins, P. (2002). Estimated moments at L5/S1 level and muscular activation of back extensors for six prone back extension exercises in healthy individuals. *Scandinavian Journal of Medicine and Science in Sports*, Vol.12, No.2, pp. 81-89.

Plamondon, A.; Trimble, K.; Lariviere, C. & Desjardins, P. (2004). Back muscle fatigue during intermittent prone back extension exercise. *Scandinavian Journal of Medicine and Science in Sports*, Vol.14, No.4, pp. 221-230.

Pollock, M.; Graves, J.; Leggett, S.; Young, G.; Garzarella, L.; Carpenter, D.; Fulton, M. & Jones, A. (1991). Accuracy of counter weighting to account for upper body mass in testing lumbar extension strength. *Medicine and Science in Sports and Exercise*, Vol.23, No.4, pp. S66.

Pullman, S.L.; Goodin, D.S.; Marquinez, A.I.; Tabbal, S. & Rubin, M. (2000). Clinical utility of surface EMG: report of the therapeutics and technology assessment subcommittee of the American Academy of Neurology. *Neurology*, Vol.55, No.2, pp. 171-177.

Rainville, J.; Hartigan, C.; Jouve, C. & Martinez, E. (2004). The influence of intense exercise-based physical therapy program on back pain anticipated before and induced by physical activities. *Spine Journal*, Vol.4, No.2, pp. 176-183.

Rantanen, P.; Penttinen, E.; Rinta-Kauppila, S. & Ruusila, T. (1995). Cardiovascular stress in isokinetic trunk strength test. *Spine*, Vol.20, No.4, pp. 485-488.

Rantanen, T.; Era, P. & Heikkinen, E. (1997). Physical activity and the changes in maximal isometric strength in men and women from the age of 75 to 80 years. *Journal of the American Geriatrics Society*, Vol.45, No.12, pp. 1439-1445.

Rashiq, S.; Koller, M.; Haykowsky, M. & Jamieson, K. (2003). The effect of opioid analgesia on exercise test performance in chronic low back pain. *Pain*, Vol.106, No.1-2, pp. 119-125.

Raty, H.P.; Kujala, U.; Videman, T.; Koskinen, S.K.; Karppi, S.L. & Sarna, S. (1999). Associations of isometric and isoinertial trunk muscle strength measurements and lumbar paraspinal muscle cross-sectional areas. *Journal of Spinal Disorders*, Vol.12, No.3, pp. 266-270.

Reid, S.; Hazard, R.G. & Fenwick, J.W. (1991). Isokinetic trunk-strength deficits in people with and without low-back pain: a comparative study with consideration of effort. *Journal of Spinal Disorders*, Vol.4, No.1, pp. 68-72.

Robinson, M.E.; Greene, A.F.; O'connor, P.; Graves, J.E. & Macmillan, M. (1992). Reliability of lumbar isometric torque in patients with chronic low back pain. *Physical Therapy*, Vol.72, No.3, pp. 186-190.

Ropponen, A.; Gibbons, L.E.; Videman, T. & Battie, M.C. (2005). Isometric back extension endurance testing: reasons for test termination. *Journal of Orthopaedic and Sports Physical Therapy*, Vol.35, No.7, pp. 437-442.

Ropponen, A. (2006). Comparison of the roles of common constitutional and behavioural parameters in back performance estimates. *Isokinetics and Exercise Science*, Vol.14, pp. 241-250.

Roussel, N.A.; Truijen, S.; De Kerf, I.; Lambeets, D.; Nijs, J. & Stassijns, G. (2008). Reliability of the assessment of lumbar range of motion and maximal isometric strength in patients with chronic low back pain. *Archives of Physical Medicine and Rehabilitation*, Vol.89, No.4, pp. 788-791.

Roy, S.H.; De Luca, C.J.; Emley, M. & Buijs, R.J. (1995). Spectral electromyographic assessment of back muscles in patients with low back pain undergoing rehabilitation. *Spine*, Vol.20, No.1, pp. 38-48.

Rytokoski, U.; Karppi, S.L.; Puukka, P.; Soini, J. & Ronnemaa, T. (1994). Measurement of low back mobility, isometric strength and isoinertial performance with isostation B-200 triaxial dynamometer: reproducibility of measurement and development of functional indices. *Journal of Spinal Disorders*, Vol.7, No.1, pp. 54-61.

Sachs, B.L.; Ahmad, S.S.; Lacroix, M.; Olimpio, D.; Heath, R.; David, J.A. & Scala, A.D. (1994). Objective assessment for exercise treatment on the B-200 isostation as part of work tolerance rehabilitation. A random prospective blind evaluation with comparison control population. *Spine*, Vol.19, No.1, pp. 49-52.

Salminen, J.J.; Maki, P.; Oksanen, A. & Pentti, J. (1992). Spinal mobility and trunk muscle strength in 15-year-old schoolchildren with and without low-back pain. *Spine*, Vol.17, No.4, pp. 405-411.

Salminen, J.J.; Erkintalo, M.; Laine, M. & Pentti, J. (1995). Low back pain in the young. A prospective three-year follow-up study of subjects with and without low back pain. *Spine*, Vol.20, No.19, pp. 2101-2108.

San Juan, J.G.; Yaggie, J.A.; Levy, S.S.; Mooney, V.; Udermann, B.E. & Mayer, J.M. (2005). Effects of pelvic stabilization on lumbar muscle activity during dynamic exercise. *Journal of Strength and Conditioning Research*, Vol.19, No.4, pp. 903-907.

Schenk, P.; Klipstein, A.; Spillmann, S.; Stroyer, J. & Laubli, T. (2006). The role of back muscle endurance, maximum force, balance and trunk rotation control regarding lifting capacity. *European Journal of Applied Physiology,* Vol.96, No.2, pp. 146-156.

Shirado, O.; Kaneda, K. & Ito, T. (1992). Trunk-muscle strength during concentric and eccentric contraction: a comparison between healthy subjects and patients with chronic low-back pain. *Journal of Spinal Disorders,* Vol.5, No.2, pp. 175-182.

Shirado, O.; Ito, T.; Kaneda, K. & Strax, T.E. (1995a). Concentric and eccentric strength of trunk muscles: influence of test postures on strength and characteristics of patients with chronic low-back pain. *Archives of Physical Medicine and Rehabilitation,* Vol.76, No.7, pp. 604-611.

Shirado, O.; Ito, T.; Kaneda, K. & Strax, T.E. (1995b). Electromyographic analysis of four techniques for isometric trunk muscle exercises. *Archives of Physical Medicine and Rehabilitation,* Vol.76, No.3, pp. 225-229.

Simmonds, M.J.; Olson, S.L.; Jones, S.; Hussein, T.; Lee, C.E.; Novy, D. & Radwan, H. (1998). Psychometric characteristics and clinical usefulness of physical performance tests in patients with low back pain. *Spine,* Vol.23, No.22, pp. 2412-2421.

Sjolie, A.N. & Ljunggren, A.E. (2001). The significance of high lumbar mobility and low lumbar strength for current and future low back pain in adolescents. *Spine,* Vol.26, No.23, pp. 2629-2636.

Smeets, R.J. & Wittink, H. (2007). The deconditioning paradigm for chronic low back pain unmasked? *Pain,* Vol.130, No.3, pp. 201-202.

Smeets, R.J.; Vlaeyen, J.W.; Hidding, A.; Kester, A.D.; Van Der Heijden, G.J. & Knottnerus, J.A. (2008). Chronic low back pain: physical training, graded activity with problem solving training, or both? The one-year post-treatment results of a randomized controlled trial. *Pain,* Vol.134, No.3, pp. 263-276.

Smith, D.; Bruce-Low, S. & Bissell, G. (2008). Twenty years of specific, isolated lumbar extension research: a review. *Journal of Orthopaedics,* Vol.5, No.1, pp. e14.

Stokes, I.A.; Henry, S.M. & Single, R.M. (2003). Surface EMG electrodes do not accurately record from lumbar multifidus muscles. *Clinical Biomechanics,* Vol.18, No.1, pp. 9-13.

Suni, J.H.; Miilunpalo, S.I.; Asikainen, T.M.; Laukkanen, R.T.; Oja, P.; Pasanen, M.E.; Bos, K. & Vuori, I.M. (1998). Safety and feasibility of a health-related fitness test battery for adults. *Physical Therapy,* Vol.78, No.2, pp. 134-148.

Suter, E. & Lindsay, D. (2001). Back muscle fatigability is associated with knee extensor inhibition in subjects with low back pain. *Spine,* Vol.26, No.16, pp. E361-366.

Swezey, R.L.; Swezey, A. & Adams, J. (2000). Isometric progressive resistive exercise for osteoporosis. *Journal of Rheumatology,* Vol.27, No.5, pp. 1260-1264.

Szpalski, M.; Federspiel, C.F.; Poty, S.; Hayez, J.P. & Debaize, J.P. (1992). Reproducibility of trunk isoinertial dynamic performance in patients with low back pain. *Journal of Spinal Disorders,* Vol.5, No.1, pp. 78-85.

Taimela, S. & Harkapaa, K. (1996). Strength, mobility, their changes, and pain reduction in active functional restoration for chronic low back disorders. *Journal of Spinal Disorders,* Vol.9, No.4, pp. 306-312.

Taimela, S.; Kankaanpaa, M. & Airaksinen, O. (1998). A submaximal back extension endurance test utilising subjective perception of low back fatigue. *Scandinavian Journal of Rehabilitation Medicine,* Vol.30, No.2, pp. 107-112.

Takemasa, R.; Yamamoto, H. & Tani, T. (1995). Trunk muscle strength in and effect of trunk muscle exercises for patients with chronic low back pain. The differences in patients with and without organic lumbar lesions. *Spine,* Vol.20, No.23, pp. 2522-2530.

Tekin, Y.; Ortancil, O.; Ankarali, H.; Basaran, A.; Sarikaya, S. & Ozdolap, S. (2009). Biering-Sorensen test scores in coal miners. *Joint Bone Spine,* Vol.76, No.3, pp. 281-285.

Thomas, J.S.; France, C.R.; Sha, D. & Wiele, N.V. (2008). The influence of pain-related fear on peak muscle activity and force generation during maximal isometric trunk exertions. *Spine,* Vol.33, No.11, pp. E342-348.

Udermann, B.E.; Graves, J.E.; Donelson, R.G.; Ploutz-Snyder, L.; Boucher, J.P. & Iriso, J.H. (1999). Pelvic restraint effect on lumbar gluteal and hamstring muscle electromyographic activation. *Archives of Physical Medicine and Rehabilitation,* Vol.80, No.4, pp. 428-431.

Udermann, B.E.; Mayer, J.M.; Graves, J.E. & Murray, S.R. (2003). Quantitative Assessment of Lumbar Paraspinal Muscle Endurance. *Journal of Athletic Training,* Vol.38, No.3, pp. 259-262.

Van Dieen, J.H.; Heijblom, P. & Bunkens, H. (1998). Extrapolation of time series of EMG power spectrum parameters in isometric endurance tests of trunk extensor muscles. *Journal of Electromyography and Kinesiology,* Vol.8, No.1, pp. 35-44.

Vanderthommen, M.; Demoulin, C.; Jacques, P.-A. & Crielaard, J.-M. (2007). Muscular recruitment during instrumental evaluation of the trunk extension torque: influence of a pelvic stabilization system, In: *6th Interdisciplinary World Congress on Low Back & Pelvic Pain,* 350-351, Abstract book (poster), Barcelona, Spain.

Verbunt, J.A.; Seelen, H.A.; Vlaeyen, J.W.; Van De Heijden, G.J.; Heuts, P.H.; Pons, K. & Knottnerus, J.A. (2003). Disuse and deconditioning in chronic low back pain: concepts and hypotheses on contributing mechanisms. *European Journal of Pain* Vol.7, No.1, pp. 9-21.

Verbunt, J.A.; Seelen, H.A.; Vlaeyen, J.W.; Bousema, E.J.; Van Der Heijden, G.J.; Heuts, P.H. & Knottnerus, J.A. (2005). Pain-related factors contributing to muscle inhibition in patients with chronic low back pain: an experimental investigation based on superimposed electrical stimulation. *Clinical Journal of Pain,* Vol.21, No.3, pp. 232-240.

Verbunt, J.A.; Smeets, R.J. & Wittink, H.M. (2010). Cause or effect? Deconditioning and chronic low back pain. *Pain,* Vol.149, No.3, pp. 428-430.

Viljanen, T.; Viitasalo, J.T. & Kujala, U.M. (1991). Strength characteristics of a healthy urban adult population. *European Journal of Applied Physiology and Occupational Physiology,* Vol.63, No.1, pp. 43-47.

Vlaeyen, J.W.; Kole-Snijders, A.M.; Boeren, R.G. & Van Eek, H. (1995). Fear of movement/(re)injury in chronic low back pain and its relation to behavioral performance. *Pain,* Vol.62, No.3, pp. 363-372.

Vollestad, N.K. (1997). Measurement of human muscle fatigue. *Journal of Neuroscience Methods,* Vol.74, No.2, pp. 219-227.

Walsworth, M. (2004). Lumbar paraspinal electromyographic activity during trunk extension exercises on two types of exercise machines. *Electromyography and Clinical Neurophysiology,* Vol.44, No.4, pp. 201-207.

Wang, M.; Leger, A.B. & Dumas, G.A. (2005). Prediction of back strength using anthropometric and strength measurements in healthy females *Clinical Biomechanics,* Vol.20, No.7, pp. 685-692.

Section 2

Treatment Approach

8

Conservative Management of Low Back Pain

Marcia Miller Spoto
Nazareth College of Rochester, USA

1. Introduction

Low back pain is a common human experience. Especially in developed countries, low back pain has become a health condition with significant socio-economic implications. The costs of treating back and neck pain disorders in the US have increased substantially over the past 15-20 years, with the majority of these costs attributed to relatively invasive medical procedure such as injections and surgery. Despite the increased cost, there does not appear to be a corresponding improvement in function among individuals reporting spine pain over this same time period, nor improved general health outcomes (Martin BI et al, 2008).

Back pain is a symptom and not a specific health condition or disease. There are many musculoskeletal and non-musculoskeletal causes of low back pain. Health care providers who treat back pain must engage in differential diagnosis as a first step in addressing a person with a back complaint. When back symptoms are caused by visceral or systemic disease, the patient must be referred to an appropriate medical specialist. Similarly, when back symptoms are caused by serious musculoskeletal pathology, the clinician should refer the patient appropriately. There conditions involving pathophysiologic changes in the lumbosacral spine, however, which can be successfully managed with more conservative approaches to care (Weinstein JN et al, 2006). Importantly, in many cases back pain can be considered *non-specific* and unrelated to pathologic change (Savage RA et al, 1997). Movement impairments can underlie both pathoanatomic and non-pathoanatomic causes of low back pain and these impairments are often the focus of conservative management (Sahrmann SA, 2002).

Beyond the first step of differential diagnosis, the major challenge for health care professionals involved in the treatment of back pain is diagnosing the problem in ways that will direct appropriate treatment and establish a more accurate prognosis. The International Classification of Disease (ICD) system (World Health Organization, 2005), which is universally accepted as a classification system for health conditions, has not been found to be particularly helpful from a prognostic standpoint or in directing interventions for back pain (Riddle DL, 1998). One of the reasons for this is that there is often a weak relationship between pathologic changes noted on imaging and an individual's level of symptomotolgy or function (Boos N et al, 200). Another reason is that again, by far, the majority of cases of low back pain can be considered non-specific and are not attributable to serious underlying pathology. So there is a need for new models of diagnosis that are more meaningful.

One of the themes of this chapter is that the diagnostic process is central to the overall management of back pain. It is a pivotal point around which clinical decisions are rendered.

Diagnostic classification systems for back pain have been developed within various health professions due to the need to look beyond the pathology-based orientation and for the purpose of guiding clinical decisions for spine management. For example, the McKenzie system, utilized most extensively in physical therapy, places patients with back pain into one of several categories or subcategories based upon their response to specific spinal movements (McKenzie RA, 1981). The selection of intervention is based upon the patient category. There are numerous other systems that have been developed as well. Each system possesses its own set of rules and each will direct different types of interventions. The end result of having so many different approaches to treating back pain is that it creates considerable clinical variance in back pain management. Nonetheless, the diagnostic process is the key to effectively treating back pain.

A second theme of this chapter is that a comprehensive diagnostic system for back pain must be consistent with a biopsychosocial model of healthcare and it must incorporate a person's level of function. The International Classification of Functioning, Disability and Health (ICF) provides an expanded system of classification and offers a broader perspective on the inter-relationships between health conditions and function (World Health Organization, 2008). Although the ICF is not currently being widely used as a diagnostic system for back pain, the codification scheme found in the ICF may help the health care community better understand the relationships between health conditions and functioning in the future. This system will be discussed in more detail later in the chapter.

There is a growing body of evidence that for most people who experience back pain, conservative care should placed front and center in the overall management of their problem. In addition, patient response to conservative care is being used more and more in the decision-making process relative to the need for surgical intervention (Chou R et al, 2011). In other words, people that fail to improve after a course of conservative care are more likely to benefit from surgery.

So how is conservative care defined? Conservative care may be viewed differently depending upon the orientation or discipline of the health care practitioner. For the conservative care practitioner, it would likely include only non-surgical treatment options. For the purposes of this chapter, conservative care will be defined as follows: *conservative care is the least invasive treatment for a given condition that can be justified based upon a preponderance of the evidence.*

Conservative care for back pain can take many forms, especially if one considers complimentary and alternative medicine options. If only licensed health care professionals are considered, physical therapists and chiropractors together account for the largest groups of providers that offer comprehensive conservative care. Although the two professions differ in many significant ways, especially with regard to philosophic underpinnings, there is at the same time considerable overlap in the types of treatment rendered by these providers. As will be discussed, conservative management is more than just specific treatment approaches; it is the entire framework for understanding back pain, evaluating and diagnosing back problems, and directing treatment.

Conservative care practitioners are in the best position to help reverse the trend in developed countries to over-treat back pain. These practitioners are less likely to believe that back pain is a symptom in need of treatment and more likely to view back pain as a common human experience that involves the whole person - including the individual's perceptions about their condition. With the exception of cases that involve serious pathology, people with back pain need to learn how to help themselves. To this end, education is singularly the most important "treatment" for the conservative care provider.

This chapter will explore the various elements of comprehensive conservative management of back pain. There are three general elements of patient management that comprise comprehensive care for the health care practitioner:

- Patient Examination
- Diagnostic Process
- Intervention

These elements are sequential and inter-related. In addition, to complete the cycle, outcomes of care must be assessed. An episode of care is complete when outcomes are favorable and treatment goals are met. When goals are not met, any or all elements of patient management may have to be revisited.

2. Patient examination

A comprehensive patient examination is essential for conservative management of back pain. The art and science of the clinical exam has been lost for many health care practitioners, which seems to parallel the advancement in technology - especially technology related to diagnostic imaging. Far too often when a person with back pain seeks medical care, emphasis is placed upon symptomology and imaging findings. It is imperative that both symptoms and imaging findings are interpreted within the context of a thorough clinical examination (Chou R et al, 2011). This will not only lead to a more accurate diagnosis, but will also help to limit unnecessary medical tests and procedures.

Table 1 provides an overview of the major components of a comprehensive patient examination.

Exam Item	Example
Medical Screening	General Health Assessment, R/O Serious Pathology
Review of Paraclinical data	Medical reports, imaging results
Functional Outcomes Measures	Oswestry Disability Index, Rolland Morris Scale
History of Current Condition	Oral History, Follow-Up Questions From Medical Screening
Observation & Postural Assessment	Standing and Sitting
Active Movement Testing	Cardinal Plane Movements, Repeated Movements
Neurological Screening	Reflexes, Myotomes, Dermatomes
Muscle Performance Testing	Abdominal/Back Extensor Strength , Gluteal Strength
Muscle Length Testing	Hamstring, Hip Flexors, Hip Adductors
Orthopedic Special Tests	Straight Leg Raise, Slump Test, Prone Lumbar Instability Test
Joint Mobility Assessment	P-A Vertebral Pressures
Palpation	Lumbar Paraspinal Muscles, Myofascial Pain

Table 1. Comprehensive Patient Examination

2.1 Medical screening

Medical screening begins as part of the general patient intake process. Health questionnaires provide the most efficient way to collect this information. Figure 1 is an example of a health questionnaire that can be used in an outpatient care setting, which provides detailed information on the patient's health status. The clinician will review this information prior to taking an oral history of the current complaint. Health conditions that are identified on the screening tool may require follow-up questions by the clinician. In addition, in cases where there is suspicion of possible visceral or systemic involvement in the current complaint, the clinician can use this information to investigate the problem in greater depth. There will be one of three possible outcomes from the medical screening process: (1) medical referral, (2) medical consultation, (3) patient is deemed appropriate for conservative care

PAST MEDICAL HISTORY

Please checkmark "√" if you or anyone in your immediate family (specify whom) has had any history of the following:

Condition	Personal	Family	Condition	Personal	Family
Acid Reflux (GERD)	☐	☐	Hepatitis (any type)	☐	☐
Alcoholism	☐	☐	HIV/AIDS	☐	☐
Allergies (any)	☐	☐	Huntington's Disease	☐	☐
Anemia	☐	☐	Inflammatory Bowel	☐	☐
Asthma	☐	☐	Kidney Disease	☐	☐
Autoimmune Disease	☐	☐	Kidney Stones	☐	☐
Bleeding disorders	☐	☐	Latex Sensitivity	☐	☐
Blood Pressure Problem	☐	☐	Liver Disease	☐	☐
Bronchitis	☐	☐	Lupus	☐	☐
Cancer (any type)	☐	☐	Mental illness	☐	☐
Chest Pain/Angina	☐	☐	Multiple Sclerosis	☐	☐
Cholesterol problems	☐	☐	Osteoarthritis	☐	☐
COPD	☐	☐	Osteoporosis/Osteopenia	☐	☐
Deep Vein Thrombosis	☐	☐	Ovarian Cysts	☐	☐
Diabetes	☐	☐	Parkinson's Disease	☐	☐
Diverticulitis	☐	☐	Peptic Ulcer	☐	☐
Drug Addiction	☐	☐	Pneumonia	☐	☐
Emphysema	☐	☐	Prostate Disease (males)	☐	☐
Endometriosis (females)	☐	☐	Rheumatoid Arthritis	☐	☐
Epilepsy/seizures	☐	☐	Skin problems	☐	☐
Fibromyalgia	☐	☐	Sexually Transmitted Disease	☐	☐
Glaucoma	☐	☐	Stroke/TIA	☐	☐
Gout	☐	☐	Thyroid Disorder	☐	☐
Guillain-Barré	☐	☐	Tuberculosis	☐	☐
Headaches	☐	☐	Urinary Incontinence	☐	☐
Heart Attack	☐	☐	Urinary Tract Infection	☐	☐
Heart Disease	☐	☐	Vascular Disease	☐	☐

Please list any additional family or personal past medical history information here ____________

Current Medical Symptoms *(Please check if you are currently having any of the following…)*

☐ Fever/chills/sweats (day or night)
☐ Unexplained weight loss or gain
☐ Unusual fatigue/drowsiness
☐ Sudden weakness
☐ Confusion/memory loss
☐ Nausea/vomiting/loss of appetite
☐ Changes in bowel or bladder function
☐ Numbness or tingling
☐ Trouble sleeping
☐ Other ____________

Medical/Surgical History

Do you have a pacemaker? ☐ Yes ☐ No
Have you ever had a joint replacement? ☐ Yes ☐ No
Have you ever been hospitalized? ☐ Yes ☐ No If yes please specify____________

____

____

Medical/Surgical History *(continued)*

Please list any operations you have had and the date(s):

	Date of Surgery	**Reason for Surgery**
1.)		
2.)		
3.)		
4.)		
5.)		

Prescription Medications ***(Please list all prescription medications you are currently taking)***

Medication	Dosage	Medication	Dosage

Over-the-Counter Medications ***(Please list all over the counter medications you are currently taking. This includes vitamins, minerals, pain relievers, cold medicines, supplements.)***

Medication	Dosage	Medication	Dosage

Living Environment

Please specify your current living situation. I currently live:
☐ Alone ☐ With family, spouse, partner ☐ Assisted living ☐ Other ____________
Do you have any stairs/steps in your home? ☐ Yes ☐ No
If yes, how many?____________
Do you exercise regularly? ☐ Yes ☐ No
If yes, what kinds and how often?____________
What types of sports/recreational activities do you participate in?____________
What do you hope to get out of physical therapy?____________
Do you have any other concerns that you would like your physical therapist to be aware of? ☐ Yes ☐ No
If yes, please specify:____________
EMERGENCY CONTACT:____________ RELATION:____________ PHONE____________
PRIMARY CARE PHYSICIAN: ____________ PHONE: ____________

Fig. 1 Medical Screening Questionnaire

2.2 Review of paraclinical data

Many people with back pain have sought care from a number of different health care providers and have already undergone diagnostic testing. Medical reports generated from this prior care can be very useful to the clinician conducting the patient examination. The clinician should make an effort to obtain this information and review it as part of the examination process. Any conflicting information should be rectified. Otherwise, the data can be added to the rest of the clinical findings during the course of the patient examination and ultimately corroborated during the diagnostic process.

2.3 Functional outcome measures

It is very important to assess the level of disability associated with an episode of back pain. The standard way to obtain this information is through self-report disability scales. Several of these types of scales have been established as both reliable and valid measures, such as the Oswestry Disability Index (Vlanin M, 2008). Scores derived from these measures can be used to determine a level of disability ranging from mild to severe. The Roland Morris Disability Index is another self-report disability tool that is clinically useful (Roland M, Morris R, 1983). A simple scale that can be used for any patient with back pain is the *Patient Specific Functional Scale*. This scale has been studied for its psychometric qualities more for cervical spine conditions (Cleland JA et al, 2006), however use of this scale insures that the function being measured is meaningful to the patient. These scales can complement one another (Beurskens AJHM et al, 1996). There are other ways of evaluating a patient's level of function. Direct measures, or performance tests, can also be conducted. Examples of performance tests for back pain include assessment of bending and lifting tasks. All of these tests should be utilized to evaluate treatment outcomes, and may be the most valuable measures of treatment effectiveness.

2.4 History of current condition

The health care provider must obtain an accurate and complete history from the patient seeking care for back pain. The patient interview can provide pivotal information that is then used by the clinician to diagnose the patient problem. This interview is both an art and a science. Good communication skills are essential. The history usually begins as an open-ended question such as "so tell me about your problem". The value of an open-ended question is that the patient has an opportunity to tell their "story" and often it is an efficient way to collect critical information. Follow-up questions can then begin. Sometimes patients provide extraneous information and may need to be directed by the clinician. Table 2

Mechanism of onset/injury
Length of time since onset of symptoms for current condition
Previous history of back pain
If recurrent, number and typical length of time of episodes
Location and characteristics of symptoms
Symptom behavior (24 hour)
Aggravating/Relieving factors
Previous diagnostic tests
Previous treatment
Occupation/Work environment
Level of physical activity

Table 2. Essential Information Obtained in History

contains the essential information that is to be collected during the history. At the completion of the interview, it can be very insightful for the clinician to query the patient on their own views of what is causing their back pain. This is particularly important when the patient has sought care from a number of different providers. Many times, the patient has received opinions from these providers that reflect a variety of perspectives on back pain and this can lead to confusion as the patient attempts to resolve conflicting information. Patients also often misinterpret information. A person's beliefs about their problem can be a significant factor in their overall prognosis for recovery.

2.5 Observation & postural assessment

Observation and postural assessment is where the physical examination of the patient begins. The primary objectives of observation/postural assessment in a person with back pain is to determine: (1) the general orientation of the spine and extremities in space, (2) if there are impairments related to structural alignment, (3) if there is muscle atrophy, joint or tissue swelling, or skin discoloration, and (4) how posture may be contributing to the patient problem. In many, if not most cases of back pain, the condition is caused by accumulated stress on the spine, which is in turn due to the way in which the individual functions day in and day out. For example, work demands for many people entail prolonged sitting or standing postures. If the orientation of the body in space or alignment of body segments lacks efficiency from a movement health standpoint, tissues are exposed to excessive loading. Accumulated stress can overload body tissues, which can lead to tissue breakdown and eventually symptoms of back pain. The clinician should note any significant findings, then correlate these findings with the patient's symptoms and other physical findings.

2.6 Active movement testing

Assessment of the patient's range of motion and symptomatic response to trunk movement contributes a great deal to a movement system diagnosis of back pain. For some clinicians, it is the most critical aspect of the physical examination for both diagnosis and treatment. Figure 2 contains the most basic trunk movements assessed. Single plane, multi-plane, and repeated movements are performed during this portion of the exam. Most of the time, active movement testing begins in the standing position. Baseline pain level, utilizing the numeric pain rating scale, and location is established before active movement is performed. Symptomatic responses can include: increased, decreased, no effect, and produced. The clinician should note whether pain occurs through the range of movement or only at end range. Range of motion measurement in the clinic setting is most reliable and valid when obtained with an Inclinometer (Saur PM et al, 1996). The quality of the movement is also noted. Aberrant movement, such as the presence of a painful arc or frontal plane deviations associated with trunk flexion, can indicate lumbar instability (Hicks GE et al, 2005). Quality of movement can be assessed in other ways as well. For example, does the patient flex primarily at the hip joint and avoid thoraco-lumbar flexion? Or, is there excessive lumbar flexion? Upon return to neutral from the flexed position, does the patient initiate the movement with the hip extensors, or the trunk extensors? Quality of movement assessment reveals a great deal about movement strategies (Sahrmann SA, 2002).

In addition, the clinician may evaluate how extremity joint movement impacts back symptoms and spine movement in order to obtain more detailed information. For example, in standing can the patient perform unilateral hip and knee flexion without rotating the lumbar spine and without pain? If the examiner controls the impaired spine movement, can the corrective movement be performed without provoking symptoms? Test items can be chosen based upon the most frequent functional movements the patient performs, or those that are reported to reproduce symptoms.

TRUNK MOVEMENTS (STANDING)	ROM Loss	Symptomatic Response	Quality of Movement
Flexion			
Extension			
Right Lateral Flexion			
Left Lateral Flexion			
Right Rotation			
Left Rotation			
Right Side-Glide			
Left Side-Glide			
Supine Flexion			
Prone Extension			
Comments:			

COMBINED MOVEMENTS:

REPEATED MOVEMENTS:

PERIPHERAL JOINT SCREEN:

Fig. 2. Active Movement Testing

Limitations in range of movement and/or joint mobility, and altered motor control contribute to altered movement patterns of the spine. A movement system diagnosis relies heavily on the clinical picture that emerges during active movement testing. These findings are then correlated to the information gleaned during the history, particularly with symptom behavior during functional tasks, as well as muscle performance testing. Indeed, the result of this portion of the examination helps in the planning for muscle strength/length testing.

2.7 Neurological screening

A neurological screen can be considered a basic component of the physical examination of the patient with back pain. It is especially important when the patient presents with extremity pain, or with neurological symptoms such as numbness or paraesthesia. It is the discretion of the clinician to forego a neurological exam when the patient's complaint is local spine pain in the absence of neurological symptoms. A summary of neurological tests can is presented in figure 3.

Neurological impairments need to be considered in the context of the patient's mechanism of onset, symptoms and other clinical findings. Positive neurological signs must be considered in the differential diagnosis, and may serve to prompt appropriate medical referral.

REFLEXES	RIGHT	LEFT
Patellar		
Achilles		

LUMBAR MYOTOMES	RIGHT	LEFT
Hip Flexion (L2)		
Knee Extension (L3)		
Ankle Dorsiflexion (L4)		
Great Toe Extension (L5)		
Ankle Plantarflexion/Eversion (S1)		
Knee Flexion (S2)		

SENSATION: L1/L2/L3/L4/L5/S1/S2 Dermatomes

Light Touch

Other

Fig. 3. Neurological Testing Lumbar Spine

2.8 Muscle performance testing

There are many ways to evaluate muscle strength, including dynamometry, manually applied resistance, EMG and isokinetic testing. The most practical and common method in the outpatient clinic setting is manual muscle testing. It is important to be selective in this portion of the patient examination since muscle strength tests can be provocative; in some cases muscle testing should be deferred if the patient's condition is irritable. The determination of specific tests is based upon information gleaned primarily from the posture and active movement assessments. Muscle atrophy and left versus right muscle asymmetries can be observed during the static standing posture analysis. During active movement, motor recruitment patterns can lead the examiner to identify both weak and dominant muscles or muscle groups. The examiner can then confirm these findings through direct assessment of muscle function. Most muscles or muscle groups can be isolated during manual testing to a reasonable degree, (Kendall FP et al, 1993) although complete isolation is not possible. For people with back pain there are key muscle groups that should be given consideration, including the back extensors, abdominals (upper and lower divisions), hip extensors, hip abductors and hip flexors. Figure 4 provides a list of muscles typically considered during examination of a person with back pain.

Knowledge of impairments of muscle performance contributes substantially to the diagnosis of movement system impairment. In addition, impaired muscle function is targeted specifically in the plan of care for the patient through corrective exercise.

MANUAL MUSCLE TEST/ MUSCLE LENGTH TEST	RIGHT	LEFT	RIGHT	LEFT
Erector Spinae			Normal / short / stiff	
Gluteus Maximus			Normal / short / stiff	Normal / short / stiff
Gluteus Medius			Normal / short / stiff	Normal / short / stiff
Psoas			Normal / short / stiff	Normal / short / stiff
Hip Adductors			Normal / short / stiff	Normal / short / stiff
Hamstrings			Normal / short / stiff	Normal / short / stiff
Quadriceps			Normal / short / stiff	Normal / short / stiff
Piriformis			Normal / short / stiff	Normal / short / stiff
Quadratus Lumborum			Normal / short / stiff	Normal / short / stiff
Gastroc/Soleus			Normal / short / stiff	Normal / short / stiff

Fig. 4. Muscle Strength and Length Tests

2.9 Muscle length testing

Adaptive muscle shortening can either be a consequence of impaired movement, or a contributing factor in movement dysfunction. Muscle length deficits will limit joint movement, and the joints spanned by the muscle will not be able to achieve a neutral position. Alternatively, muscles can develop stiffness, which can be defined as an increased resistance to passive movement. For muscle length testing, the examiner generally attempts to passively lengthen a muscle over the joint(s) that it crosses while ensuring stabilization of the proximal bony lever. A short muscle will be incapable of lengthening fully across the joint(s); a stiff muscle will achieve adequate length but will demonstrate increased resistance to passive stretch. In either case, the consequence of short or stiff muscles is altered and inefficient movement patterns. Further, muscle length and strength deficits tend to be interdependent and reflect, and contribute to, an imbalance of forces across joints.

As with the results of muscle performance testing, the identification of muscle length deficits will assist in the diagnosis and treatment of movement impairment.

2.10 Orthopedic special tests

The primary purpose of special tests in an orthopedic spine examination is to selectively expose the tissues to mechanical stresses in order to rule in or rule out specific musculoskeletal causes of back pain. Tissue sources of pain can then be identified. The clinician must be aware of the limitations of special tests and mindful that in many cases, a specific tissue source of pain cannot be accurately determined.

Figure 5 contains a list of special tests frequently used in the examination of the lumbar spine. This list is only representative of the numerous tests that currently exist (Magee DJ, 2002). Sensitivity and specificity data can be found in the literature for some but not all of these tests, which helps the clinician evaluate the utility of each test. Selection of tests is based upon information obtained in the history, including results of diagnostic imaging, and the clinician's hypothesis generated by the collective information from the rest of the examination. It is beyond the scope of this chapter to analyze individual tests; this information can be found in standard orthopedic evaluation texts.

SPECIAL TESTS	RIGHT	LEFT
SLR	+ / -	+ / -
Bragard's Test	+ / -	+ / -
Lindner's Sign	+ / -	+ / -
Slump Test	+ / -	+ / -
Well Leg Raise	+ / -	+ / -
Bowstring Test	+ / -	+ / -
Bechterewis Test	+ / -	+ / -
Quadrant Test	+ / -	+ / -
Prone Knee Flexion	+ / -	+ / -
McKenzie's Slide Glide	+ / -	+ / -
Stork Standing Test	+ / -	+ / -
Prone Lumbar Instability	+ / -	
Valsalva Maneuver	+ / -	

Fig. 5. Orthopedic Special Tests

When a tissue source of pain can be discerned, it is important to include this in the diagnostic complex. This enables the health care provider to be as specific as possible in assigning an ICD code to the patient problem. It also can lead the clinician to request follow-up tests or may lead instead to an appropriate medical referral.

2.11 Joint mobility assessment

Impairments of joint mobility frequently accompany active range of motion (AROM) deficits, however joint mobility is considered a distinct aspect of joint movement and therefore impaired joint mobility can be present when AROM is normal. Joint mobility is assessed through passive movements imparted by the examiner. These movements can be physiologic, meaning there is a corresponding active movement associated with the passive movement, or accessory, meaning there is no associated physiologic movement. Examples of physiologic movements in the lumbar spine extension and flexion; examples of accessory movements include posterior-to-anterior glide and lateral glide.

Clinical findings during joint mobility assessment that would be indicative of impairment are reproduction of the patient's symptoms, altered mobility (too much are too little movement), and/or the production of involuntary muscle guarding. Joint mobility can be categorized as: (1) Hypomobile, (2) Normal, or (3) Hypermobile. This is determined based upon what is considered normal for the individual; a "within person" reference standard is used as opposed to a "between person" reference standard. The 3-point scale has been found to have adequate validity and reliability (Landell R et al, 2008).

Joint mobility impairments can contribute to abnormal and inefficient active joint movement. The clinical findings during joint mobility assessment are used in the diagnostic process and to help direct treatment. In particular, decisions about whether or not the patient is a candidate for joint mobilization and manipulation are often based upon this aspect of the patient examination. Figure 6 is representative of the common accessory and physiologic movements examined in the lumbar spine.

JOINT MOBILITY ASSESSMENT	**RIGHT**	**LEFT**
P-A Central Vertebral Pressure	Normal / hypo / hyper	Normal / hypo / hyper
P-A Unilateral Vertebral Pressure	Normal / hypo / hyper	Normal / hypo / hyper
Transverse Vertebral Pressure	Normal / hypo / hyper	Normal / hypo / hyper
Flexion	Normal / hypo / hyper	Normal / hypo / hyper
Extension	Normal / hypo / hyper	Normal / hypo / hyper
Side Flexion	Normal / hypo / hyper	Normal / hypo / hyper
Rotation	Normal / hypo / hyper	Normal / hypo / hyper

Fig. 6. Joint Mobility Assessment

2.12 Palpation

Palpation of accessible body structures is often performed last in the physical examination due to the potential for the provocation of symptoms, particularly in more acute conditions. If symptoms are produced, increased or worse following palpation, this may influence the accuracy of other tests and measures. On the other hand, for subacute and chronic conditions, the clinician may want to start with palpation in order to better direct the remainder of the exam.

When the clinician is knowledgeable in surface anatomy and skilled in the art of palpation, this portion of the exam can provide important information relative to the tissue source of symptoms. This is particularly true for tissues that, when irritated or inflamed, produce pain that is well localized.

2.13 Summary

In the patient exam, essentially the clinician is asking a series of questions through a thoughtful selection of tests and measures. The intake data, medical screening process and history all inform this selection of tests for the physical examination. It is very important that the examination is systematized and consistent in a general way from one patient to the next. This helps to ensure that the exam is thorough and that all critical data is collected. Figure 7 provides a collection of signs and symptoms of common clinical conditions obtained through the patient examination process. This information can assist the clinician in determining specific health conditions that are contributing to the patient's low back complaints.

Condition	Presenting Symptoms/History	Clinical Findings
Lumbar Strain	Acute trauma/microtrauma Pain localized to lumbar spine Pain relieved by rest	Pain with active movement multidirectional Trunk ROM pain limited Segmental Hypomobility/ palpatory tenderness Negative neurologic signs
Disc Herniation	Acute or insidious onset Unilateral back and/or leg pain Flexion positions/postures aggravate	Spinal tilt may be evident Pain with active trunk flexion Centralization of pain with trunk extension + neurological signs with nerve root compromise + nerve tension signs (SLR, Slump Test)
Lateral Stenosis	Long history of back pain Leg pain > back pain Extension positions/postures aggravate	Pain with active trunk extension/lateral flexion + neurological signs with nerve root compromise + nerve tension signs (SLR, Slump Test)
Central Stenosis	Bilateral leg pain/paresthesia Extension positions/postures aggravate Flexion positions/postures relieve	Loss of active trunk extension ROM + neurological signs + quadrant test
Facet Joint Sprain	Acute trauma/microtrauma Unilateral back pain Extension positions/postures aggravate	Pain with active trunk extension Negative neurological signs Segmental hypomobiltiy (subacute phase)
SI Joint Syndrome	Pain in lumbosacral region/buttock Flexion postures/positions aggravate Common in women after childbirth	Pelvic asymmetries noted with palpation Pain with active trunk flexion Negative neurological signs + SI provocation tests (Thigh Thrust, Distraction) Palpatory pain in sacral sulcus Hypo or hyermobility of SI joint

Fig. 7. Musculoskeletal Differential Diagnosis

At the completion of the examination phase of management, the patient data must be interpreted and a treatment plan can then be established. The critical link between analysis and intervention is diagnosis. Diagnosis is the central element of patient management and will be discussed next.

3. Diagnosis

Diagnosis can be considered both a process, and a label that is generated from this process. In medicine, the *International Statistical Classification of Disease and Related Health Problems* (ICD) is utilized extensively by health care providers and most medical diagnoses are expressed as ICD codes. The ICD is a hierarchical system, whereby the most specific diagnosis is rendered that can be supported by diagnostic testing. For many musculoskeletal conditions, and especially back pain, the reliability of assigning diagnostic codes has not been studied extensively. Therefore, the reliability and validity of the coding system as a whole has not been established. The lack of consistency in categorizing patient conditions leads to clinical variance in managing conditions.

The dilemma surrounding diagnosis of back pain has significant implications, since diagnosis drives treatment decisions. Further, accurate diagnosis is essential to evaluating the effectiveness of treatments, which is a core value in evidence-based practice.

In addition to the challenges of accurate application of the ICD system, the system itself is considered inadequate in directing conservative treatment. Back pain is a largely a problem of the movement system. Back pain can occur in the absence of pathology. Many times a specific pathology cannot be identified in a person with back pain, so constructs other than pathology have to be considered in a clinically useful diagnostic system.

There are many ways in which clinicians can categorize back pain that fall outside the traditional ICD system. Numerous systems have been developed over the years within the professions involved in managing back pain, including medical primary care, physical therapy and chiropractic. Physical therapists in particular are on the front lines of conservative musculoskeletal care. In the physical therapy profession, a practical need exists to find a way to create subgroups of patients for the purpose of determining the most targeted interventions. Diagnostic systems have been developed to help fill this need. These methods of classification all vary in the constructs that serve as a basis for the categories, however there are also points of convergence. For example, patient response (symptomatic) to active movement is used to categorize patients in several of the more common systems. As expected, since the focus in conservative care is more functionally oriented, patient data derived from movement or functional testing is utilized in clinical decision-making.

The existing diagnostic classification models all have merit, however the diversity found in these systems creates variability in the way that clinical decisions are rendered. The lack of a standardized taxonomy has led to challenges not only for clinicians, but also the research community and ultimately people experiencing back pain.

Much of the research on diagnostic systems for back pain has been quantitative in nature. Several of the more common systems have undergone analysis of both reliability of assigning diagnostic categories to people with back pain, and validity of the systems. Validity has been investigated by determining if a targeted intervention is more likely to be effective when it is matched to the patient subgroup (Childs JD, 2004). These studies have begun to build a case for the usefulness of at least 3 systems used in physical therapy practice: (1) McKenzie, (2) Treatment-based, and (3) Movement System Impairment. All of these systems are structured and have explicit inclusion criteria. However little is known about how these are being used in clinical practice.

Since one point of agreement among health care professionals and researchers is that classification systems must be clinically pragmatic, there is a need for qualitative studies to explore what clinicians are actually doing in practice with regard to diagnosis. In order to fulfill this need, the author conducted a survey of physical therapists in clinical practice (Spoto MM, Collins J, 2008). A purposeful sample of physical therapists that are certified specialists in orthopedic practice was obtained. The participants were recognized for having a depth of knowledge and skill in orthopedic practice beyond that required for general practice. The general characteristics of the subjects can be found in table 3. These subjects were asked to answer both open and close-ended questions about how they approach diagnosis.

Primary Practice Setting		**Secondary Practice Setting**		**Years in Practice**	
Patient Care	84%	*Patient Care*	16%	3-8	18%
Teaching: Graduate	8%	*Teaching: Graduate*	25%	9-14	23%
Teaching: Postgraduate	1%	*Teaching: Postgraduate*	8%	15-20	26%
Management	6%	*Management*	40%	21-26	21%
Research	5%	*Research*	3%	>26	11%
Consultant	0%	*Consultant*	3%		

Table 3. Subject characteristics for physical therapists

The results of this study demonstrate that considerable variability is found in the way in which physical therapists classify back conditions. This is not surprising given the existence of numerous diagnostic systems in practice. In addition, over one-half of the physical therapists surveyed used more than one classification system. All of this contributes to the lack of consistency in the labels used by physical therapists to name the patient condition. Several themes emerged from this study and are summarized in figure 8. The first two themes reflect the need to move beyond the ICD and incorporate other constructs in the diagnosis. Psychiatrists and psychologists, for example, utilize a multi-axial system of diagnosis for psychological disorders in the *Diagnostic and Statistical Manual of Mental Disorders*. For back disorders, constructs such as impairments and functional limitations should be considered and incorporated with the ICD.

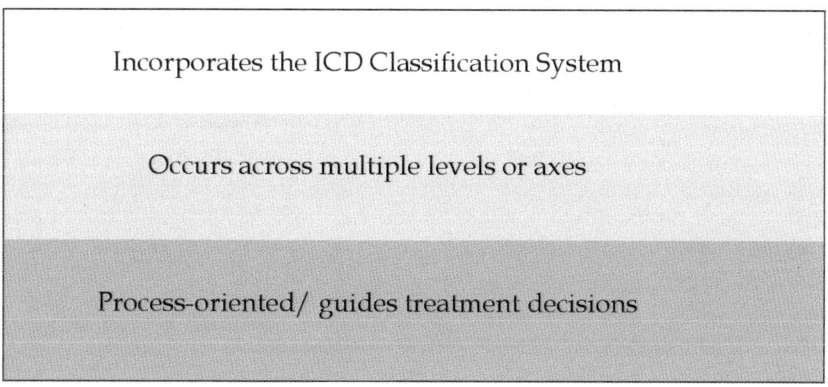

Fig. 8. Diagnosis by Physical Therapists

For physical therapists, diagnosis tends to be process-oriented. The various classification systems all have rules for interpreting patient data in ways that direct treatment. Until a more standard system is developed, with explicit criteria for selecting diagnostic categories, physical therapists engage in clinical reasoning to derive treatment decisions. Clinical reasoning, supported by the rules that govern the diagnostic system, is essentially the diagnostic process. Further, physical therapists indicate that they believe the primary role of diagnosis is to determine appropriate treatment. Since the overarching goal of treatment is to restore function, diagnosis must address (movement) function.

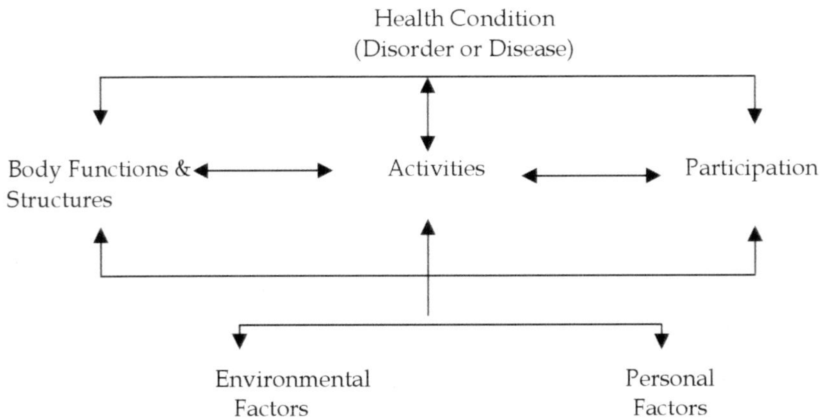

Fig. 9. ICF Model of Functioning & Health

A multidisciplinary model of functioning has been established in the *International Classification of Functioning, Disease and Health* (ICF). The ICF framework includes multiple factors or components that contribute to human functioning and health (WHO, 2008). Health conditions or diseases comprise one aspect of a person's health, however health conditions interact with body functions, both at the individual parts (tissues, joint, body part) and whole person levels, and these in turn interact with personal and environmental factors. The ICF framework is an expanded and more accurate way to define and address both health and disability. There are efforts ongoing in the health care professions to incorporate this new model into diagnostic classification systems for musculoskeletal conditions (Childs JD et al, 2008).

It is clear that health care providers recognize the need for a more meaningful way to approach diagnosis of back problems. Given that the ICD and ICF coding systems are universal, it seems reasonable that the constructs expressed in these systems could be integrated so that all components of health and disability are captured, and meaningful subgroups of back problems can emerge. In the meantime, conservative care practitioners will continue to use clinical subgroups, comprising clusters of signs and symptoms, to categorize patients in order to direct appropriate treatment.

4. Conservative intervention (Non-pharmacologic)

The conservative practitioner generally employs a combination of interventions in the treatment of back pain. A multi-modal approach is most common. Many of the research studies investigating the effectiveness of non-pharmacologic conservative treatments are designed to compare one intervention to either another intervention, or to no treatment. Since a single type of intervention is not likely to demonstrate a large treatment effect, especially when compared to another single-modal intervention, there is a need to develop a larger pool of high-quality studies investigating overall conservative management strategies. Another challenge is that in clinical trials investigating effectiveness of interventions for people with back pain, research subjects are often heterogeneous - reflecting the lack of a standard way to categorize back conditions. There is a growing pool of evidence that when similar groups are studied, and interventions are matched to treatment subgroups, outcomes are better (Childs JD et al, 2004). Figure 10 provides common treatment categories and the patient characteristics that would predict success with the specific types of conservative interventions.

Treatment Group	Patient Profile
Manipulation	Relatively acute pain Lumbar intersegmental hypomobility Local Pain Low FABQ Score
Lumbar Stabilization	< 40 years of age Episodic/recurring pain Aberrant trunk movements Lumbar intersegmental hypermobility
Specific Exercise	Directional preference (extension/flexion) Centralization with active movement tests
Traction	Radicular pain No directional preference Peripheralization with active movement

Fig. 10. Treatment-based classification: matching interventions to patient subgroups

Parallel to the challenge of providing high quality evidence supporting the effectiveness of conservative interventions for back pain, however, is the growing speculation about the role of invasive medical procedures in treating back pain. A recent study that investigated treatment outcomes of injured workers found that back patients that underwent spinal fusion had worse outcomes at 2 years compared to those receiving conservative care (Nguyen TH et al, 2011). These findings should be taken within the context of the considerable increase in both risk and cost for invasive treatments. Martin and Deyo have recently provided an interesting cost analysis of spine care in the US. They found that costs associated with spine care have risen substantially over the past decade and that there is no corresponding improvement in health status for people with spine problems (Martin BI, Deyo RA, 2008). The medical profession needs to develop evidence-based criteria for surgical intervention, in particular, by identifying the patient characteristics that predict success with surgical management. With ever increasing medical costs associated with musculoskeletal care, the current focus should be on finding the most cost effective treatments.

There is growing support in the literature for multi-modal, conservative treatment of spine pain (UK BEAM Trail Team, 2004). With the pursuit of more meaningful ways to categorize back disorders combined with more pragmatic clinical trials - where the focus is on studying overall management strategies rather than specific interventions - there is likely to be higher quality evidence in support of conservative intervention for the majority of people with back disorders.

Conservative interventions considered here will include the most common treatments utilized in practice: (1) Joint Mobilization/Manipulation, (2) Exercise Interventions, (3) Patient Education, (4) Physical Modalities, (5) Cognitive-Behavioral Interventions, and (6) Traction. A description of each intervention and a summary of the evidence on effectiveness will follow.

4.1 Joint mobilization/manipulation

Joint mobilization can be defined as: "a manual therapy technique comprising a continuum of passive movements to the joints and/or related soft tissues that are applied at various speeds and amplitudes, **including a small amplitude, high velocity therapeutic movement**" (APTA, 1997). Joint mobilization encompasses manipulation since manipulation is generally considered specifically the small amplitude, high velocity movement imparted to a joint. Another way of expressing this is to distinguish between "Non-Thrust" and "Thrust" techniques, the former referring to mobilization and the latter manipulation.

Joint mobilization is utilized to treat primarily impairments of joint mobility, range of motion and pain. Many disciplines employ joint mobilization, including the professions of chiropractic, physical therapy, osteopathy and medicine. Manipulative therapy has been studied extensively and therefore a high volume of information can be found on the topic. There has been great interest in better understanding the mechanisms of action of manipulation, and in investigating the effectiveness of manipulation in treating back pain.

The mechanisms of action of spine manipulation can be broadly divided into (1) mechanical and (2) non-mechanical effects. Although there have been many theories relative to the mechanical effects of manipulation over the years, recent evidence based upon more direct measurement of spine movement supports the conclusion that thrust techniques result in multi-axial intervertebral displacements. These displacements increase in association with the applied force and occur at multiple segmental levels (Keller TS et al, 2003). This suggests that a manipulative force will impact an entire spinal region as opposed to a specific segmental level. However it is common practice to apply the force to the most restricted segmental level, determined by joint mobility assessment findings. Non-mechanical effects of manipulation are thought to be related to altered pain processing, both at the peripheral and central nervous system levels. A Hypoalgesic effect has been found to occur immediately following joint manipulation (Bialosky JE et al 2008). Also of interest is the somewhat paradoxical effect of manipulation to either increase motorneuron firing, when it is desirable to facilitate deep segmental muscle activity for example, or decrease motorneuron firing when heightened muscle activity is unwanted (Colloca CJ et al, 2006).

Numerous clinical trials have been conducted investigating the effectiveness of manipulation for treating back pain. In a systematic review of non-pharmacologic interventions for back pain, Chou suggests that manipulation, along with cognitive behavioral therapy, exercise and interdisciplinary rehabilitation, is moderately effective in reducing pain and improving function in people with acute or chronic back pain (Chou R , Huffman LH, 2007). A recent systematic review, however, concludes that spinal manipulation has a small effect on pain and function compared to other interventions, and that this difference is not clinically significant (Rubinstein SM et al, 2007).

A clinical prediction rule has been established to better predict which patients respond favorably to manipulation (Flynn T A, 2002). Predictors of success with manipulation can be found in table 4. The positive Likelihood Ratio (LR) for the presence of 4 or more patient characteristics is 24, indicating that when patients meet the criteria, they have a very good chance of responding positively to manipulation. This rule has undergone validation studies, which support the contention that when patients are placed in subgroups based upon their presenting signs/symptoms and exam findings, treatment can be better targeted to their condition and outcomes will improve (Childs et al, 2004).

It is worthy to note that all national clinical guidelines for low back pain address spinal manipulation, although the recommendations vary. The majority of countries recommend manipulation for the treatment of acute low back pain (Bigos S et al, 1994).

Patient Characteristics
Duration of symptoms < 16 days
No symptoms distal to the knee
Hypomobility of at least one lumbar segmental level
At least one hip with >35 degrees of internal rotation
Fear-Avoidance Belief Questionnaire work score <19

Table 4. Clinical Prediction Rule for Spinal Manipulation

Spinal manipulation is a safe, conservative care option for the treatment of back pain. There are few contraindications, however: the presence of serious underling pathology, advanced osteoporosis, infection and cauda equina syndrome would be considered absolute contraindications to spinal manipulation. The mechanisms of action of manipulation are not fully understood, however currently it is believed that there are both mechanical and non-mechanical effects.

In general, manipulation has been found to have a small to moderate effect on decreasing pain and improving function in people with back pain. Most conservative care practitioners who perform spinal manipulation employ other types of interventions when treating back pain. Finally, clinical decision rules can be used to help identify which patients are likely to respond favorably to manipulation. Table 4 summarizes the patient characteristics that would predict success with a treatment program that includes spinal manipulation. The likelihood of the patient benefiting from manipulation increases in relation to the number of criteria met; if patients meet all or most criteria they have a high probability of improving with manipulation.

4.2 Exercise

Exercise interventions, along with patient education, are foundational in the conservative approach to treating musculoskeletal conditions of the spine. It is through exercise that body tissues adapt to the stresses and demands of everyday living, and recover from injury. The majority of cases of back pain are mechanical in nature, and ultimately a functional approach will produce the greatest long-term benefit. Exercise also requires active participation on the part of the patient, and therefore helps to foster self-efficacy.

There are many types of exercise and exercise programs for the back. The terminology used to describe these types of exercise can be confusing, and there is overlap in their descriptors. Examples of exercise types include: strengthening, flexibility, endurance (aerobic), motor control, stabilization, corrective, posture retraining, and functional. It is important in analyzing research on the effectiveness of exercise to understand what type of exercise was employed in the study because exercise is not a single entity. Ideally, exercise is prescribed and specifically targeted to the patient's movement impairments. For example, there are a subset of people with back pain who may not demonstrate strength deficits, however they demonstrate faulty patterns of muscle recruitment in the performance of functional tasks. For these individuals, motor control exercises - which emphasize the correct execution of the movement - will best address the patient problem.

In addition to specific categories of exercise, several exercise programs exist which are directed at treating low back pain. For example, William's flexion exercises were developed in the 1930's and consist of a series of exercises designed to improve the strength and flexibility of the trunk and pelvic girdle. These exercises favor flexion-based spinal movements. Later, The McKenzie approach to treating back pain was developed and the "extension principle" was established (McKenzie RA, 1981). This principle is in turn based upon the general concept of *directional preference,* whereby the prescription of exercise is dependant upon the patient's symptomatic response with specific trunk movements. The McKenzie approach is inclusive of the diagnostic procedures used to determine the type of mechanical problem causing the patient's symptoms. Interpretation of the many clinical trials conducted relative to the efficacy of the McKenzie system (Machedo LAC, 2006). Other more general exercise programs, those designed for the general population, have been incorporated into conservative management strategies; examples of these programs include yoga (Chou R, 2007) and Pilates.

There have been numerous clinical trials investigating the effectiveness of exercise in the treatment of back pain. A randomized control trial involving patients who had undergone microdiscectomy compared the effectiveness of lumbar stabilization exercise to general exercise and to no exercise. The lumbar stabilization subgroup demonstrated the most significant improvement in pain and function (Yilmaz A et al, 2003). Koumantakis also found that lumbar stabilization was effective in decreasing pain and improving function in people with non-specific low back pain (Koumantakis GA, 2005). In another systematic review, Ferreira found that spine stabilization exercise has a modest benefit for people with spine pain. Generally, outcomes of treatment are better with spine stabilization compared to no treatment, "usual care", and patient education. Further, spine stabilization is more effective in treating chronic pain than acute pain, although it does help prevent recidivism after acute pain episodes (Ferreira PH, 2006). In a systematic review of clinical trials that involved subjects with various stages of back pain, acute, subacute and chronic, Hayden found exercise to be effective in reducing pain in people with chronic pain . A particular approach to exercise, graded activity, was found to result in fewer absences from work in people with subacute pain. For the acute population, exercise was as effective as other conservative interventions in treating back pain (Hayden JA et al, 2005).

A clinical prediction rule has been developed to help identify back pain patients who are likely to respond favorably to spine stabilization exercise (Hicks GE et al, 2005). This clinical decision-making tool can be found in table 5. Relatively younger patients that demonstrate aberrant movements during active movement testing, who have a SLR of at least 91 degrees and who test positive on the prone instability test are more likely to benefit from spine stabilization exercise.

Patient Characteristics
Age < 40 years
Positive Prone Instability Test
Aberrant movement observed
Straight Leg Raise > 91 degrees

Table 5. Clinical Prediction Rule for Spine Stabilization Exercise

It appears that there is more support in the literature for exercise interventions in the chronic versus acute back pain population, however as the research community refines methodology in studying treatment for acute pain, there is promise that exercise will gain support in certain subgroups of patients. For example, there is evidence that on active movement testing, when patients demonstrate decreased symptoms with select trunk movements, prescribing exercise that is consistent with the directional preference improves outcomes (Long A et al, 2004).

Of all interventions for back pain, exercise is the one most directly oriented to improving the structural integrity of the spine. For many people with back pain, not only can skilled movements help to control pain, but most importantly if performed regularly, they will maintain function and prevent re-occurrence.

4.3 Patient education

Educational interventions have always been an integral part of the conservative approach to treating musculoskeletal conditions. Patient education for back patients should address, among other things, the importance of maintaining an active life and avoidance of bed rest, activity modification, and prevention. There is evidence that empowering patients with knowledge of their condition and fostering a sense of self-efficacy improves health outcomes. It is especially important in the acute phase to emphasize the need to stay active (Liddle SD, 2007).

When addressing patient education, it is important to distinguish between acute injury and chronic pain. In acute injury states, patients should be instructed to control forces on the spine as a first measure. This may mean a short period of rest. Then the patient can begin an *active rest* phase, where they modify activities as needed to control pain but stay active and move throughout the day. Following this phase, they can gradually return to normal activity.

For people with chronic or chronic recurring back pain, it is important for the health care practitioner to evaluate the patent from a pain management perspective. This may include the utilization of scales to assess pain response, such as the *Fear-Avoidance Belief Questionnaire* and the *McGill Pain Questionnaire*. Elevated fear- avoidance beliefs have been associated with poorer health outcomes for musculoskeletal conditions, so it is important to include strategies to address these beliefs (Nicholas MK, George SZ, 2011).

Individual education appears to be most effective, although it is not clear what mode of education is best (Engers AJ, 2008). In a large prospective controlled trial, patients that were given an educational pamphlet in a medical care setting demonstrated decrease pain and improved satisfaction with care compared to patients that did not receive the educational intervention (Coudeyre E et al, 2007). A simple back booklet has been developed that de-emphasizes back pain as a medical problem and promotes self-efficacy. When tested in a randomized controlled trial, investigators found that for back pain patients with elevated fear-avoidance beliefs, there was a significant improvement in self-report disability scores compared to a control group who were given a more traditional educational intervention (Burton AK et al, 1999).

Patient Education for Back Pain
Pain mechanisms & pain control
Advice on staying active/Avoidance of bed rest
Emphasis on back pain as a common human experience
Risk factors for chronic pain
Activity modification/ Joint protection
Promote self-efficacy
Role of anxiety and stress

Table 6. Components of patient education for people with back pain

Patient education should be part of a comprehensive program of care for people with back pain. This needs to be considered when analyzing the research on patient education. As with other conservative interventions, the impact of patient education on pain and function is small to moderate. However, the costs associated with patient education are relatively low and therefore worth the time investment for the patient and health care provider.

4.4 Physical modalities

The role of physical agents in the treatment of low back pain is primarily for pain control and to aid in the healing response in the presence of acute injury. The most common physical modalities are: heat, cold, ultrasound and electrotherapy (including TENS). Although many clinical guidelines for low back pain do not recommend passive therapies, this is generally due to the small effect size of individual physical modalities on improving outcomes for people with back pain (Bigos S et al, 1994). This is especially true for chronic pain. In acute pain, the use of heat has relatively stronger support than the other modalities (Chou R, 2007). In contemporary practice, modalities are used in conjunction with active therapies. When patients present with acute back pain that impacts their quality of life and interferes with their ability to function, early pain control can speed recovery. There is evidence that the inclusion of physical agents to standard treatment approaches has added benefit and improves treatment outcomes (Hurwitz EL et al, 2002).

4.5 Cognitive behavioral interventions

Cognitive behavioral therapy has long been used in the mental health arena to treat a variety of psychological conditions such as anxiety disorders and depression. This psychotherapeutic approach is structured, requires a step-by-step progression, and is time-intensive. The cognitive-behavioral approach has also been found to benefit people with back pain. Cognitive-behavioral strategies have been applied especially to the chronic pain population in recognition of the strong role that patient's beliefs, thought processes and behaviors have on their experience of back pain. A patient's cognition interacts with their movement system and can influence the level of disability and the intensity of the pain experience (Nicholas MK, George SZ, 2011). The physical therapist is in a good position to help modify patient's belief systems to enhance functional recovery due to the relatively long relationship physical therapists develop with their patients.

A list of common strategies used in conservative management of musculoskeletal condition can be found in table 7.

Pain mechanisms & pain control
Advice on staying active/ Avoidance of bed rest
Emphasis on back pain as a common human experience
Risk factors for chronic pain
Activity modification/ Joint protection
Promote self-efficacy
Role of anxiety and stress

Table 7. Cognitive-behavioral strategies utilized in the treatment of back pain

Cognitive behavioral interventions have been found to be effective in decreasing pain and improving function in patients with low back pain - either alone or in combination with active exercise. (Smeets RJ, 2006). In a systematic review of behavioral interventions for chronic low back pain, the authors found moderate-level evidence in support of behavioral interventions for short-term pain control (Henschke N et al, 2011).

It is likely that cognitive-behavioral interventions will become more integrated into conservative back pain management as knowledge of the role of psychosocial factors in the pain experience increases. Identification of yellow flags in back pain patients helps the healthcare provider select patients most likely to benefit from a cognitive behavioral approach. Likewise, recognition of yellow flags in the acute pain population has the potential to prevent future episodes of back pain.

4.6 Traction

There is almost no treatment for back pain that can claim greater longevity than traction. However, despite this long history and the many innovative ways that have been developed to apply traction forces to the spine, there is little evidence to support its use in practice. A systematic review based upon an analysis of 25 randomized controlled trials involving traction concludes: "the results of the available studies involving mixed groups of acute, sub-acute and chronic patients with LBP with and without sciatica were quite consistent, indicating that continuous or intermittent traction as a single treatment for LBP is not likely effective for this group" (Clarke JA et al, 2010).

There is some evidence that a subgroup of patients, those that experience leg pain, signs of nerve root compression and either perpheralization of symptoms with trunk extension movements or display a positive well leg raise have better outcomes with traction. In addition, a clinical prediction rule has been developed that can help identify patients that are more likely to respond favorably to tractions: (1) FABQ score < 21, (2) absence of neurological signs, (3) age > 30 years, and (4) does not perform manual labor (Cai C et al, 2009).

5. Conclusion

The conservative approach to treating back pain encompasses all elements of patient management from the initial examination, through the diagnostic process and finally to the prescription of the most appropriate interventions. It is based upon principles that are now well supported in the literature, including selection of the least invasive treatments that can be supported by the current scientific evidence, the orientation toward helping patients help themselves, and utilizing an active program of care. These principles reflect a biopsychosocial model of healthcare, where the experience of pain is viewed as a multi-faceted phenomenon. The best hope for reversing the trends toward ever more costly care for back pain is to focus treatment on the underlying factors that contribute to it, and to encourage people to take responsibility for their health.

6. References

American Physical Therapy Association. Guide to physical therapist practice. Physical Therapy. 1997; 77 (11): 1163-1674.

Beurskens AJHM, de Vet HCW, Koke AJA. Responsiveness of functional status in low back pain: a comparison of different Instruments. *Pain.* 1996; 65 (1): 71-76.

Bialosky JE, Bishop MD, Robinson ME, et al. The influence of expectation on spinal manipulation induced hypoalgesia: an experiemental study in normal subjects. *BMC Musculoskeletal Disorders.* 2008; 9: 19.

Bigos S, Bowyer O et al. Acute low back pain problems in adults. Clinical practice guidelines, No 14. Rockville, Maryland. US Department of Health and Human Services Public Health Service Agency for Health Care Policy and Research. Publication No. 95-0642; December, 1994.

Boos N, Semmer N, Elfering A et al. Natural history of individuals with asymptomatic disc abnormalities in magnetic resonance imaging: predictors of low back pain-related medical consultations and work incapacity. *Spine.* 2000; 25: 1484-1492.

Brontfort G, Maiers MJ, Evans RL et al. Supervised exercise, spinal manipulation, and home exercise for chronic low back pain: a randomized clinical trial. *The Spine Journal.* 2011; 11: 585-598.

Burton AK, Waddell G, Tillotson KM, Summerton N. Informatiom and advice to patients with low back pain can have a positive effect: A randomized controlled trial of a novel educational booklet in primary care. *Spine.* 1999; 24: 2484-2491.

Cai C, Pua YH, Lim KC. A clinical prediction rule for classifying patients with low back pain who demonstrate short-term Improvement with mechanical lumbar traction. *Eur Spine J.* 2009; 18: 554-561.

Childs JD, Fritz JM, Flynn TW, et al. A clinical prediction rule to identify patients with low back pain most likely to benefit From spinal manipulation: a validation study. *Ann Intern Med.* 2004; 141: 920-928.

Childs JD, Cleland JA, Elliot JM, Teyhen DS et al. Neck Pain: Clinical Practice Guidelines Linked to the International Classification of Functioning, Disability and Health. *JOSPT.* 2008; 38 (9): A1-A34.

Chou R, Huffman LH. Nonpharmacologic therapies for acute and chronic low back pain: a review of the evidence for an American Pain Society/American College of Physicians clinical practice guideline. *Annals of Internal Medicine.* 2007; 147 (7): 492-504.

Chou R, Qaseem A, Snow V et al. Diagnosis and treatment of low back pain: a joint clinical practice guidelne from the American College of Physicians and the American Pain Society. *Ann Intern Med.* 2007; 147: 478-491.

Clarke JA, van Tulder MW, Blomberg SEI et al. Traction for low back pain with our without sciatica. *Cochrane Database of Systematic Reviews.* 2010, Issue 5. Art. No: CD003010.

Cleland JA, Fritz JM, Whitman JM, Palmer JA. The reliability and construct validity of the Neck Pain Disability Index and the Patient Specific Functional Scale in patients with cervical radiculopathy. *Spine.* 2006; 31 (5): 598-602.

Colloca CJ, Keller TS, Harrison DE et al. Spinal manipulation force and duration affect vertebral movement and Neuromuscular responses. *Clinical Biomechanics.* 2006; 21 (3): 254-62.

Deutscher D, Horn SD, Dickstein R et al. Associations between treatment processes, patient characteristics, and outcomes in Outpatient physical therapy practice. *Arch Phys Med Rehabil.* 2009; 90: 1349-1363.

Engers AJ, Jellema P, Wensing M, van der Windt DAWM, Grol R, van Tulder MW. Individual patient education for low back pain. Cochrane Database of Systematic Reviews 2008, Issue 1. Art. No.: CD004057.

Ferreira PH, Ferreira ML, Maher CG et al. Specific stabilisation exerice for spinal and pelvic pain: a systematic review. *Australian J of Physiotherapy.* 2006; 52: 79-88.

Flynn T et al. A clinical prediction rule for classifying patients with low back pain who demonstrate short-term improvement with spinal manipulation. *Spine.* 2002; 27: 2835-43.

Fritz JM, Lindsay W, Matheson JW et al. Is there a subgroup of patients with low back pain likely to benefit from mechanical traction? Results of a randomized clinical trial and subgrouping analysis. *Spine.* 2007; 32: E793-800.

Hayden JA, van Tulder MW, Malmivaara A, Koes BW. Exercise therapy for treatment of non-specific low back pain. *Cochrane Database Syst Rev.* 2005; CD000335.

Henchke N, Ostelo RW, van Tulder MW et al. Behavioral treatment for chronic low back pain. *Cochrane Database of Systematic Reviews.* 2010. Issue 7. Art. No: CD002014.

Hicks GE, Fritz JM, Delitto A, McGill SM. Preliminary development of a clinical prediction rule for determining which patients with low back pain who will respond to a stabilization program. *Arch Phys Med Rehabil.* 2005; 86: 1753-62.

Hurwitz EL, Morgenstern H, Harber P et al. A randomized trial of medical care with and without physical therapy and chiropractic with and without physical modalities for patients with low back pain: a 6 month follow-up outcomes from the UCLA low back pain study. *Spine.* 2002; 27 (20): 2193-2204.

Keller TS, Colloca CJ, Gunzburg R. Neuromechanical characterization of in vivo lumbar spinal manipulation. Part I. *Journal of Manipulative & Physiol Ther.* 2003; 26 (9): 567-578.

Kendall FP, McCreary EK, Provance PG. Muscles: testing and function. ed 4, Williams & Wilkens, Baltimore, MD: 1993.

Koumantakis GA. Trunk muscle stabilization training plus general exercise versus general exercise only: randomized control trial of patients with recurrent low back pain. *Physical Therapy.* 2005; 85: 209-225.

Landel R et al. Intertester reliability and validity of motion assessments during lumbar spine accessory motion testing. *Physical Therapy.* 2008; 88: 43-49.

Liddle SD, Gracey JH Baxter JD. Advice for the management of low back pain: a systematic review of randomized controlled Trails. *Man Ther.* 2007; 12: 12:310-327.

Long A., Donelson R, Fung T. Does it matter which exercise? A randomized control trial of exerise for low back pain. *Spine.* 2004; 29: 2593-2602.

Machedo LAC, Souza MS, Ferreira PH, Ferreira FML. The McKenzie method for low back pain: a systematic review of the literature with a meta-analysis approach. *Spine.* 2006; 31 (9): E254-E262.

Magee DJ. Orthopedic Physical Assessment. 4th ed. W.B. Saunders Co: Philadelphia, PA: 2002.

Martin BI, Deyo RA, Marza SK et al. Expenditures and health status among adults with back and neck problems. *JAMA.*2008; 299 (6): 656-664.

McKenzie RA. *The Lumbar Spine.* Spinal Publications; Waikanae, New Zealand, 1981.

Nguyen TH, Randolph DC, Talmage J, et al. Long-term Outcomes of Lumbar Fusion Among Workers' Compensation : A Historical Cohort Study. Spine. 2011(Feb 15);36(4) :320-331.

Nicholas MK, George SZ. Psychologically informed interventions for low back pain: an update for physical therapists. *Pain.* 2011. 91 (5): 765-776.

Riddle DL. Classification and low back pain: a review of the literature and critical analysis of selected systems. Physical Therapy. 1998; 78 (7):708-737.

Rubinstein SM, van Middlekoop M, Assendelft WJJ, de Boer MR et al. Spinal manipulative therapy for chronic low-back Pain. *Cochrane Database of Systematic Reviews.* 2011, Issue 2. Art No: CD008112. DOI: 10.1002/14651858.CD008112.pub2.

Sahrmann SA. Diagnosis and Treatment of Movement Impairment Syndromes. Mosby, Inc., St. Louis, MO: 2002.

Saur PM, Ensink FB, Frese K, et al. Lumbar range of motion: reliability and validity of the inclinometer technique in the clinical measurement of trunk flexibility. *Spine.* 1996; 21:1332-1338.

Savage RA, Whitehouse GH, Roberts N. The relationship between the magnetic resonance imaging appearance of the lumbar spine and low back pain, age and occupation in males. *Eur Spine J.* 1997; 6: 106-114.

Stausberg J, Lehmann N, Kaczmarek D et al. Reliability of diagnosis coding in ICD-10. *Int J Med Inform.* 2008; 77: 50-7.

Smeets RJ, Vlaeyen JW, Hidding A et al. Active rehabilitation for chronic low back pain: cognitive-behavioral, physical or both? *BMC Musculoskeletal Disord.* 2006: 7:5.

Spoto MM, Collins J. Physiotherapy diagnosis in clinical practice: a survey of orthopedic certified specialists in the USA. *Physiotherapy Research International.* 2008; 13: 31-41.

Stanton TR,Fritz JM, Hancock MJ et al. Evaluation of a treatment-based classification algorithm for low back pain: a cross-sectional study. *Phys Ther.* 2011; 91: 496-509.

UK BEAM Trial Team. United Kingdom back pan exercise and manipulation (UK BEAM) randomized trial: effectiveness of physical treatments for back pain in primary care. *BMJ.* 2004; 329; 1377.

Vlanin M. Psychometric properties and clinical usefulness of the Oswestry Disability Index. *Journal of Chiropractic Medicine.* 2008; 7 (4): 161-163.

Weinstein JN, Tosteson TD, Lurie JD et al. Surgical versus non-operative treatment for lumbar disk herniation. *JAMA.* 2006;296 (20): 2441-2450.

World Health Organization. *International Classification of Disease.* ICD-10. Geneva, Switzerland: 2005.

World Health Organization: *International Classification of Functioning, Disability and Health: ICF.* Geneva, Switzerland: World Health Organization; 2008.

Yilmaz, A. Yilmaz, F. Merdol, D. et al: Efficacy of dynamic lumbar stabilization exercise in lumbar microdiscectomy. *The Internet Journal of Minimally Invasive Spinal Technology.* 2008. Volume 2 Number 3.

Therapeutic Exercises in the Management of Non-Specific Low Back Pain

Johnson Olubusola Esther
Department of Medical Rehabilitation,
Obafemi Awolowo University, Ile-Ife,
Nigeria

1. Introduction

Low back pain (LBP) is neither a disease nor a diagnostic entity of any sort (Ehrlich, 2003). It is a common problem which affects the majority of adults at least once in a life time. It is irksome, of global concern, as common as headache affecting all age groups and races (May, 2001; Hazard, et al, 1996). It is a prevalent musculoskeletal condition, and a common cause of disability especially in its chronic/recurrent state. The majority of LBP episodes resolve spontaneously while a significant minority becomes recurrent and a small percentage remain persistent (Dunn and Croft, 2004). LBP has a point prevalence of about 7 to 33% and lifetime prevalence of nearly 85% (Walker, 2000). Frank et al, (1996); Vollin, (1997) reported similarly that it affects about 70-85% of individuals once in their lifetime.

Management of LBP is costly; accounting for a large and increasing proportion of health care expenditures without evidence of corresponding improvements in outcomes (Martin et al, 2008). Frymoyer, (1988) reported that the major costs of LBP can be identified with the chronic and recurrent LBP. Low back pain occurs in a wide variety of medical, musculoskeletal, and neurologic conditions (Roach et al, 1997, Cypress, 1983). Most individuals reporting at the clinic for management of excruciating LBP have experienced pain in the low back many times before the episode that brings them to the hospital. Low back pain accounts for serious job absenteeism in industrialized societies, a case that would have been similar in most parts of Africa except that there is hardly any financial compensation for sick leave, hence less report of LBP in clinics.

Low back pain was defined as pain and discomfort, localised below the costal margin and above the inferior gluteal folds, with or without leg pain (sciatica) (Omokhodion et al, 2002), and as "pain limited to the region between the lower margins of the 12th rib and the glutei folds" with or without leg pain (sciatica) (Manek and Macgregor, 2005). It is specifically an aggregation of symptoms of pain/discomfort originating from the lumbar spine apparatus with or without radiation of pain to the gluteal fold and legs. It is regarded as a symptom from impairments in the structures in the low back which originates e.g. from muscles, ligaments, intervertebral disc. Low back pain is a symptom of myriads of causes ranging from mechanical causes; accounting for about 90% of cases and non-mechanical causes i.e. secondary to an underlying pathology in the rest of the population. It is a symptom which appears in the clinic as a disease entity because it is highly reported. It can be primary i.e.

mechanical/non-specific and also secondary with an underlying pathology i.e. non-mechanical. Non-specific LBP appears to be commoner affecting mostly individuals between ages 30 and 50years; in children and adolescents however, LBP appears to be usually secondary to an underlying pathology.

2. Classification

Low back pain can be acute, sub-acute or long-term; acute-on-chronic, with recurrence rearing its head among a significant minority. Acute low back pain is usually defined as the duration of an episode of low back pain persisting for less than 6 weeks; sub-acute as LBP which lasts between 6 and 12 weeks and long-term LBP as persisting for 12 weeks or more; chronic LBP is defined as LBP persisting for 12 weeks or more. Recurrent low back pain is defined as a new episode after a symptom-free period of 6 months, but not an exacerbation of chronic low back pain (van Tulder et al, 2004). Walker, 2000 estimated that 70-95% of any adult population will suffer at least one episode of back pain in its lifetime, while Truchon, 2001 proposed 60-80%. Fifty per cent of such cases will recur within 3 months (Lawrence et al, 2006). Recurrent and chronic LBP accounts for more than 70% of cases reported at clinics. Acute LBP is a common presentation of back pain and it is usually self-limiting; lasting less than 3 months and may not need any medical intervention. About half of those individuals who experience acute LBP will have recurrences within the first year of the first episode, leading to a possible history of chronic low back pain (Moffroid, 1997). Waddell and Bry-Jones (1994) submitted that LBP not settled within 8–12 weeks is likely to result in chronic disabling pain.

Acute LBP tends towards becoming a complex chronic pain disorder, involving anatomical, physiological, psychological and social aspects (Roach et al, 1997). Chronic/recurrent LBP is a chief source of incapacitation, suffering and expense frequently resulting in significant worry and interference with daily activities leading to significant level of disability. It is a tremendous burden on patients and health service providers. It usually results from acute pain of muscular or connective tissue origin, which persists in approximately 30% of cases in adults and 20% of cases in adolescents.

3. Schools of thought

There are several schools of thoughts regarding the management of LBP that have thrived through decades of physiotherapy practice, ranging from the crude methods of tying a patient to a ladder and dropping him, James Mennell, Cyriax and Kaltenborn schools of thoughts, the William's flexion exercise, Richardson and other researchers spinal stabilization theory and McKenzie's standardized basis of classification of LBP with its extension and flexion protocols of treatment. Other schools of thought include Nwuga's vertical and transverse oscillatory manouevres of treatment of disc lesion, also Alexander and Mulligan's technique of management of LBP. James Mennell pointed at the facet joints, postural strain, and adhesions as causative factors in back pain. He proposed treating low back pain with manipulations designed to restore joint play in joints for the relief of pain and restoration of normal voluntary movement and functions (Nwuga, 2007). In 1933 Mixter and Bar reported that the intervertebral disc as a major factor in back pain with or without sciatica. James Cyriax also agreed with this school of thought and identified two types of disc lesion, viz: nuclear protrusion and annular protrusion. He applied a rotational torsion stress on the spine. His treatment has been criticized over the years as being non specific with massive tractive force. Maitland distinguished between mobilization and manipulation and puts emphasizes on mobilization where oscillatory movements are performed on a chosen joint and within the available range of movement within the limit of the patient's tolerance, mobilization was better accepted as being milder and easy to learn. Nwuga in 1976 worked on integrating the thoughts of these authors with some innovations of his own and came up with his own vertical and transverse oscillatory pressure. He came up with the Nwugarian institute for back pain management in 1996 to promote the training of Nigerian physiotherapists in the art and science of manipulative therapy (Nwuga, 2007). His technique is popularly employed by physiotherapists in Nigeria in treating low back pain.

The concept of spinal stability was introduced in medical research in 1970 (Barr et al, 2005). It was theorized that back injury and therefore pain could be caused by the gradual degeneration of joints and soft tissue over time from repetitive microtrauma, which was caused by poor control of spinal structures (Farfan, 1975). This theory has evolved and conclusions are that spinal stability is a dynamic process that includes both static positions and controlled movement which includes both an alignment in sustained postures (Figure 1) and movement patterns that reduce tissue strain, trauma to the joints or soft tissue, and allows for efficient muscle action (Sahrmann, 2002). It was also theorized that movement patterns that were altered by faulty strength and flexibility, fatigue from poor endurance, or abnormal neural control would eventually cause tissue damage. Tissue damage would lead to decreased stability of spinal structures, increased challenges to the already inefficient muscles, and the perpetuation of a degenerative cascade (Magee, 2002).

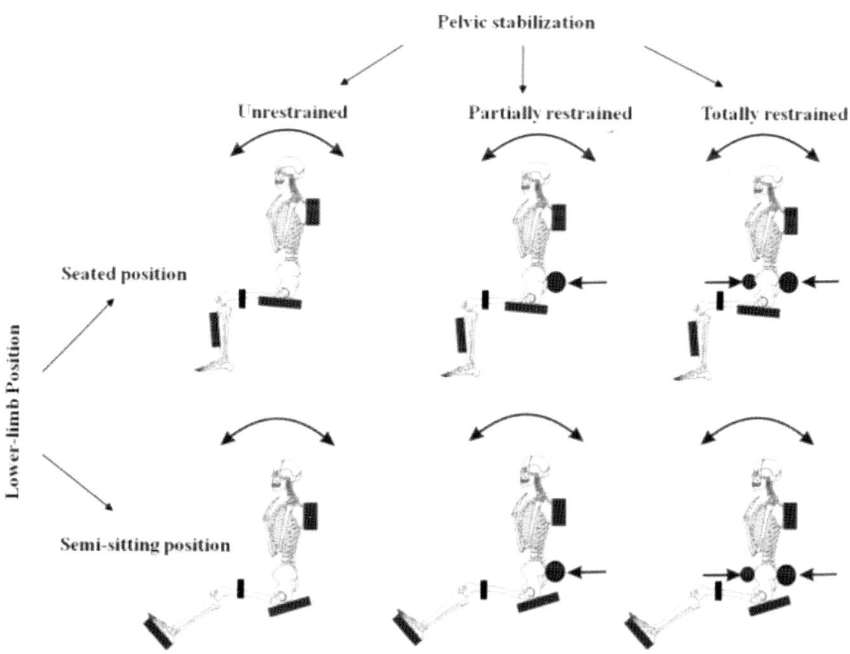

Fig. 1. Pelvic Stabilization in Sitting Positions (da Siva et al, 2009)

The lumbar multifidi and abdominals especially the transversus abdominis have been implicated in LBP and in face of muscle deactivation subsequent to recovery from an episode of LBP. Furthermore evidences by Hides et al (1992, 2008) are in support of the positive role of the lumbar multifidus muscle in segmental stabilization of the lumbar spine. Barr et al, (2005) in their review on lumbar stabilization submitted that the multifidi and transversus abdominus muscles are major stabilizers of the spine. Biomechanical studies have also highlighted the role of the multifidus muscle in provision of segmental stiffness (Keifer and Shirazi, 1995; Wilke et al, 1995), control of the spinal segment's neutral zone (Panjabi et al, 1989; Panjabi 1992) and its capacity to stabilize the spine when spinal stability is challenged. It has been reported that within a day subsequent to the first episode of LBP, the lumbar multifidus muscle showed ipsilateral pain related decrease in muscle bulk and this loss of bulk is not recovered even after recovery from back pain (Hides et al, 1994, 1996).

Panjabi (1992) reported evidences of lumbar instability, low muscular strength and endurance among subjects with LBP. Instability according to him could be a result of tissue damage, making the segment more difficult to stabilize, low muscular strength or endurance, or poor muscular control; bone and ligaments: lumbar instability is usually a combination of all three. These three components are interdependent, and one system could compensate for deficits in another. The multifidi extend along the entire length of the spine and is much thicker at the low back and waist (Johnson, 2002), comprising superficial and deep fibers (Figure 2). The transverses abdominus is the chief abdominal stabilizer of the spine (Figure 3). The quadratus lumborum (Mc Gill, 2002), pelvic floor muscles (Sapsford and Hodges, 2001), internal and external oblique, rectus abdominus, iliopsoas and paraspinal muscles are other muscles that contribute to stability of the spine.

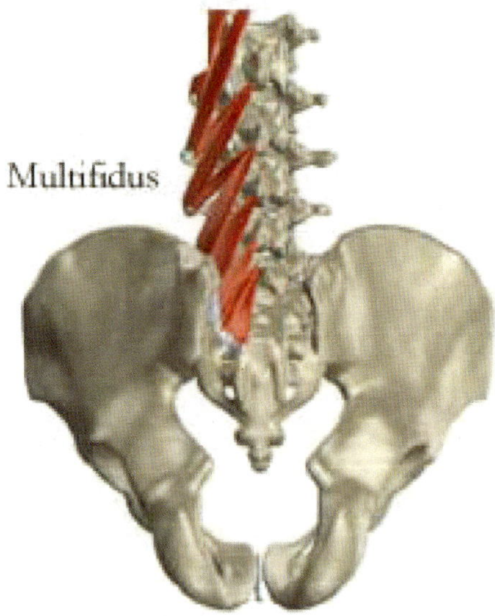

Fig. 2. Multifidus Muscles
Source: coreconcepts.com.sg. Accessed 23rd December, 2011

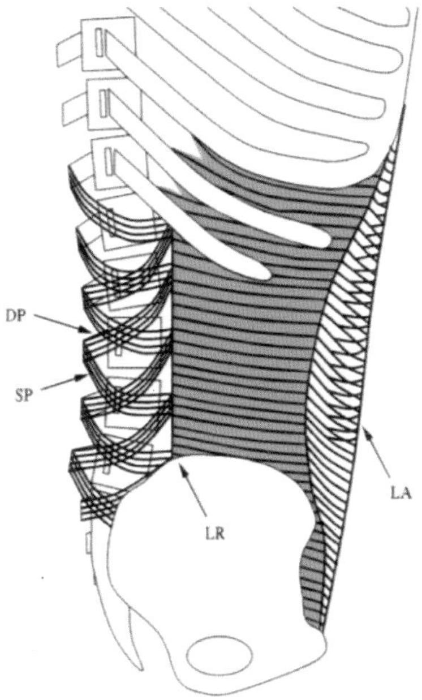

Fig. 3. Anatomy of transversus abdominis. The attachments of tranversus abdominis to the lumbar vertebrae via middle ananterior layers of the thoracolumbar fascia are not shown. Todemonstrate the bilaminar fascial attachment of the posterior layer of the thoracolumbar fascia it is shown connecting only to the spinous processes. LR ± lateral raphe, LA ± linae alba, SP ± superficial lamina of the posterior layer of the thoracolumbar fasica, DP ± deep lamina of the posterior layer of the thoraco-lumbar fascia.
Source: Hodges, (1999)

McKenzie purported the use of repeated movements and sustained positions in the examination and treatment of low back disorders (The McKenzie Institute, 2001). McKenzie subsequently classified mechanical LBP into three syndromes; postural, dysfunction and derangement syndromes (McKenzie, 1981). Patients with postural syndrome are individuals who have intermittent episodes of pain believed to be the result of prolonged stress on soft tissues (bad posture) around the lumbar spine. They have full range of movements, no deformity and they are treated with postural advice (McKenzie, 1981; Porter, 1993). Patients with dysfunctional syndrome are individuals who are believed to have had trauma or a postural problem producing adaptive shortening of the soft tissues. Pain is triggered by over use, posture is poor, movement in the spine is restricted and there is pain at the end-range (McKenzie, 1981; Porter, 1993). Patients with derangement syndrome of the intervertebral disc may be with or without kyphotic or scoliotic deformity. There are two types of derangement, posterior derangement D1 to D6 and anterior derangement D7. Treatment for these derangements is usually to move the individual to D1 where they can manage themselves (McKenzie, 1981; Porter, 1993). Pain is usually centralised, after which, patients can care for themselves with extension activity and maintain lumbar lordosis and subsequently obtain functional recovery (Mckenzie, 1981; Donelson et al, 1990; Porter, 1993). All these theories addressed the intervertebral disc and or the facet joint as probable sources of problem in non-specific back pain. Mulligan (2004) however submitted a theory that incorporates the intervertebral discs and facet joints. He opined that facet joint mobility brings improvement in minor cases of LBP. He reported on sustained natural apophyseal glides (SNAGS) which are a combination of sustained facet glide with movement. This he reported improves mobility of the facet joint and simultaneously heals the intervertebral disc.

A large number of muscles cross the spine, and all contribute to the modulation of lumbar stability and movement to some extent. This is a complex system consisting of deep muscles that have their origin or insertion on the lumbar vertebrae, which theoretically are responsible for the control of stiffness and intervertebral relationships, and the global muscle system that encompasses the large superficial muscles of the trunk that are the torque generators for spinal motion and handle external loads applied to the spine (Bergmark, 1989; Barr et al, 2005). Weakness of abdominal and back muscles especially the back extensors, muscular dysfunction in the low back, and abdominal muscles, and poor joint flexibility in the back and hamstring are reported as precursors for LBP (Biering Sørenson, 1984, Pollock and Wilmore, 1990, Robinson, 1992, Richardson and Jull, 1995, McArdle et al, 1996,). Several tests have been developed to identify individuals with weak abdominal and leg muscles with the aim of preventing low back pain. Kraus Weber test of minimum fitness is a series of exercises that measure strength and flexibility of the back, abdominal, psoas and hamstring muscles, it was developed by Kraus and Hirschland in 1954 from their clinical experience that majority of back disorders could have been prevented by maintaining a certain level of fitness. Persons who could pass this test were considered to be unlikely candidates for developing low back problems (Safrit and Wood, 1995). The Kraus Weber test addressed strength and flexibility and not muscular endurance. Muscular endurance capabilities of back muscles may be as important as or even more important than strength in the prevention and treatment of low back pain. Moffroid (1997) submitted that lack of endurance of the trunk muscles is an important factor in LBP. Evidences are in literature linking weaknesses of abdominal and back extensor weakness with low back pain or and its susceptibility in, adults and children (Holmstrom et al, 1992, Mannion and Dolan, 1994, Luoto et al, 1995, Adegoke and Babatunde, 2007; Mbada and Ayanniyi, 2008; Johnson et al, 2009), and the Biering Sørenson's back muscles endurance tests of back pain susceptibility uphold this submission (Biering Sørenson, 1984). Biering Sørensen test of Static Muscular Endurance (BSME) is a simple clinical tool for the assessment of low back muscular endurance. It has been reported to be valid, reliable, safe, practical, responsive, easily administered and inexpensive (Alaranta, 2000; Udermann et al, 2003). The BSME either in its original version or as variants is believed to provide a global measure of back extension endurance capacity (Moreau et al, 2001).

4. Management

Low back pain is a costly quality of life-related health problem (Selkowitz, 2006), and its management has remained a formidable challenge in medical practice all over the world (Feurstain and Battie, 1995). It is also a complex multivariate problem that has been known to be resistant to simple solutions (The Back Letter, 2001) and its management has remained an unending task for health service providers especially because quite a sizeable proportion of the population will attend the clinic sometime in their lifetime complaining of LBP.

Efforts have hence been exerted to improve the efficacy of its treatment especially in its recurrent or chronic nature (Feurstain and Battie, 1995). Physiotherapy is probably the treatment most widely used for back complaints of mechanical origin especially in the sub-acute and chronic states. Spinal manipulation for patients who are failing to return to normal activities have however been suggested among patients with LBP (van Tulder et al, 2009).

Several approaches of management have been used in managing non-specific low back pain with varying degrees of success. Drugs have been widely accepted in managing acute LBP. Physiotherapy is central to the overall management of LBP in the sub-acute and chronic phases. Physiotherapy management of long term low back pain favours active low back treatment programmes involving improving aerobic fitness, increasing the strength and flexibility of the lumbar musculature and ensuring lumbar stability (Shiple, 1997). Physiotherapy modalities including cryotherapy, Transcutaneous Electrical Nerve Stimulation (TENS) and heat therapy, back care education, back school, biofeedback, and functional restoration are used as adjunct to physiotherapy regimens including massage, heat, traction, ultrasound, short wave diathermy, back care education. It also involves the use of physical agents and modalities in physiotherapy to manage LBP. These include rest using supports e.g lumbar corsets, heat therapy, cold therapy, spinal manipulation and electro analgesia (Low and Reed, 1994; Foster et al, 1999; Li and Bombardier, 2001; Gracey et al, 2002). These rehabilitative and physical treatments can be helpful and with the aim of combating relapse, however when LBP become complex, the psychological components become an important part of the treatment. Pain management programme/pain clinics are used in managing psychological aspect of pain. Work hardening is also introduced to restore physical, behavioural and vocational functions facilitating return to work.

5. Exercise therapy

Several treatment strategies, for instance, joint mobilization and manipulation, soft tissue massage techniques, electrotherapy, acupuncture, and traction, are utilized in clinical practice to treat low back pain, with varying degrees of effectiveness. Exercises are commonly prescribed for LBP by physiotherapists, but only seem to be supported as an intervention by evidence for patients with chronic LBP further more conclusions from systematic reviews are that exercises are effective in managing chronic LBP Hayden, (2005); Liddle, (2004). Lewis et al, (2008) in their systematic review also reaffirmed that exercises were effective in reducing pain in people with CLBP. Most studies concluded that active exercises were a valuable therapeutic approach in managing LBP, despite the lack of consensus on the optimal exercise techniques, intensity or active intervention (Abenhaim, 2000).

Exercise therapy appears to be the most often-used physical therapy intervention in treating people with back pain (Nachemson, 1990). It aims at abolishing pain, restoring and maintaining full range of motion, improving the strength and endurance of lumbar and abdominal muscles, thereby contributing to early restoration of normal function (Nachemson, 1990; Brukner and Khan, 1993). Additionally mechanical support to the low back which helps to obtain recovery with minimal chance of relapse is provided. Exercise training are often used improve function in low back rehabilitation and to prevent deconditioning of lumbar musculature, to prevent persistent low-back pain (Chok et al, 1999; Shiple, 1997). Jackson and Brown (1983) opined that exercises will decrease pain, strengthen muscles, decrease mechanical stress to spinal structures, improve fitness level, prevent injury, and improve posture and mobility in patients with low back pain. The exercise modes used by physiotherapists managing LBP patients include aerobic exercise, range of motion and stretching exercises and strengthening exercises for the trunk musculature (Brukner and Khan, 1993). Also balance training for better trunk and abdominal control, stabilization exercise and endurance exercises (Biering Sorenson, 1984; Foster and Fulton, 1991; Panjabi, 1992). In a study by Franca et al (2010) segmental stabilization and strengthening exercises effectively reduced pain and functional disability in individuals with chronic low back pain. Additionally segmental stabilization further improved transversus abdominus muscle activation capacity.

The role of exercise in back pain transcends all the phases of medical or health management namely preventive, curative and rehabilitative phases. It is probably the cheapest physiotherapeutic intervention and which gives the patient some measure of direct control over her treatment (Brukner and Khan, 1993). Exercise and movements cause alternate compression and relaxation of the articular cartilage, and ensure the movement of the synovial fluid into the articular cartilage as the area of pressure changes over the surface (Twomey, 1992). This allows for good health and optimal functioning of the articular cartilage. It also results in thicker, stronger ligaments that maintain their compliance and flexibility and that also become stronger at the bone-ligament-bone complex. The nutrition and health of the intervertebral discs is equally enhanced by exercises. Exercise also reduces the risk of developing osteoarthritis and osteoarthritic changes have been shown to begin only in areas where collagen is not often stressed by movement and pressure (Twomey, 1992). Exercises are done as mainstay of treatment to improve trunk stabilization. Exercises which results in proper muscle function will compensate for structural damages in spinal structure (Barr et al, 2005); nevertheless the deficits that have been defined in lumbar stabilization in patients with LBP seem to be mostly related to muscular and neurologic function.

Bone and muscle are both dynamic structures that respond positively to exercises and adversely to disuse (Mernard and Stanish, 1991). A strong inverse relationship exists between muscle mass and osteoporosis such that a decline in muscle mass is matched by an increasing fragility of bone. However the loss of muscle mass due to disuse can be substantially reversed by exercise training programme (Shepard, 1988, Menard and Stanish, 1991). It has hence been suggested that physiotherapists have the responsibility to include exercise as an essential part of prophylaxis and treatment in addition to other more passive treatment modalities such as massage, mobilization, manipulation and traction (Twomey, 1992).

Endurance of the back muscles is associated with LBP (Nourbakhsh and Arab, 2002). Endurance can be defined as the ability to perform prolonged bouts of work without experiencing much fatigue or exhaustion (Wilmore, 1982). It was similarly defined as the ability of a muscle to contract repeatedly or generate tension, sustain that tension, and resist fatigue over a prolong period of time (Delateur, 1982). It is probably the most underrated component of the total physical training program and is comprised of two different components (Wilmore, 1982) and is more important than strength in low back muscles training. Muscular or local endurance refers to the ability of an isolated muscle group to perform repeated contractions over a period to time (Kisner and Colby, 1996). This kind of endurance exercise is both rhythmical and repetitive in nature or static with resulting fatigue confined to the local group of muscles that is exercised (Wilmore, 1982). General or cardiovascular endurance is the ability to perform large dynamic exercise for long periods of time (Kisner and Colby, 1996). Muscular strength is to muscular endurance as development of the cardiovascular and respiratory system is to cardiovascular endurance (Wilmore, 1982). Endurance is mechanically defined as either the point of isometric fatigue, where the contraction can no longer be maintained at a certain level or as the point of dynamic fatigue, when repetitive work can no longer be sustained at a certain force level (Alaranta, 2000)

Endurance exercises incorporating the back extensors and the abdominal muscles have been proposed for use in the management of low back pain (Biering Sorenson, 1984; Foster and Fulton, 1991). This is possibly because individuals with greater levels of muscular strength and endurance and cardiovascular fitness tend to have fewer spinal problems (Cady et al, 1979; Mayer and Gatchel, 1988; and Nelson et al, 1995), and that trunk muscle endurance has been identified as a potential risk factor for the development of back pain (Biering Sorensen, 1984).

Chok et al (1999) reported that trunk endurance training reduced pain and improved function at 3 weeks after the onset of treatment in their study to evaluate the effectiveness of trunk extensor endurance training on pain and disability in subjects with sub-acute low back pain of 7 days - 7 weeks onset. Johannes et al (1995) compared the effects of intensive training of muscle endurance and a treatment protocol that emphasized coordination in the trunk and found that the two groups studied, improved in pain, disability and spinal mobility. Johnson et al (2010) compared the efficacy of McKenzie exercise, endurance training and endurance training and back care education and concluded that McKenzie exercise was effective in modulating long-term LBP and proposed that a combination therapy involving McKenzie exercise, endurance training with McKenzie exercise was more effective. Exercise training increases endorphins and alter perception of pain, perhaps by reducing anxiety and depression (Blumenthal et al, 1982). Identifying high or low muscular endurance has been reported to alert the patient and clinician to a need for possible modifications to the usual treatment regime (McIntosh et al, 1998).

Figures 4-12: Low Back Core Stabilization Exercises; 4-9 level one exercises; 10-12, level two exercises; Source: Dr. Douglas M.G. DC; http://www.chirogeek.com

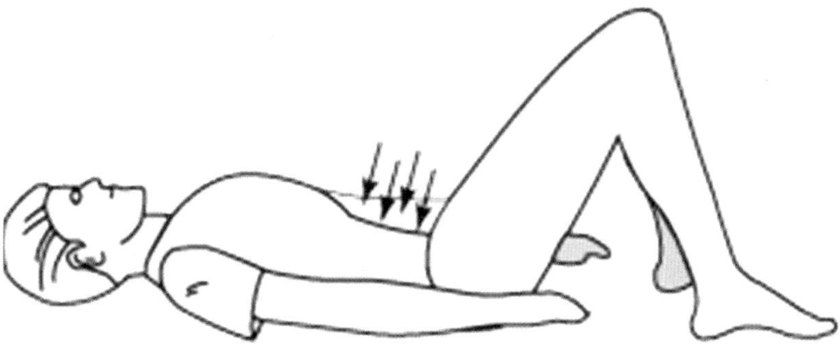

Fig. 4. Pelvic tilt: Exercise for the core spinal stabilizer transversus abdominus muscle

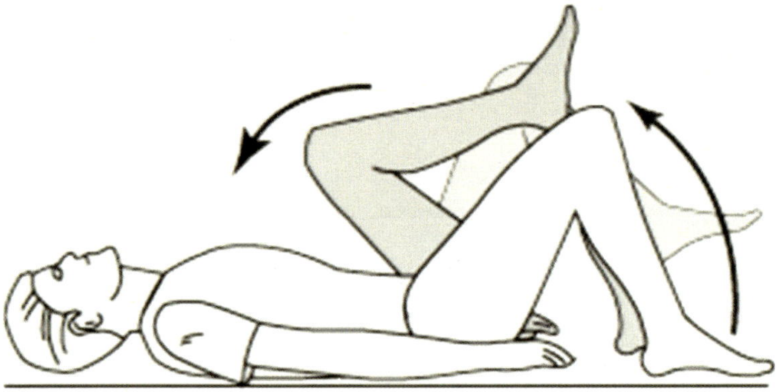

Fig. 5. Supine leg drag to the chest

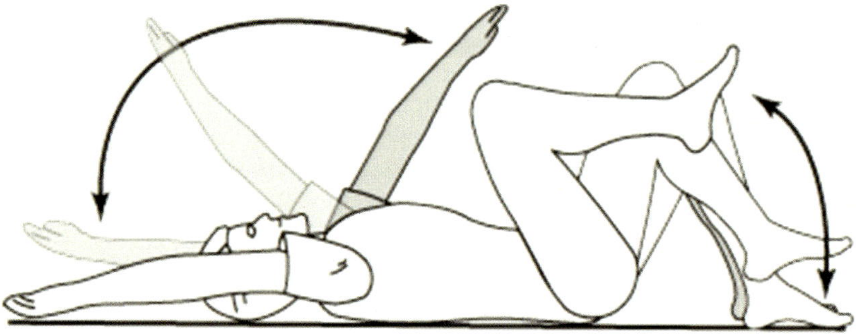

Fig. 6. Supine lying alternate arm and leg

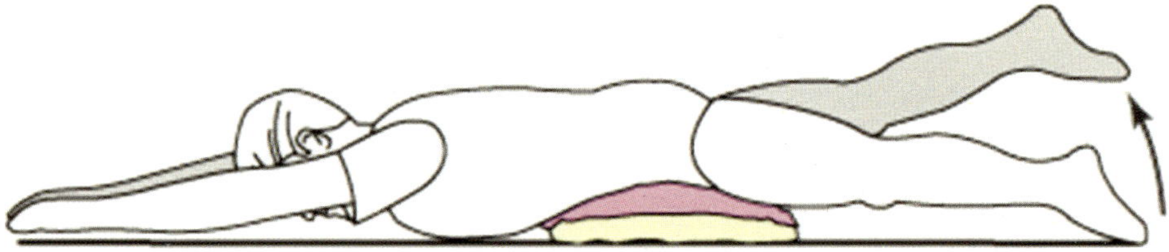

Fig. 7. Prone leg extension

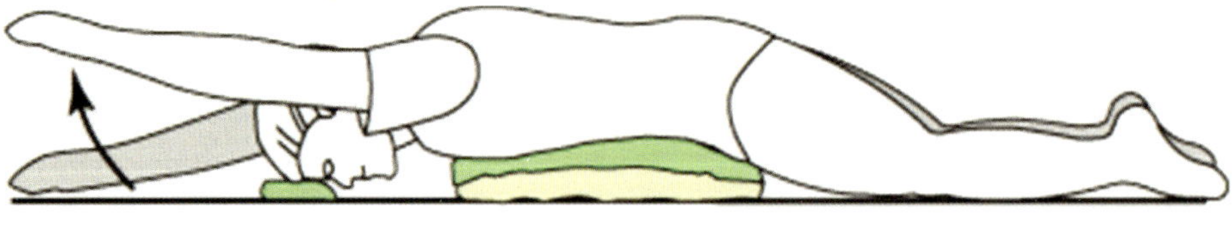

Fig. 8. Prone single arm extension

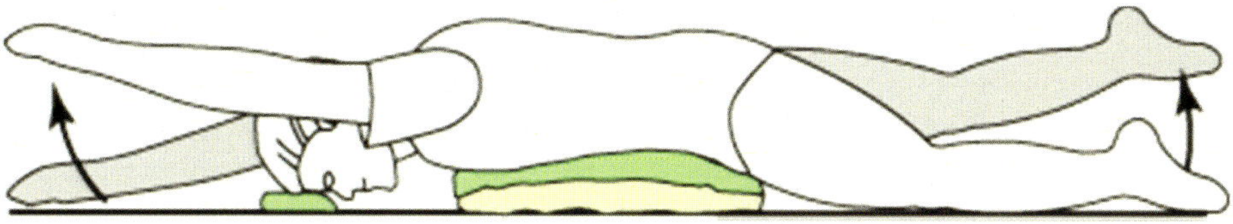

Fig. 9. Prone alternate arm and leg extension

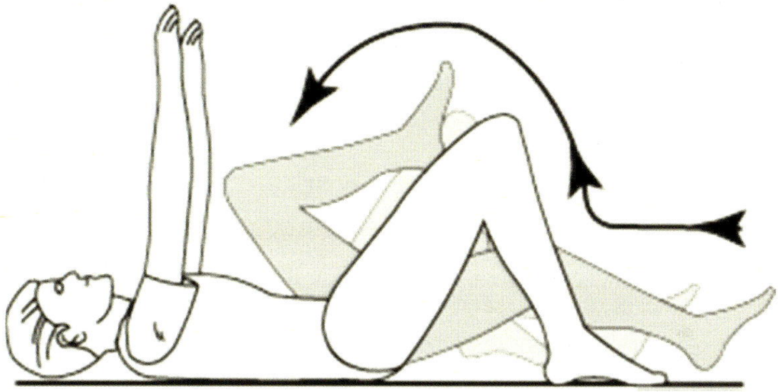

Fig. 10. Supine heel drag to extended arms

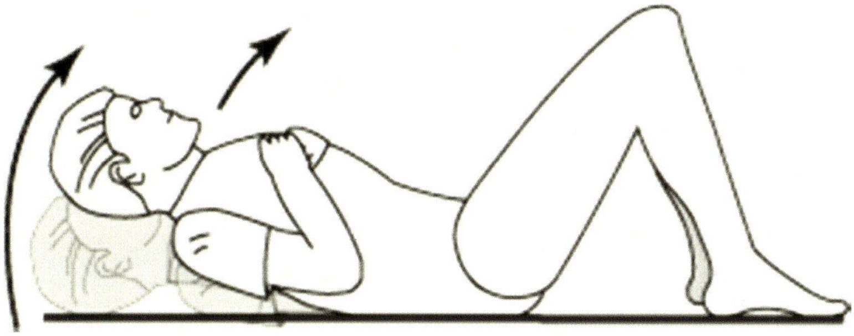

Fig. 11. Supine sit-up

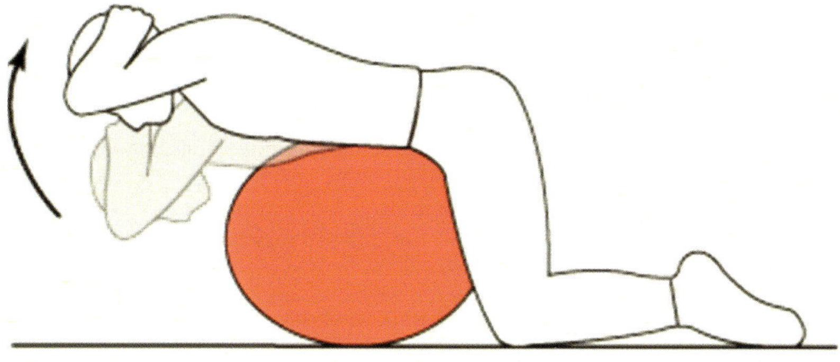

Fig. 12. Ball hyperextension

a. Manipulative Therapy

The application of controlled force to a joint, moving it beyond the normal range of motion in an effort to aid in restoring health is referred to as manipulation. It may be performed as a part of other therapies or whole medical systems, including chiropractic, massage, and naturopathy. It is a broad term encompassing massage, passive and active assisted range of motion and joint distraction or traction (Farell and Jensen, 1992). It was earlier proposed that manipulative therapy works by reducing subluxations, correcting vertebral mal-alignment, adjusting nuclear prolapse or tearing joint adhesion. However, evidence from studies reviewed by Twomey (1992) suggested a mechanism in which 'gapping' or separation of the joint surfaces by manipulation or movement would allow a piece of firm articular cartilage, caught between the articular surfaces the of the zygoapophyseal joint, blocking movements thereby returning the facet joint to its normal position. Studies have shown that spinal manipulation provides mild-to-moderate relief from low-back pain and appears to be as effective as conventional medical treatments (US DHHS, 2009). In a 2007 guidelines, the American College of Physicians and the American Pain Society included spinal manipulation as one of several treatment options to consider using when back pain does not improve with self-care. Spinal manipulation appears to provide relief from LBP at least over the short term (i.e., up to 3 months), and such effects may continue for up to 1 year. Nevertheless evidences in research are still under way to determine whether the effects of spinal manipulation depend on the duration and frequency of treatment.

Spinal manipulations are contra indicated in pateients with herniated discs resulting in or worsening cauda equina syndrome. Side effects of spinal manipulations minor discomfort in the treated area, headache, or tiredness. These effects usually go away in 1 to 2 days (US DHHS, 2009).

b. Back school

Back schools are health education programmes on back pain. Many back schools have been developed for different populations since 1969 when the first one was developed in sweden by Zachrison-forsell (Zachrison-forsell, 1980). The term "back school" implies providing information about the anatomy and function of the spine as well as advice on activities regarding prevention and self-treatment (Dihta, 1999); the teaching is carried out in group sessions. It is common to include instruction and practical guidance for exercise during back school sessions. The back school usually lasts approximately 4-6 hours. Often, the theoretical instruction is an integrated element of a comprehensive course of back rehabilitation, which also includes exercise programs. The integrated rehabilitation program is usually of 15-30 hours duration, spread over weeks to months (Dihta, 1999). Back school programs are usually led by physiotherapists, ergo therapists and relaxation therapists. The philosophy of the traditional back school was guided by "be careful" messages, such as; sit correctly, lift correctly, avoid forward bending, and so forth. In a modern back school the emphasis is to avoid fear, and the philosophy is to "ignore the pain as much as possible". This change in attitude has resulted in improved preventive results (Dihta, 1999).

A study compared high- and low-intensity back schools with usual care in occupational health care in Netherland, among workers sick-listed because of sub acute nonspecific low back pain (Heyman et al, 2006). The low-intensity back school was most effective in reducing work absence, functional disability, and kinesiophobia, and more workers in this group scored a higher perceived recovery during the 6-month follow-up. Akinpelu and Odebiyi (2004) determined the effect of a Nigerian back school model on some Nigerian industrial workers' knowledge of low back pain and back care and reported that the subjects' mean knowledge score increased significantly immediately and at 8 weeks after back school model administration. The authors therefore concluded that the back school model was effective in improving the workers' knowledge of LBP and back care. Also reports of Cochrane back reviewers (Heymans et al, 2004; Heymans et al, 2005) and a meta analysis (Maier and Harter, 2001) on the efficacy of back school versus sham diathermy and placebo was that back school was superior to sham diathermy and placebo for short term recovery and return to work and not for pain or long term recurrences. Authors have generally submitted that back school should be integrated into the other effective means of management e.g exercises. Daltroy et al (1997) designed an educational program modeled after several well-known back schools to reduce low back injuries among 4000 postal workers and observed increased knowledge among experimental unit workers, but no significant improvements in behaviours associated with back health or in proportion of workers with tired backs.

6. Back care education

An essential of physical therapy management is the education of patients with low back pain on appropriate musculoskeletal structures, functions and the basic pathology of the patient's problem, and lifestyle adaptation that may be necessary to prevent recurrence of LBP (Twomey, 1992). Teaching is necessary and professionally desirable as the active role of the physiotherapist in the management of back pain and other conditions (Sotosky, 1984). The five educational elements commonly used in physical therapy sessions are- teaching, provision of information about illness, instructions for home exercises, giving advice, information and counselling about stress related problems (Sluijis, 1991). Patients in back care programmes are made to understand age changes and their effects on the spine and the spine's vulnerability to stress under particular loading conditions. They are then given instructions on home exercises for back and advised on the best postures for activities in standing, sitting and even lying positions (Twomey, 1992).

7. Pain clinics in the management of LBP

Behavioral and cognitive behavioral, inpatient and outpatient multidisciplinary pain clinics are usually considered to be the last resort as a treatment option. This course of treatment usually is offered late in the course of chronic LBP, typically after the patient has adopted a disability lifestyle automated by refractory operant influences. True behavioral modification is most effectively accomplished in an inpatient setting, where all aspects of the patient's waking and sleeping activities can be structured and controlled. The cost of hospitalization and interdisciplinary services in this venue must be weighed against other economic factors, such as those related to further medical or surgical care, loss of productivity, and compensated disability (Wheeler, 2007). Cognitive-behavioral pain treatment programs are usually combined with a functional rehabilitation approach and prove to be a successful treatment for many (Wheeler, 2007). There are few studies on the use of pain clinics in the management of LBP, however Adam-Wilkey et al (2008) controlled trial compared outcomes in perception of pain and disability for a group of patients suffering with chronic LBP when managed in a hospital by either a regional pain clinic or a chiropractor and reported that reduction in mean pain intensity at the end of the study was 1.8 points greater for the chiropractic group than for the pain-clinic group.

I compared nineteen studies on effects of different physiotherapy regimens in the management of sub-acute and chronic mechanical LBP under the following headings viz: sample size, age and type of LBP, sampling technique and treatment methods which included duration of study, methods of treatment, and outcomes of the studies from 1985 to 2010. Two of the studies were done in the eighties, five in the nineties and nine in years two thousand and three till two thousand and ten. Sample sizes for the study were between thirty and two hundred and sixty. Most of the studies however involved approximately sixty individuals. Only one study, Petersen et al (2002) involved 148 subjects. Six of the studies were randomised clinical trials, quite a number assigned subjects into the groups randomly and four did not specify what they did. Subjects' age range fell between eighteen and seventy years. Although this is quite a wide range, most studies involved individuals from eighteen years to about forty to fifty five years. Only Risch et al (1993) involved an age range of twenty two to seventy years but a couple of other studies simply referred to their populations as adult populations. Most of the studies reviewed involved individuals with chronic LBP but , Chok et al, (1999), Petersen et al (2002) and Akosile et al (2006) involved individuals with , sub-acute, or both sub-acute and chronic LBP. Hides et al (2001) studied only individuals with acute LBP.

The least duration of any of these studies was 4 weeks; most of them took between 6-8 weeks and others above 8 weeks even up to 3 months. The vast array of the treatment methods had physiotherapy in form of exercises of different types including trunk muscle strengthening and endurance, McKenzie exercises, low impact aerobic exercise, spine stabilization. A study by (Nwuga and Nwuga, 1985), compared William's flexion exercise and McKenzie exercise and Akosile (2006) involved spine manipulation. Johnson et al, (2010) administered a combination treatment involving, McKenzie exercise, endurance training and back care education. Most studies incorporated back care education as baseline treatment and sometimes for comparison. Only four studies incorporated heat therapy in the management and only one study (Hides et al, 2001) involved medical management and this was the only study that involved subjects with acute LBP. It can be observed from these studies that most protocols of exercise were effective in the management of chronic LBP. The methods were not effective when it was either placebo or back care education solely or massage plus thermotherapy of some sort. These were however incorporated in some of the exercise protocols and the protocols were effective in the management of LBP. The only instance when exercise was not solely effective was in the study involving acute LBP (Hides et al, 2001). In this instance medical management was more effective in modulating acute LBP and stabilization exercise prevented recurrence of the LBP in the same study. Hides et al (2001) concluded that biomechanical research may explain why it is important to focus on particular muscles for their stabilizing functions in rehabilitation (Hides et al 2001). Franca et al (2010) reported superiority of segmental stabilization over strengthening exercise in combating muscle deactivation subsequent to episode of LBP. Muscle deactivation due to an episode of LBP has been implicated for recurrence of LBP.

8. Conclusion

Researchers have used exercises of various types in the management of LBP with varying degrees of successes but not many studies have been able to rate one exercise protocol over another in the management of chronic LBP and not so much is in place as to which exercise is favourable at either the sub-acute or chronic stages. Combination physiotherapy regimens involving exercise of different types, back care education, specific schools of thoughts have also been used in managing low back pain and authors have reported better clinical improvement with combination of regimens focusing not just on the disc or facet joint for pain modulation but also on muscles reconditioning and patient education. Psychosocial component of management must be in focus in chronic/long-term cases, although not much has been documented in this regard. Waddell and Watson (2004) reviewed rehabilitation interventions for LBP, analysed within a biopsychosocial framework to test the hypothesis that effective rehabilitation interventions should have all three biological, psychological and social elements to address all of the potential obstacles to recovery. They concluded that virtually all the interventions included some form of exercise or physical activity element aimed at addressing the biological problem and restore physical function. However, this physical element alone was insufficient to achieve return to work. Most successful interventions also addressed beliefs in one way or another, and many of them included some kind of occupational intervention (work hardening). Most of the programmes that did not explicitly address these latter two elements were unsuccessful in achieving return to work. This evidence appears to support the hypothesis that a rehabilitation intervention is more likely to produce successful vocational outcomes if it addresses all three bio-psycho-social elements of disability and obstacles to recovery in chronic/long term LBP. Back care education on the other hand has is accepted as an important adjunct to other physiotherapy procedures in the management of low back pain and not necessarily as solely an effective means of managing LBP (Daltroy et al, 1997; Lønn et al, 1999), and evidences supporting back school as sole treatment modality are weak. Endurance exercise however has been reported to be effective in preventing chronic/long-term LBP but has not been investigated in many randomized controlled trials. Optimal functioning of the muscle system is desirable to control and protect the spinal segments following injury. Despite initial resolution of painful symptoms, failure to protect spinal segments could increase the likelihood of a recurrence of symptoms. Specific exercise training targeting the back and abdominal muscles including the multifidus and transversus abdominus muscles have been shown to decrease pain and disability in chronic low back pain patients.

McKenzie's classification is a standardized approach of assessing LBP as it identifies a directional preference for spinal movement which can form basis for classification in treating LBP. When this approach like any other mobilization is used in combination with rehabilitation of the abdominal; and back muscles, much better outcomes may be realized in combating LBP, especially when it is sub-acute, chronic/long-term. Treatment should be individualized, and where group treatment is considered, classification should form the basis of grouping. Group exercise will improve patient interaction and participation which may further ensure better and more specified outcomes and forestall recurrence. Prevention strategies should be introduced early in life, hence more studies to look into low back pain in children and adolescents.

9. References

Abenhaim, L.; Rossignol, M.; Valat, J.P.; Nordin, M.; Avouac, B.; Blotman, F.; Charlot, J.; Dreiser, R.L.; Legrand, E.; Rozenberg, S.; Vautravers, P. (2000): The role of activity in the therapeutic management of back pain: report of the international Paris task force on back pain. *Spine*, 25(Suppl 4), S1–33.

Adam- Wilkey, D.C.; Michael-Gregory, M. B; David-Byfield, D.C.; Peter, W. M. (2008): A comparison between chiropractic management and pain clinic management for chronic LBP in a National Health Service Outpatient Clinic. *The Journal of Alternative and Complementary Medicine*, 14, 465–473.

Adegoke, B.O.A.; Babatunde, F.O. (2007): Effect of an exercise protocol on the endurance of trunk extensor muscles: a RCT. *Hong Kong Physiotherapy Journal*, 25, 2-9.

Akinpelu, A.O.; Odebiyi, D.O. (2004): Nigerian back school model: development and effect on industrial workers knowledge of back pain and back care. *African Journal of Medicine and Medical Sciences*, 33, 201-5.

Akosile, C. O.; Nwankwo, E. I.; Johnson, O.E.; Raji, F. S. (2006): Comparative Effect of Different McKenzie Extension Exercise - Based Protocols on Spinal Flexibility of Low Back Pain Patients. *Journal of International Council for Health, Physical Education Recreation, Sport and Dance* (*African Journal*), 1, 14-18.

Alaranta, H. (2000), Strength and Endurance testing, in: *The ClinicalApplication of Outcomes Assessment*, S.G. Yeoman Ed., Appleton and Lange, Stamford, Connecticut,158–162.

Barr K.P.; Griggs M.; Cadby T. (2005): Lumbar stabilization: Core concepts and current literature, part 1. *American Journal Physical Medicine and Rehabilitation*, 84:473–480.

Bergmark, A. (1989): Stability of the lumbar spine: A study in mechanical engineering. Acta *Orthopaedica Scandinavica Supplementum*, 230:1–54.

Biering-Sorenson, F. (1984): Physical Measurements as Risk Indicators for low back trouble over a one-year period. *Spine*, 9, 106 - 119.

Blumenthal, J. A.; Williams, R. S., Needels, T. L. (1982): Psychological Changes accompany aerobic exercise in healthy middle-aged adults. *Psychosomatic Medicine*, 44, 529-536.

Brukner, P; Khan, K. (1993): *Clinical Sports Medicine*. Sydney, McGraw-Hill, 264-289.

Cady, L.D, Bischoff, D.D.; O'Connell, E.R. (1979): Strength and fitness and subsequent back injuries in firefighters *Journal of Occupational Medicine*, 21(4):269-272.

Chok, B., Lee, R., Latimer, J.; Tan, S. (1999): Endurance training of the trunk extensor muscles in people with sub-acute LBP. *Physical Therapy*, 79 (11), 1032-1042.

Chou R. (2007): Nonpharmacologic therapies for acute and chronic low back pain: a review of the evidence for an American Pain Society/American College of Physicians clinical practice guideline. *Annals of Internal Medicine*, 147(7):492–504.

Daltroy, L.H., Iversen, M.D., Larson, M.G. Ryan, J. Zwerling, C. Fossel, A.H. ; Liang, M.H. (1997): A controlled trial of an educational program to prevent low back injuries. *New England Journal of Medicine* , 337, 322-328.

Da Silva, R.A.; Lariviere C.;Arsenault, A.B.,Nadeau S.,Plamondon, A. (2009): Pelvic stabilization/semi sitting position increase the specificity of back exercises. *Medicine and Science in Sports and Exercise*, 41,435-443

Delateur, B.J. (1982): Therapeutic exercise to develop strength and endurance, in: *Handbook of Physical Medicine and Rehabilitation*, 3rd ed., F.J. Kottke, G.K. Stillwell and J.F. Lehmann, Eds., Krusen's, WB Saunders, Philadelphia.

DIHTA, (1999): Low Back Pain; Frequency, management and prevention from an health technology assessment perspective. *Danish Health Technology Assessment*. 1,73,182-191.

Deyo, R.A.; Mirza, S.K.; Martin, B.I. (2006): Back pain prevalence and visit rates: estimates from U.S. national surveys, 2002. *Spine*, 31, 2724-7.

Donelson, R.; Silva, G; Murphy, K. (1990): Centralisation phenomenon, its usefulness in evaluating and treating referred pain. *Spine*, 15, 211-213.

Dunn, K.M., Croft, P.R. (2004): Epidemiology and natural history of low back pain. *Eur Med* 40(1):9–13.

Ehrlich G.E. (2003): Low back pain. *Bulletin of the World Health Organization*, 81 (9)

Farell, J.P.; Jensen, G.M. (1992): Manual therapy factors affecting pain and disability in low back pain: mechanism and assessment. *Physical Therapy*, 72, 843-852.

Farfan H.F. (1975): Muscular mechanism of the lumbar spine and the position of power and efficiency. *Orthopaedic Clinics of North America*, 6, 135–44

Feurstein, M.; Battie, P. (1995): Behavioral factors affecting pain and disability in low back pain: mechanism and assessment. *Physical Therapy*, 75, 267-280.

Foster, N.E.; Thompson, K.A.; Baxter, G.D.; Allen, J.M. (1999): Management of nonspecific low back pain by physiotherapists in Britain and Ireland: a descriptive questionnaire of current clinical practice. *Spine*, 24, 1332-1342.

Franca, F.R.; Burke, T.N.; Hanada, E.S.; Marques, A.P. (2010): Segmental stabilization and muscular strengthening in chronic low back pain-a comparative study. *Clinics*, 65, 1013-1017.

Frank, J.W.; Kerr, M.S.; Broker, A.S. (1996): Disability resulting from occupational low back pain, part 1 what do we know about primary prevention? A review of the scientific evidence on prevention before disability begins. *Spine*, 21, 2908-2917.

Frymoyer, J.W. (1988): Epidemiology. In: Frymoyer JW, Gordon SL, ed. New Perspectives in Low Back Pain. Illinois: *American Academy of Orthopaedic Surgeons*, 26–27

Furlan, A.D., Imamura, M., Dryden, T., Irvin, E. (2008) Massage for low back pain. *Cochrane Database Systematic Review*, 4, CD001929.

Gracey, J.H.; McDonough, S.M.; Baxter, G.D. (2002) Physiotherapy management of low back pain: a survey of current practice in Northern Ireland. *Spine*, 27, 406-11.

Hazard, R.G. (1996): Chronic low back pain and disability. The efficacy of functional restoration. *Bulletin of Hospital Joint Disease*, 55, 213-6.

Hayden, J. A.; van Tulder, M.W.; Malmivaara, A.V.; Koes, B.W.(2005): Meta analysis: exercise therapy for nonspecific low back pain. *Annals of Internal Medicine*, 142, 765–75

Heymans, M.W.; van Tulder, M.W.; Esmail, R.; Bombardier, C.; Koes, B.W. (2004): Back schools for non-specific low-back pain. *Cochrane Database Systematic Review*, CD000261.

Heymans, M.W.; van Tulder, M.W.; Esmail, R.; Bombardier, C.; Koes, B.W. (2005): Back schools for nonspecific low back pain: a systematic review within the framework of the Cochrane Collaboration Back Review Group. *Spine*, 30:2153-63.

Heymans, M.W.; de vet, H.C.; Bongers, P. M.; Knol, D.L.; Koes, B.W.; van Mechelen, W. (2006): The effectiveness of high-intensity versus low-intensity back schools in an occupational setting: a pragmatic randomized controlled trial. *Spine*, 31, 1075-82.

Hides, J.A.; Cooper D.H.; Stokes M.J. (1992): Diagnostic ultrasound imaging for measurement of the lumbar multifidus in normal young adults. *Physiotherapy Practice*, 8:19-26

Hides JA, Stokes MJ, Saide M, et al. (1994) Evidence of lumbar multifidus muscle wasting ipsilateral to symptoms in patients with acute/subacute low back pain. *Spine*,19,165–72.

Hides, J.A., Richardson, C.A., Jull, G.A. (1996): Multifidus muscle recovery is not automatic after resolution of acute first episode low back pain. *Spine*, 21, 2763–9.

Hides, J.A.; Jull, G.A.; Richardson, C.A. (2001): Long-term effects of specific stabilizing exercises for first-episode low back pain. *Spine*, 26, E243–8.

Hides J.; Stanton W.; McMahon S., Sims K. (2008): Effect of stabilization training on multifidus muscle cross-sectional area among young elite cricketers with low back pain *Journal of Orthopaedic and Sports Physical Therapy*, 38,101-108.

Hilde, G.; Hagen, K.B.; Jamtvedt, G.; Winnem, M.(2006): Advice to stay active as a single treatment for low-back pain and sciatica. *Database Systematic Review*, 2, CD003632.

Hodges, P.W.; Richardson C.A. (1996): Inefficient muscular stabilization of the lumbar spine associated with low back pain: a motor control evaluation of transversus abdominis. *Spine*, 21, 2640±2650

Hodges, P.W. (1999): Is there a role for the abdominis in lumbo-pelvic stability. *Manual therapy*, 4, 74-86.

Holmstr¨om, E., Moritz, U.; Andersson, M. (1992): Trunk muscle strength and back muscle endurance in construction workers with and without low back disorders, *Scandinavian Journal of Rehabilitative Medicine*, 24, 3–10.

Jackson, C.P.; Brown, M.D. (1983): Is there a role for exercise in the treatment of patients with low back pain? *Clinical Orthopaedics*, 179, 39-45.

Jackson, C.P.; Brown, M.D.(1983): Analysis of current approaches and a practical guide to prescription of exercise. *Clinical Orthopaedics*, 179, 46-54.

Jenkins, E.M.; Borenstein, D.G.; (1994): Exercise for low back patient: *Ballieres Clinical Rheumatology*, 8, 191-197.

Johannes, F; Remvig, L; Kryger, P.; Beck, P.; Warming, S.; Lybeck, K. Dreyer, V.; Larsen, L.H. (1995): Exercise for chronic low back pain: a clinical trial. *Journal of Orthopaedic and Sports Physiotherapy*, 22, 52-9.

Johnson, J. (2002): The Multifidus. Back Pain Solution. Canada, New Harbinger Publications Inc., 1—33.

Johnson, O.E., Mbada, C.E., Akosile, C.O., Agbeja, O.A. (2009): Isometric Endurance of the Back Extensors in School-Aged Adolescents with and without Low Back Pain. *Journal of Back and Musculoskeletal Rehabilitation*, 22, 205-211.

Johnson, O.E., Adegoke, B.O.A.; Ogunlade, S.O. (2010): Comparison of four Physiotherapy Regimens in the Treatment of Long -Term Mechanical Low Back Pain. *Japanese Journal of Physiotherapy Association*, 13, 9-16.

Kiefer A, Shirazi-Adl A, Parnianpour M. (1998): Synergy of the human spine in neutral postures. *European Spine Journal*,7,471-479.

Kent, P.M.; Keating J.L. (2005): *Chiropractor Osteopath*, 13, 13.

Kisner, C.; Colby, L.A. (1996): *Therapeutic Exercise*. New Delhi; India. Jaypee Brothers, 13-17, 113.

Lawrence, J.P.; Green, H.S., Grauner, J.N.(2006): Back pain in athletes. *Journal of American Academy of Orthopaedic Surgeons,* 14:726–35.

Lewis, A.; Morris, M.E.; Walsh, C. (2008): Arc physiotherapy exercises effective in reducing chronic low back pain *Physical Therapy Reviews*, 13, 37-44.

Li, L.C.; Bombardier, C. (2001): Physical therapy management of low back pain: an exploratory survey of therapist approaches. *PhysicalTherapy*,81, 1018-1028. Liddle, S.D.; Baxter, .G.D.; Gracey, J.H. (2004): Exercise and chronic low back pain: what works? *Pain*, 107, 176–90

Lønn, J.H., Glomsrød, B., Soukup, M.G., Bø, K., Larsen, S. (1999): Active back school: prophylactic management for low back pain: a randomized controlled 1-year follow-up study. Spine, 24: 865–871.

Luoto, S. Heliovaara, M., Hurri H.; Alaranta, H. (1995): Static back endurance and the risk of low-back pain, *Clinical Biomechanics*, 10, 323–324.

Low, P.R; Reed, A. (1994): *Electrotherapy Explained and Pactice*. 2nd ed., Oxford Butterworth Heinemann, 134-137.

Magee, D.J. (2002): *Lumbar spine, in: Orthopedic Physical Assessment*, 4th ed.Philadelphia, Elsevier Sciences, 467–566

Maier-Riehle, B.; Härter, M. (2001): The effects of back schools—a meta-analysis. *International Journal of Rehabilitation Res.*, 24, 199-206.

Manek, N.J.; MacGregor, A.J. (2005): Epidemiology of back disorders: prevalence, risk factors, and prognosis. *Current Opinion in Rheumatology*, 17, 134—140

Mannion, A.F.; Dolan, P. (1994): Electromyographic median frequency changes during isometric contraction of the back extensors to fatigue, *Spine*, 19(11), 1223–1229.

May, S.J. (2001): Patient satisfaction with management of back pain (Part 1). *Physiotherapy*, 187, 4-9.

Mayer, T.; Gatchel, R. (1988): Functional Restoration for Spinal Disorder: The Sport Medicine Approach Philadelphia. Lea 8 Febiger, 3-308.

Mbada, C.E.; Ayanniyi, O. (2008): Static back endurance in apparently healthy Nigerian adults, *Fizyoterapi Rehabilitasyon* 19, 30–36.

McGill, S. M. (1998): Low back exercises: Evidence for improving exercise regimens. *Physical Therapy*, 78, 754-765

McGill, S.M. (2002): Developing the exercise program, in: Low Back Disorders: Evidence-Based Prevention and Rehabilitation.Champaign, IL, Human Kinetics, 239–57.

McIntosh, G., Wilson, L., Affieck, F.; Hall, H. (1998): Trunk and lower extremity muscle endurance: normative data for adults, *Journal of Rehabilitative Outcome Measures*, 2, 20–39.

McKenzie, R. A. (1981):*The Lumbar Spine: Mechanical Diagnosis and Therapy Spinal Publication*. Waikanae; New Zealand. Spinal Publication Limited, 8- 120.

McArdle, W.D., Katch, F.I.; Katch, V.L. (1991): Training muscles to become stronger. *Exercise Physiology, Energy, Nutrition and Human Performance*. 4th ed., U.S.A., Lippincot; Williams and Wilkins, 429-430.

Menard, D.; Stanish, W.D. (1991): The aging athlete. *America Journal of Sport Medicine*, 17, 187-196.

Moffroid, M.T. (1997): Endurance Of Trunk Muscles In Persons With Chronic Low Back Pain: Assessment, Performance,Training. *Journal of Rehabilitation Research and Development*,

Moreau C.E., Green B. N., Johnson C.D.; Moreau S.R. (2001): Isometric back endurance tests: a review of the literature, *Journal of Manipulative and Physiological Therapeutics*, 24(2) 110–120.

Mulligan, B.R. (2004): Spinal mobilizations. *Manual Therapy*, 5th ed. New Zealand, APN Print Limited, 9-66.

Nachemson, A.L. (1990): Exercise; Fitness and Back Pain. In Bouchard R; and Shepherd R.J. (Eds). Exercise Fitness and Health: Consensus of Current knowledge; Campaign 111. Human Kinetics Incorporation.

Nelson, B.; O' Reilly, E.; Miller, M.; Hogan J.M.; Wegner, J.; Kelly, C. (1995): The clinical effects of intensive specific exercise on chronic low back pain: a controlled study of 895 consecutive patients with 1 yr follow-up. *Orthopaedcis*, 18,971-981.

Nourbakhsh, M.R.; Arab, A.M. (2002): Relationship between mechanical factors and incidence of low back pain. *Journal of Orthopaedic and Sports Physical Therapy*,32,447-460.

Nwuga, V.C.B. (1976): Manipulation of the spine. Baltimore, Williams and Wilkins, 99–105.

Nwuga, G.; Nwuga, V. (1985): Relative therapeutic efficacy of the Williams and McKenzie protocols in back pain management. *Physiotherapy Practice*, 1, 99–105.

Nwuga, V.C.B. (2007): A review of history and schools of thought. *Manual Treatment of Back Pain*. 2nd ed. Nigeria, Williams Publishers, 4-18.

Omokhodion, F.O. (2002): Low back pain in a rural community in South West Nigeria. *West African Journal Medicine*, 21, 87–90.

Panjabi, M.M. (1989): Abumi, K.; Duranceau, J.; Oxlandn, T. (1989): Spinal stability and intersegmental muscle forces. A biomechanical model. *Spine*, 14, 194-200.

Panjabi, M.M. (1992): The stabilizing system of the spine: Part 1. Function, dysfunction, adaptation, and enhancement. *Journal of Spinal Disorders*, 5, 383–89; discussion, 397

Panjabi, M.M. (1992): The stabilizing system of the spine Part II. Neutral zone and instability hypothesis. *Journal of Spinal Disorders*, 5, 390-396; discussion 397.

Petersen, T.; Kryger, P.; Ekdahl, C.; Olsen, S.; Jacobsen, J.; (2002): The effects of Mckenzie therapy as compared with that of intensive strengthening training for the treatment of patients with sub acute or chronic low back pain. *Spine*, 15, 172-179.

Pollock, M.L.; Wilmore, J.H (1990): *Exercise in Health and Disease. Evaluation and prescription for Prevention and Rehabilitation*. Philadelphia W.B Saunders, 439-472.

Porter R.W. (1993): *The Upright Man; Management of Back Pain*.2nd Ed. Longman, Singapore Publisher (Plc)Ltd.,3-299.

Richardson, C.A.; Jull, G. A. (1995): Muscle control–pain control. What exercises would you prescribe? *Manual Therapy*, 1, 2–10.

Risch, S.V.; Norvell, N.K.; Pollock, L.M. (1993): Lumbar strengthening in chronic low back pain patients: physiologic and psychological benefits. Spine, 18, 232-238.

Roach, K. E. Brown, M. D.; Albin, R.D. (1997): The Sensitivity and Specificity of Pain response to activisty and position in categorizing patients with low back pain. *Physical Therapy*. 77(7): 730 - 738.

Robinson, R. (1992): The new back school prescription: stabilization training Part I. *Occupational Medicine: State of the Art Reviews*, 7, 17±31

Sahrmann, S.A. (2002): Movement impairment syndromes of the lumbar spine, in: *Diagnosis and Treatment of Movement Impairment Syndromes*. St. Louis, Mosby, 51–119

Safrit, M.J.; Wood, J.M. (1995): *Introduction to Measurement in Physical Education and Exercise Sciences*. 3rd ed. Missouri, Mosby, 449-50, 642-643.

Shepherd, R.T. (1998): Exercise for the elderly; cardiovascular function and aging. *Patient Management*; 1218, 103-123.

Shiple, B.J. (1997): Treating low-back pain. Exercise knowns and unknowns. *The Physician and Sports Medicine*, 25.

Sluijis, E.M. (1991): Patients education in physiotherapy towards a planned approach. *Physiotherapy*, 77, 503-508.

Sotosky, M.L. (1992): Physical Therapists attitude toward teaching. *Physical Therapy*, 64, 347-350.

The Back Letter (2001): How much of the risk of low back pain disorders is preventable. *The Back Letter*, 16, 29.

Truchon M. (2001): Determinants of chronic disability related to low back pain: Towards an integrative biopsychosocial model. *Disability and Rehabilitation*, 23, 758–767.

Twomey, L.T. (1992): A rationale for the treatment of back pain and joint pain by manual therapy. *Physical Therapy*, 72, 885-892.

Udermann, B.E., Mayer, J.M., Graves, J.E.; Murray, S.R. (2003): Quantitative Assessment of Lumbar Paraspinal Muscle Endurance,*Journal of Athletic Training*, 3, 259–262.

United States Department of Health and Human Services (2009): Get the facts; spinal manipulations for low back. *National Institute of Health; National Centre for Complementary and Alternative Medicine*, 1-6.

van Tulder, M.W.(2001):Treatment of low back pain: myths and facts.*Schmerz*,15,495-503.

van Tulder, M.W.; Tuut, M.; Pennick, V.; Bombardier, C.; Assendelft, W.J.J. (2004): Quality of primary care guidelines for acute low back pain. *Spine*, 29, E357-E362.

van Tulder, M.W.; Becker, A.; Bekkering, T.; Breen, A.; Teresa, M.; del Real, G.; Hutchinson, A.; Koes B.; Laerum, E.; Malmivaara, A. (2009): European guidelines for the management of acute nonspecific low back pain in primary care on behalf of the cost B13 Working Group on Guidelines for the Management of Acute Low Back Pain in Primary Care.

Volinn, E. (1997): The epidemiology of low back pain in the rest of the world; a review of surveys in low- and middle-income countries. *Spine*, 22, 1747–54.

Waddell, G.; Bryn-Jones, M. (1994): British sickness and invalidity benefit for back incapacities 1953–54 to 1991–92. In: Refshauge KM, Gass EM. (eds) Musculoskeletal Physiotherapy, London: Butterworth-Heinemann, 278-9.

Walker, B. F. (2000): The Prevalence of Low Back Pain: A Systematic Review of the Literature from 1966 to 1998. *Journal of Spinal Disorders*, 13, 205–217.

Wheeler, A.H. (2007): Pathophysiology of chronic low back pain. In Eds. Schneck M.J.; Talavera, F.; Halsey,J.M.; Baker,M.D.;Loernzo, N. *emedicine*, 1-53.

Wilke, H.J.; Wolf, S.; Claes, L.E.; Arand, M.; Wiesend, A. (1995): Stability increase of the lumbar spine with different muscle groups. A biomechanical in vitro study. *Spine*, 20, 192-198.

Wilmore, Y.H. (1982): *Training for Sport and Activity*. 2nd ed.; Boston Allyn and Bacon inc. 17, 34-69, 116, 236-238.

Zachrisson-Forssell, M. (1980): The Swedish back school. *Physiotherapy*, 66,112-114.

10

Physiotherapy Treatment on Chronic Non Specific Low Back Pain

A.I. Cuesta-Vargas, M. González-Sánchez,
M.T. Labajos-Manzanares and A. Galán-Mercant
Department of Psychiatry and Physiotherapy, University of Malaga, Spain

1. Introduction

1.1 Physiotherapy in acute low back pain

While it is true that back pain is defined as pain or discomfort located in the bottom of the ribcage and the top edge of the buttock, based on the time course in which you are (acute, subacute or chronic), how to act on them, bound to have different approaches for a maximization of results.

With regard to the different methods of intervention it has to comment that much has been said for years about the effect of bed rest as a strategy for improving low back pain symptoms. However, it was found that is equal or less effective than a placebo treatment or no treatment and may become a risk for chronicity process from acute low back pain [1-8].

By contrast, an active lifestyle, seems to favor the reduction of pain, time to return to work and disability rather than bed rest. It has also been shown to maintain this level of activity promotes a faster recovery, reducing the risk of relapse and more chronic pathology. However, when attempting to go beyond the trigger level, introducing therapeutic exercises as part of treatment, we observe that the results are equal to or worse than any other conservative treatment[1,8-11]. Moreover, therapeutic exercise is not advised in many clinical practice guidelines from different countries as a means of intervention in the early stages of low back pain episode[1,3,4,12-16].

On the other hand, the use of analgesics in clinical practice guidelines from different states, we recommend the use of paracetamol and NSAIDs (in that order) [1,3,17-19] for the treatment of acute low back pain, suggesting the use of muscle relaxants in cases where the other two types of drugs have not been effective[20,21].

There is a slight controversy regarding the use of spinal manipulation as a mode of intervention in acute low back pain, as it is not entirely clear whether or not it is advisable to use in this state of pathology[22]. Faced with such an open debate, we understand that it would be necessary to analyze each case individually so far there is consensus in the way of intervention.

On the other hand, there are two very well-identified interventions that suggest they are used as a treatment to be performed in a second stage of acute low back pain (LBP subacute) aimed at preventing chronicity more than the relief of symptoms of acute low back pain. These two modes of intervention are back school and multidisciplinary treatments[1,2325].

Thus, in acute low back pain, it is observed at the base of treatment are three aspects that are crucial for clinical success:

- One is to provide the patient with adequate information, an overemphasis on the fact that back pain is not too serious problem, the evolution in most cases the evolution is directed toward a rapid recovery and return to daily life . In this part of treatment is recommended to make it easier for the patient increase awareness about your pain, trying to be supportive and helps to eliminate the negative stigma of this disease skeletal muscle. This will important that there is consistency in message among all clinicians who work with the patient.
- Provide adequate control of symptoms.
- Advise patient to try to keep an active lifestyle and return to normal life, including his working life as soon as possible.

1.1.1 Identifiers in acute chronic low back pain

As defined, low back pain was defined as pain or discomfort that is located between the bottom of the ribs and the top of the buttocks, with or without radiation to the lower limbs. As in other musculoskeletal disorders, there are three stages of low back pain attending to issues of temporality, acute, subacute and chronic.

There have been several studies whose aim was to identify those signs or variables that may help predict a patient's eventual evolution toward chronicity. To this end, the authors have been gradually moving away from the biomedical model to observe the patient from a broader perspective, the bio-psycho-social.

In literature, there is a lot of factors that may influence patients with acute LBP, however, have identified a number of them appear to be correlated with increased likelihood of more chronic musculoskeletal this pathology. These factors, mainly psychological and occupational, have proved more reliable as predictors of chronic low back pain. These indicators, identified by Melloh et al. (2008)[27] (Figure 1) should be taken into account by professional therapists and clinicians working with these patients and include them as areas that should be involved in the treatment plan.

- Characteristics or working conditions.
- Impact on the role or on DLA.
- Issues related to pain.
- Medical considerations.
- Depression.
- Strategies of response to pain.
- Fear of beliefs about the disease.
- Social or emotional support.

Image 1. predictors of chronicity by Melloh.

1.2 Low back pain clasifications

85% of low back pain who are diagnosed are performed without an objective test anatomical/radiological abnormality detected[28,29]. People suffering from this disorder suffer musculoskeletal LBP.

Optimal treatment remains a great mystery, but there are some randomized trials suggest some improvement of which is scientifically proven. Nevertheless, it was found that people with LBP, have impaired motor control, which varies greatly depending on each person[30].

The approach is now more accepted in the scientific community is one that is based on the diagnosis for a classical determination, noting how the loss of motor control itself or as a result of secondary pathology.

This diagnostic process places great emphasis on the conclusion between the subject's history, radiology, pain behavior, physical examination findings as well as significant pathology (red flags) and psychological (yellow flags), including negative beliefs, stress anxiety, catastrophizing, depression[31,32], ...

One of the key that has changed the concept of LBP is to observe the musculoskeletal imbalance from a bio-psycho-social, which is currently accepted and widespread. So based on this approach, this motor response can be classified into three distinct groups[32]:

- Group 1: subjects whose response is adapted motor control and is secondary to an underlying disease process.
- Group 2: subjects with secondary response is due to a psychological and / or social, not organic.
- Group 3: subjects that offer a maladaptive response following a load on the tissue that is abnormal and leads to ongoing pain and anguish.

On the other hand, Dankaers (2011)[31] has identified some distinct patterns based on the direction where the motion is lost, where motor control is working properly motor control. This identifies the inflection patterns, active and passive extension, lateral tilt and multi-directional patterns. It has also been demonstrated as well-trained physiotherapists and doctors are able to differentiate the subjects and subclassified into these different groups.

1.3 Physiotherapy in chronic low back pain

Physiotherapy or physical therapy is a health science dedicated to study the life, health, illness and death of human beings from the standpoint of human body movement. It's characterized by search for the proper development of functions that produce the body's systems, where his performance good or bad, affects the human body or kinetic movement. It Intervene when human beings have lost or are at risk of losing or alter temporarily or permanently the proper motion and thus physical function by using scientifically proven techniques.

The World Health Organization (WHO) defines physical therapy in 1958 as "the science of treatment through: physical, therapeutic exercise, massage and electrotherapy. In addition, the Physiotherapy involves performing electrical tests and manuals to determine the value of involvement and muscle strength tests to determine functional abilities, range of joint movement and vital capacity measures and diagnostic aids for the control of evolution".

Given this reality, this discipline would possess all the credentials to treat low back pain from a conservative viewpoint successfully and safely. However, it is necessary to consider the spectrum of affection from low back pain that this disease does not always present a homogenous condition, but the severity of the condition may limit the person slightly, since this would suffer localized pain, or much more severe, preventing it to perform any work activity, with significant socioeconomic implications, particularly in developed countries. This musculoskeletal problem has an impact on many aspects of the person, such as quality of life, mobility, more likely to suffer long-term diseases, increased risk of social exclusion due to an inability to work, reduced income, isolation due to social disability.

Thus, low back pain is presented as a pathology that can be a considerable burden on the individual, their families, society and the economy (through loss of working days, or even the need to apply for retirement advance). Given this reality, the objectives of interventions and conservative treatments carried out through physical therapy, should be oriented towards reducing the symptoms of this dysfunction, such as pain management and disability, reducing anxiety states, trying to minimize the risk of recurrence and the time required for re-entry into the work.

This discipline has innumerable health tools that can be understood as a means of intervention in patients with chronic musculoskeletal disorders in general and low back pain in particular. This intervention strategies which a therapist can use are numerous: therapies, cognitive therapies that help pain management, complementary therapies, orthotics, physical therapy, electrotherapy, exercise, education, back school, some treatments invasive, such as acupuncture or postural ergonomics, for example.

While all of these alternative therapies are an option a priori for this clinician, not all these methods of intervention are equally effective. So this chapter will attempt to make a proposal for intervention based on scientific evidence demonstrating the effectiveness of each of the chosen methodologies, prompting the therapist to perform an exercise of reflection and selection techniques that may be more effective in their daily practice.

2. Patient assessment, diagnosis, prognosis and treatment: Clinical history

2.1 Introduction

An initial assessment can clarify the diagnosis of chronic low back pain or less. In the physical therapy a way that is nonspecific, ie not caused by a diagnosed disease, such as cancer, fracture, ankylosing spondylitis or other inflammation, though hardly reach the specific lumbalcias exceed six weeks of evolution, as is usually the early diagnosis of the cause of it.

2.2 History

For a complete patient assessment, it is important an adequate and exhaustive examination. The correct diagnosis depends on knowledge of functional anatomy, an accurate history of the patient, diligent observation and a complete examination. Accurate diagnosis is only established by a comprehensive assessment that includes the above factors. The purpose of the assessment must be to understand fully and clearly the patient's problems and the physical basis of the symptoms that cause them discomfort. All patients with chronic low back pain should have a history and examination that should be performed in acute and subacute stages of the disease. However, a clinical examination should be performed also in the chronic phase, the first objective should focus on the location of calls red flags, to access the yellow flags and then make a specific diagnosis. However, it is well accepted that low back pain, sometimes it is not possible to reach a diagnosis based on the pathological changes detected, because too many diagnostic systems have been proposed in which back pain is categorized based on the distribution of pain, pain behaviour, clinical signs, disability, ecc[33].

The aspect that has to be prioritized is to ensure that the pain is musculoskeletal in origin. The next step is to exclude the presence of specific pathologies of the spine. While the first suspect should appear in the medical history, we can get confirmation of the diagnosis through a thorough analysis of the individual[33]. The red flags such as neoplasms, infections, the syndrome of the cauda equina (cauda equina) are often difficult to find at this stage of the disease, however it is important to rule out a priori any of these options. The examiner should have sufficient knowledge to detect and diagnose major structural changes, deformities and serious spinal conditions. The patient should help the therapist to identify the type of pain and suffering the distribution. Clinical examination should provide confirmation that the patient complains of symptoms. If this were not the case, the type of pain should be classified as non-specific. It is also important to identify psychosocial yellow flags calls because they are factors that increase the risk of developing or perpetuating chronic pain, lengthening the time of disability suffered by the patient and, eventually, loss of working days the symptoms associated with produced by low back pain. Within these warning signs should be included inadequate skills in reference to back pain, (such as the patient to override a passive treatment by understanding that the assets will be lower), inappropriate behavior in terms of pain, being afraid to move and thus to progressively reduce the level of activity, work-related problems such as low job satisfaction or emotional problems may be clear examples of psychosocial yellow flags[34].

2.3 Physical examination

It is recommended that the diagnosis of triage in the first assessment and subsequent reassessments to exclude specific pathologies of the spine and nerve root. However, it seems advisable not spinal palpation and the use of motion tests in the diagnosis of low back pain. This recommendation is based on moderate evidence exists about the validity of the test of straight leg raising. This same level of evidence would say that there is no single test that has high sensitivity and specificity in the diagnosis of ankylosing spondylitis, a radiculopathy or spinal cancer. On the other hand, always based on moderate evidence, one could say that the pain provocation tests are more reliable than palpation tests. This has not been established as valid and reliable palpation tests, provided they are used for diagnosis, the presence of a manipulable lesion remains hypothetical[35,36].

2.4 Further exploration

Images are often used in patients with low back pain radicular pain assessment or identify any signs of serious alarm (red flag) and objective. The most common tests of diagnostic imaging in primary care centers usually plain radiography, bone scan, computed tomography (CT) and magnetic resonance imaging (MRI). In general, the reference to the image must be based on a specific indication, although it is true that sometimes the patient arrives at the physical therapist once you have completed all the diagnostic tests, but it has the opportunity to participate in this regard[37-39].

Of all diagnostic tests, radiography, its low cost and availability, is the most common, from a front, rear or side. This test allows us to precisely analyze the vertebral body height, alignment of the disc, and other morphological aspects of bone, however limited it to perform an analysis of the soft tissue structures. So despite the fact that other perspectives would be useful in the diagnosis of other rheumatic diseases, for diagnosis of low back pain, radiography would not be the best option, as it only allows an assessment of structural alterations[40].

For the evaluation of the warning signs of soft tissue, MRI is the best option for the precision it offers, in addition to be suffering a slow but steady expansion which makes it more and more evidence is available[39].

2.5 Physiotherapy diagnosis

A diagnosis is a common task for all healthcare professionals involved in treating patients, not just doctors, and in itself is not a medical act. The medical diagnosis is an important element but is not sufficient information to direct the physiotherapist. Physiotherapy diagnosis is an opinion based on rational critical analysis of all available information. It is imprencindible, therefore the incorporation of an evaluation, analysis and interpretation, own of the physiotherapist to guide him /her in planning therapeutic interventions, prevention and education and / or training the patient or user of their services. It is not, as the aforementioned decision, to "diagnose illnesses," it is an exclusive competence of the physician[36].

The physiotherapist has an important role in the functionality of the neuro - musculo – skeletal system and will need further evaluation within this framework. Thus, physiotherapy diagnosis should be formulated from the significant data on the patient's problems, as reflected in the common history. This history bio-psycho-social help each multidisciplinary team with the patient care. In addition and from a specific perspective, the diagnosis should be based also on an examination or assessment to assess the level of functional impairment of the patient as well as an explanation for the origin of such involvement.

Professional practice in physiotherapy involves processes and procedures among which the evaluation process, through which the therapist organizes its resources to learn and understand the patient's health condition from a motor and functional[36].

2.6 Prognosis

When speaking of prognosis in patients with low back pain, it is necessary to refer to those factors that help predict the evolution of the pathology and, therefore, those variables that help to predict future trends or events such as the return to work, the cost of the intervention, disability or the evolution of pain the patient suffers. Among these factors, the individual character and psychosocial professionals play an important role in the persistence of symptoms and disability. Thus, after analyzing several studies, one could argue with strong evidence that workers who suffer acute back pain and work in places where they have to bend over constantly, have a higher risk of more chronic such alteration. Also, with the same degree of evidence, one could argue that people with low back pain for at least 4 weeks, have more trouble working back to normal and the lower the effectiveness of clinicians when the patient been absent during that period of his job.

It can be said, moreover, that there is moderate evidence that specific evidence of the physical examination are of great prognostic value in chronic low back pain Thus, a prognosis of evolution of acute low back pain sub-acute to chronic, with moderate evidence, there are greater expectations of this happening when the patient psychosocial distress, depressive mood, severity of pain and functional impact and extreme symptom report, patient expectations, and previous episodes of back pain. And also maintaining the level of evidence could be considered predictors of chronicity the shorter length of labor, radicular or performing heavy work without modification[35].

2.7 Physiotherapy treatment

In a patient who suffers chronic back pain, a physiotherapist must do an exercise of reflection and try to plan your intervention based on two fundamental aspects: the symptomatological and functional. This could open a small internal debate about what should the clinician prioritize and possess both relative and absolute importance very important.

The wide range of therapeutic options held by the therapist, makes the customization of treatment as long as possible, should be a priority to tackling and improve musculoskeletal disorder that led to that person to the therapist.

As has been shown that chronic musculoskeletal involvement has a spectrum of influence that goes far beyond his own person, with repercussions on the family, society and employment. This problem should not go unnoticed by the physiotherapist and delegate, as far as possible in other health professionals if the situation closely, try to give a solution born of the subject and affect their environment but also to walk the opposite direction, the environment impact on the subject itself.

2.8 Ultrasound and low back pain

In recent years, the use of ultrasound (U.S.) has been progressively extended, due to its economy, reliability, relative ease of use and accessibility. Specifically in the back, although it has shown the importance of the deep back muscles by neurophysiological and biomechanical. Ultrasound is gradually taking a greater presence and are identifying themselves as a very useful tool for the assessment and treatment of patients with low back pain[41-47].

This instrument has been used for quantitative assessments using static and dynamic images to understand the morphology and behavior during muscle contraction on both parasespinal and abdominal belt muscles. They have observed changes in muscle architecture based on the intensity and duration of the contraction, allowing use by a researcher to analyze the behavior of muscle as well as instruments of feedback to the patient[49,50].

While there has been the usefulness of this instrument, it is important to consider the location, the positioning of the operator with respect to the patient to make a record and therefore a correct interpretation of the image[51].

Studies on a static muscle is important for different important aspects of it, such as differences in the edges of the muscle, so that it can be studied by analyzing the relationship between cross-sectional area, and other aspects like morphology, subject's BMI, pennation angle, shape, thickness ... These same records can be made in the same way during both isometric and isotonic contraction, being able to see how it changes as the muscle changes the intensity of contraction, the time of the same or the angle of the two bones in which it is inserted[49-52].

Ultrasound has proven to be a tool with reliability comparable to that of nuclear magnetic resonance, however, the latter does not have the ability to analyze the muscle during an isokinetic contraction. Reference has been used as electromyography, showing a curvilinear relationship on parameters that can be obtained with ultrasound, as the muscle thickness or pennation angle, so that it could be possible suggest the use of ultrasound, in both the clinical and research[51].

3. Evidence based physiotherapy: What are most effective interventions?

3.1 Introduction

The evidence-based physiotherapy (EBP) is a current focus on teaching and health practice, which emphasizes the importance of examining the evidence from research, careful interpretation of clinical information derived from unsystematic observations, and where understanding of the pathophysiology of disease is insufficient for quality clinical practice[53,54]. "The practice of evidence-based physical therapy should be informed primarily by the research of high quality, patient preferences and knowledge of physical therapists"[55].

Under the current definition of the FBE there are some additional factors that interact with the quality research, knowledge and practice of patient preferences, these factors are culture, politics, resources, ecc. So they are who will determine the specific context on which the decision applies.

The FBE clinical practice is an attempt to respond to this new situation, mainly through three strategies: learning methodology, the pursuit and implementation of abstracts and scientific information gathered by others and the acceptance of protocols and guidelines developed tested by third parties. The exercise of the FBE would not be such without the consideration of each situation and each scenario. On the other hand, the roles in the relationship between professionals and patients are variable, and there is a clear demand for direct participation of patients in decision making[55].

The FBE can be applied in daily work with any type of physiotherapy intervention, whether diagnostic, therapeutic or preventive and may be a useful tool for assessing the results of these interventions (Herbert, 2000), because it helps optimize the time of professional application criteria can accumulate in different scenarios and / or patients, improving accessibility to information and helps to reduce uncertainty. Also, when our expertise and daily practice does not follow the recommendations of the literature, the decision finally will be more likely to adopt proven and reasoned. The suggestions will be stronger if one is aware of the extent and strength of recommendations regarding an intervention.

3.2 Evidence-Based Physiotherapy (EBP)

Different scales have been used when classifying the different types of studies consulted. Thus, those involving an intervention, we used the proposed assessment by PEDro, which classifies studies according to internal validity on a scale of 0 to 10, which uses the following evaluation points, which add a point to the validity of the study for each one that is confirmed. The trials achieved a score equal to or greater than 5 were considered high quality[57]. The criteria used were:

1. Subjects Were Allocated randomly to groups (in a crossover study, subjects randomly Were Allocated an Treatments Which Were in order received)
2. Allocation concealed WAS
3. Were the groups similar at baseline regarding the Most Important Prognostic Indicators
4. There Was blinding of all subjects
5. There Was blinding of all therapists Who Administered the therapy.
6. There Was blinding of all Assessors Who Measured at least one key outcome.
7. Measures of outcome at least one key Were Obtained from More Than 85% of the subjects initially allocated to groups.
8. All subjects for Whom Were available Outcome Measures The Treatment Received or Allocated as condition or control, where, This Was not the case, data for at least one key outcome WAS analyze by "intention to treat"
9. The results of between-group Statistical Comparisons are at least one report for key outcome
10. The study Provides Both point Measure and Measures of variability for at least one key outcome

Thus, the quality of the methodology used in a systematic review (SR) was evaluated by Oxman and Guyatt index. On a scale of 0 to 7, those who scored higher than 5 were considered high quality, while its value was less than the index, were classified as low quality.

Thus, it is classified according to levels of evidence based on evidence levels for the treatments are classified according to the following classification[58]:

- Level A (strong): the results are drawn from a high quality systematic review consists of multiple randomized controlled trials (RCT) of high quality.
- Level B (moderate evidence): results of a systematic review consists of randomized controlled trials (RCT) of low quality.
- Level C (limited or conflicting evidence): derived from a clinical trial (high or low quality) or a systematic review of several RCT inconsistent results.
- Level D (without evidence): No RCTs were identified.

Thus, taking as base the strength of evidence consulted, there have been a series of statements in which roughly suggests the use of a particular methodology or intervention technique.

3.3 Clinical evidence of physical agents in physiotherapy

- **Interferential Therapy**. Defined as the surface application of medium frequency alternating current to cause low frequencies to 150 Hz There is no evidence on the effectiveness of using this therapy compared with placebo treatment in low back pain, although there is limited evidence about the similarity of effects caused by lumbar traction, massage and interferential therapy in chronic low back pain[59,60].

- Laser therapy: surface application of laser wavelength of 632-904 nm. Optimal treatment parameters (wavelength, dose, dose intensity) are uncertain. When analyzing the effect of this therapy as a means of reducing low back pain there is conflicting evidence about it[61,62].
- Lumbar support, brace or corset used to give passive support to the back. This type of instrument lacks scientific evidence when compared with placebo treatment or other treatments for low back pain intervention[63,64].
- Shortwave diathermy: Therapeutic elevation of the temperature of deep tissues by application of short wave electromagnetic radiation with a frequency range between 10 and 100 MHz This intervention methodology lacks scientific evidence when compared with a placebo or other treatment as a means of intervention in low back pain[65].
- Therapeutic ultrasound: Therapeutic application of high frequency sound waves up to 3 MHz evidence that this technique is limited in treating back pain when compared to placebo and no treatment when considering other methods of intervention[66].
- Thermotherapy: superficial heat in the lower back. There is a lack of scientific evidence of this methodology when compared to placebo treatment or other treatment as an instrument of intervention on chronic low back pain[66,67].
- Traction: pulling intervention that aims to stretch the lumbar spine. ExSite a variety of methods can be used with this technique, but usually involve the use of a harness around the lower rib cage and revolves around the iliac crest, using free weights and pulleys, a motorized mechanism, inverse techniques or headband to cause traction. As evidence of this methodology of intervention, it is limited to say that lumbar traction is not more effective than sham traction and zero when compared with other methods of intervention in low back pain[67,68].
- Transcutaneous electrical nerve stimulation (TENS) using surface electrodes, using electrical impulses seeking to relieve symptoms by changing the perception of pain. The evidence that this methodology is no better than placebo treatment of low back pain is strong, being moderate when compared to the electro-axial decompression, or acupuncture[66,69-72].

3.4 Clinical evidence of manual therapy in physiotherapy

- Manipulation / mobilization, manual therapy techniques used in the short or long levers to move back. This move pushes the spinal joint beyond its range of motion, by a pulse of high velocity low amplitude. Those made with large amplitude, low velocity and passive movements often remain within the joint range.

With moderate evidence, one might argue that the mobilization of the spine gets better results in the treatment of low back pain a simulated mobilization, but get the same effect as standard medical practice through the use of analgesics.

The level of evidence becomes moderate when mobilization and standard medical practice are combined and is more effective than medical treatment in isolation. Evidence is also moderate when viewed equal effects produced by therapeutic exercise and manipulation in low back pain[73,74].

- Massage: Soft tissue manipulation with the hands or a mechanical device through a variety of specific methods. As evidence, it seems that there is limited evidence when talking about the fact that massage causes on subjects suffering chronic back pain by saying that there is no difference between this technique and the use of a corset, that massage is more effective in symptomatological treatment of low back pain when compared to acupuncture, physical therapy, self-management education, the placebo treatment, postural education, relaxation therapy. There are also limited evidence that massage is as effective as manipulation in low back pain but, however, functional improvement is greater in spinal manipulation[75-78].

3.5 Clinical evidence of therapeutic exercise in physiotherapy

As for the therapeutic exercise, there is moderate evidence that short-term improvements achieved over the reduction of pain and disability than passive treatments. There is strong evidence that treatment with therapeutic exercise is more effective than standard medical practice for both the reduction of pain, disability and the average time to return to work. This level of evidence is maintained when you try to say that strength training - conditioning, there are more effective than other exercises in the treatment of chronic low back pain[73, 79-83].

4. Manual therapy as an intervention on chronic low back pain

4.1 Massage

Massage is the technique used for longer physical therapists in history. Instinctive mode makes use has been used by almost every culture in history, like the Greeks and Romans (where, among other uses, was used to retrieve the athletes and gladiators, respectively, after the shows), the ancient Egypt, where priests were using it in conjunction with other therapeutic techniques and even in China, where emperors of the best massage therapists available to treat their musculoskeletal complaints.

Although massage is socially understood as a technique of intervention whose focus is the muscle, it must have a broader definition because it is the set of soft tissues the main beneficiaries of this technique, for which the therapist can use both hands like some kind of mechanical device. In clinical practice, massage is often applied in combination with other therapies such as exercise and other interventions, but also sometimes as a single treatment.

A common way of using this technique is to combine the rules of physical medicine massage and neural therapy through acupuncture, where, without the insertion of the needle, but by using a specific instrument (vibrating) is achieved stimulation of acupuncture point superficial. Moreover, within the classical techniques of massage effleurage should be discarded, friction, kneading or pettrissage. If we make an analysis of the evidence of this technique as a routine therapeutic practice can see how there is limited evidence that massage gets the same effects as spinal manipulation and the use of the corset. More effective than spinal manipulation, exercise therapy and postural education, relaxation therapy, physical therapy and acupuncture are less effective than the use of therapeutic physical exercise combined with health education when discussing the effect upon the symptoms of people suffering from chronic LBP.

4.2 Spinal manipulation / mobilization

It is important to distinguish between what is manipulation and mobilization. Manipulation of the column is defined as an impulse of high velocity low amplitude that exceeds the limited range of motion but always runs within the anatomical limits of the joint. However, mobilization is understood as a low speed drive range of movement and manipulation, although in both cases remains the rule of not exceeding the anatomical limit of the joint.

Although the distinction between both methodologies, most studies that have been consulted didn`t made a clear distinction between each technique, but usually defined as "spinal manipulation package."

While these manual techniques are widely used as a tool in daily clinical practice, there are no randomized trials that allow too many draw firm conclusions about the effect that spinal manipulation leads.

While these manual techniques are widely used as a tool in daily clinical practice, there are no randomized trials that allow too many draw firm conclusions about the effect that spinal manipulation leads. Still, in recent years some trials have been developed that have allowed the increased strength of the conclusions, as they have increased the intrinsic quality of it and thereby allowing some light to the effect that these techniques lead to people with chronic LBP.

As for the evidence can be provided on the effect of manual therapy can bring to their use in the treatment of LBP symptomatological chronic, there are two limits that must be considered when interpreting the same. The first is that all interventions that have been observed allowing an evolution of the effects of manipulaición / mobilization in the short term, however, be important to determine how this technique can provide after long term intervention protocols, especially in this type of patients. On the other hand, there is also a problem regarding the unification of criteria in the different streams of existing manual therapy (manual medicine, osteopathy, physiotherapy, chiropractic ...) when defining a person qualified to perform such maneuvers. Based on these two aspects and based on the studies consulted, one could argue based on moderate evidence that manipulation / mobilization achieves better effects on symptoms of back pain than placebo treatment. Similarly, manipulation / mobilization used as a complement to standard medical treatment manage to increase the effect of this short term. On the other hand, it has found the same effects in the treatment of chronic low back pain when a therapist uses spinal manipulation when using a therapeutic exercise program, a program of back school or when compared with standard medical practice, although in the latter case, the evidence is strong rather than moderate [35,36,84,85].

Thus it's possible to see how the manipulation / mobilization vertebral have an effect simimar that could be seen in other health interventions in the treatment of chronic low back pain symptomatological. However, one of the aspects which would need to answer is to identify, within the range of possibilities that have qualified physical therapist to intervene, using manipulation / mobilization, subjects suffering from chronic back pain, what exercises are most effective in treatment of this disease, since there is no criterion when identifying them, the term is too imprecise.

5. Active treatment in chronic low back pain: Exercise therapy

5.1 introduction

Chronic low back pain, as defined previously, back pain is defined as pain and discomfort, located between the costal margin and the inferior gluteal folds, with or without referred pain from the leg. Chronic back pain defined as pain in this location for at least 12 weeks. This means we try to chronic sub-acute pain maintained for periods longer than 12 weeks or the appellants, where the current episode lasts at least this time.

Therapeutic physical exercise (TFE), can be defined as any program in which, during the sessions participants are required to perform static or dynamic movements and where the exercises were intended as a treatment for chronic low back pain, with supervised exercise and / or prescribed.

Being a chronic musculoskeletal disorder, therapeutic exercise, seems to be a good treatment option, however, some doubt is normal in this type of assault interventions such as exercise intensity, number of sessions per week, if you get the same effects regardless of the environment where the intervention takes place or whether the intervention should be group or individual. In any of these questions we will try to answer in this section.

5.2 Exercise intensity and cumulative exercise: Number of weekly sessions

So far has always been measuring the use of physical activity account for these two variables independently, however, for several years, a new concept is gaining prominence when speaking of exercise weekly. This idea comes from the fusion of both and has an own unit of measurement, METs (metabolics equivalents). One MET is equivalent to the expenditure of an individual who sits for a minute. Thus, an adult walks One MET Represents an individual's energy while sitting quietly Expenditure per minute. An adult walking at 4.82 km / h in flat terrain and hard consumes about 3.3 METs, whereas if the speed go up to 8.05, also spending would amount to 8 METs or so. As the end of a week, accumulating energy expenditure a person will be the summation of everything he has accomplished during that time period, being able to make an estimate of cumulative effort by the patient[86].

The concept of dose is often used to describe physical activity, but can be interpreted in many ways (cumulative, intensity, frequency, duration, physical activity ...). This idea gradually being introduced into clinical practice of a physical therapist to intervene on patients with chronic musculoskeletal disorders such as back pain, yet there is not much literature that has used this form of measurement in the low back pain. However, if there are some published studies comparing the optimal frequency of intervention on these patients through exercise. Thus there is strong evidence that all those interventions that make a subject and at the end of the week it has accumulated a minimum of two hours of treatment and a maximum of two hours and forty-five minutes of treatment on this type of pathology[86-88].

5.3 Individual or group exercise?

The physical factor is a priori, the most influential within the therapeutic effects of EFT as, individually planned and ensuring consistency in the precocity, the training effect will achieve the objectives previously established. Therefore, the key lies in the design of achievable objectives for each condition and adapted to the evolutionary process.

Thus, based on the objective pursued by each patient, we can differentiate between: planning treatment for recovery training, when we try to restore or improve impaired function, and therapeutic planning training for compensation, when we try to compensate or improve global function, because the current problem is not improved.

On the other hand, and understanding that an EFT program conducted as a means of intervention on chronic low back pain means that the duration of such treatment is usually not less than two months, so that, taking into account the cost of a physiotherapist for each hour of work, would be difficult for all patients who suffer from chronic back pain, could make an intervention where the therapist-patient ratio was 1:1. Thus, a way to save the expense would increase this ratio to reach heights that range between 1:8 and 1:12.

For its part, the therapist could make an identification of the active treatment of the person based on this initial assessment. Thus, tracking group, but a search of the objectives individually get very interesting balance between the cost of services received by the patient and increasing symptomatic improvement by the patient[89,90].

5.4 Environment where the exercise should be performed: Is the water always a good option?

More and more frequent the facilities they offer services that can be performed physiotherapy intervention for chronic musculoskeletal disorders in the aquatic environment, partially or completely carried out within it. Conducting the activity in the water, has a number of advantages such as decompression of the lumbar spine validated with accurate measurements of body height, changes in all functional parameters of mobility, strength and endurance as well as improved cardio-metabolic disorders negatively and significantly correlated with the degree of pain and disability and provide for adequate monitoring and follow-up after individual assessment through indicators with heart rate and subjective scales of effort. However, it also presents some limitations, especially in deep pools, such as feelings of insecurity in those who are not fluent in the aquatic environment.

It found, however, studies show that exercise performed in water treatment is more effective than EFT made out of it or vice versa, so it will be a patient choice and / or choosing a therapist use a certain methodology or another.

However, if you have found in clinical trials has been shown that the same treatment carried out of water but with water running supplementation produces better results in symptomatic improvement in patients with chronic LBP[91,-93].

In conclusion of this section and articles based on the respondents, one could say with strong evidence that strengthening exercises are more effective than other types of exercises. Likewise, and maintaining this level of evidence has shown that exercise is more effective than general medical practice to reduce pain, disability, and return to work in the medium term (3-6 months), but not is more effective than conventional physical therapy intervention.

The level of evidence when it comes down to that moderate exercise is more effective than passive treatment in reducing pain and / or disability[1,3,35,73]. On the other hand, and already with a limited level of evidence has been found that intensive multidisciplinary programs face can not be said which of these is most effective. Furthermore, while maintaining that level of evidence, differences were no differences between aerobic and strength exercises, in terms of pain and the degree of long-term disability, no differences between the effects on the reduction pain, to perform the exercise in just 4 sessions, compared to 8 sessions, aerobic exercises are superior to lumbar flexion, in terms of pain immediately after the program and a program for individualized home exercise is more effective than general exercises.

6. General supplement to chronic low back pain treatment: Brief advice and health education

6.1 What is the brief advice

When talking about brief advice, it is difficult to define this definition in terms of content, time and form.

From a temporal point of view, there are two types of interventions that target different. One aims to ease concerns, worries and doubts that early intervention would address the initial short questions and fears that the patient suffers. On the other hand, there are some interventions that are longer and requiring more profound impact on aspects of the problem by helping the integration of the pathology of the patient.

While there are different ways to provide brief advice to the patient (in person, by telephone, with a booklet written, using internet ...), has not been able to show which method is most effective when the patient integrate such training, although they can identify some problems that can affect certain methodologies, such as internet use, as in older people, who are not familiar with the use of this medium can be an insurmountable limit.

We are talking about a process in which a person gives to another or other information about a specific problem, chronic low back pain. Here's beliefs, the communication skills by the physiotherapist, the material available are some aspects that could influence the determinants of credibility and effectiveness of the intervention.

On the other hand, it would be important to consider those who have a paid position and it is absent due to any pressure that they may suffer by changing their employment status is experiencing, it would be important to monitor absenteeism labor is causing low back pain in the patient.

So it appears that brief advice delivered by a physiotherapist or clinical staff is a promising tool that can help save significant time and resources which can benefit both the patient and the clinician. This statement could be shot by studies that demonstrate strong evidence that brief advice is as effective as aerobic exercise routine or physical therapy in reducing disability, shortening time to return to work or patient's daily activities. Furthermore, with moderate evidence, we can say that brief advice is more effective than usual care in reducing the time of return to employment and the promotion of self-care helps reduce the typical symptoms of lumbar pain as pain or disability. However, there is limited evidence that the transmission of information through internet use is more effective than no intervention in reducing pain or disability of a person who suffers chronic back pain[94-98].

6.2 Cognitive behavioral methods of treatment

It is important to consider that treatment of low back pain is not solely focused on eliminating chronic underlying pathology, but the reduction in symptoms and disability that it causes by changing the contingencies that the environment of the patient may have and through cognitive processes. Of these, the cognitive processes can be divided into three different styles of intervention depending on the therapeutic approach is desired to give. This may be operant, cognitive and respondent. Each of them focuses on the modification of one of the three response systems that characterize emotional experiences that are the behavior, cognitions and physiological reactivity.

The first is based on the principles of operant conditioning of Skinner (1953)[99], where healthy behaviors are reinforced positively and to all those aspects that relate to negative symptoms like pain, is stripped of patient care. The assistance of the people around them as partner, family, friends, have an important role in this process.

Cognitive therapy for its part has as its objective the identification and modification of the cognitive aspects of patients on pain and disability. This change in the definition of pain or expectations of control over it is achieved with cognitive restructuring techniques (directly) or by changing beliefs, feelings and thoughts[100].

Finally, the defendant treatment which aims to achieve is a change in the direct physiological response, such as by muscle relaxation, for which the patient seeks to provide a model of relationship between stress and pain, teaching himself to use the relaxation in response to accumulated muscle tension. To achieve this, it uses material that may help the patient understand what is happening, such as biofeedback or EMG.

As you can see, these methods seek to cognitive and behavioral changes in both behavior and cognition on the basis of treatment being offered. The main approach used by these techniques is that both pain and disability that this condition creates are the result of psychological and social factors, not just because of a somatic pathology.

Although they appear several objectives and methodologies used by cognitive and behavioral therapies, these two techniques have several things in common:

- The behavior and emotions of individuals are influenced by your thoughts.
- The patient is able to acquire skills to solve various problems.
- To get a change maladaptive thoughts, feelings and behaviors, you can make use of structured techniques to help identify, control and change these conditions.

Different studies have demonstrated the effectiveness of behavioral treatment in chronic low back pain. Thus, one could argue with strong evidence that this intervention is more effective than no treatment or placebo. On the other hand, always with the same level of evidence, we can say that there are no differences in results obtained with the three streams of treatment. In addition, the behavioral approach is demonstrated more effective than traditional treatments in facilitating the return to work by patients.

The evidence comes down to moderation for that treatment to cognitive-behavioral treatment has joined other effects of long and medium term chronic low back pain. In addition, there is limited evidence that intervention on pain, disability, functional status, depression or therapeutic exercise and behavioral therapy are equally effective[100-104].

7. Multimodal treatment in chronic low back pain

7.1 Introduction

The current concept of man does that is defined beyond its own anatomic barrier. Your life will be determined by biological, psychological and social. The response and adaptation to each individual contribution they will determine your state of health. Thus, the therapeutic approach should contain different proportions depending on the case, a portion of each of these perspectives.

The content of multidisciplinary treatment programs usually consists of a broad mix of the physical, social and behavioral modification and drug use. Usually, these programs are held for a considerable number of hours a week, sometimes even on an inpatient basis. The content of these programs and how they are labeled or described is very variable. For example, multidisciplinary biopsychosocial rehabilitation, rehabilitation programs, behavioral programs, back schools, or functional restoration programs (FR) may involve one or more of these components. True multidisciplinary treatment program that includes medical (drug treatment, education), physical (exercise), vocational and behavioral components must always be at least three health professionals with clinical backgrounds (doctor, physiotherapist, psychologist), although the intensity and content of interdisciplinary therapy varies widely.

Based on the evidence we have seen in the preceding paragraphs, it appears that the most effective combination, a priori, would be to combine therapeutic exercise, manual therapy and health education and behavioral programs. Each one of which could be developed as follows:

- Individual therapeutic exercise program fully supervised, organized and run as a group (8 patients per therapist). With an initial assessment for planning of therapeutic exercise, looking at the bio-pathomechanics functional assessment as a starting point to set the exercise individually, including assessment of mobility (goniometry), strength and muscular endurance (dynamometry) and motor control system of local spine stabilization.
- Brief interventions for spinal manipulation and mobilization for the normalization of hypomobile identified areas through integrated manual therapy, exercise program.
- Health education integrated into the exercise program and behavioral strategies of adherence, as well as brief educational interventions, which may be provided by a physiotherapist to encourage a return to normal activities.

7.2 Combined or add effects

A priori one might tend to think that this question does not make much sense, because a multimodal program should be based on evidence offering a combination of those therapies that are most effective, ensuring a summation of effects, however, failed to show that as a result of a multimodal treatment intervention to obtain the sum of the effects of each of the interventions separately. It is very likely not the case because there may be variables that are improved with an intervention or another. It is also important to remember that physiotherapy intervention is aimed at symptomatic improvement of this alteration of the musculoskeletal system, and the patient support in assessing the patient's results will play an important role.

7.3 Multimodal treatment: When you do when not

From a health policy, to where it shifts the balance of costs and benefits, as these multimodal intervention programs can make a way out of health care resources. However, always committed and difficult to assign economic value to the quality of life, function, disability and / or pain, so to complete the analysis of cost-benefit can be tricky. On the other hand, would be included in this analysis are trials that can determine whether the effects on employment status, in terms of availability or fitness for patients who suffer from chronic back pain, in addition to a comparison of the response mode with the subjects on the basis of gender or age.

Although, as noted above, is necessary to deepen the results that can provide treatment multidiscipliananar subjects suffering chronic back pain be stipulated that some evidence (strong and moderate) have been obtained in this regard. Thus, strong evidence, one could argue that a treatment that combines intense physical training and behavioral therapies integrated within the same treatment protocol, is able to reduce absenteeism in workers who suffer from chronic back pain. Likewise, one could say with strong evidence that those subjects who suffer chronic back pain have reduced pain and disability, improving the function by a multidisciplinary program of physiotherapy intervention[105-112].

On the other hand, there is moderate evidence that intensive rehabilitative multidisciplinary program is more effective in reducing pain than non-multidisciplinary outpatient therapy or even the usual treatment.

8. How to increase the effect of chronic low back pain treatment? Intervention in subgroups

8.1 Introduction

When asked how to increase the effect of treatment in low back pain can be considered two types of responses. The first comes from an actual increase of the effect that treatment can bring to a particular type of patients, which would require the division of patients with low back pain whose treatment in specific subgroups specifically consideration of its characteristics making a proposed intervention much tighter to the subject in particular and the general group.

On the other side and to a very heterogeneous reality to which therapists have to face the world, another perspective that could provide a valid answer to this question would be to seek maximum efficiency of resources available to the professional clinician, not only referring to the material, but also time and space available.

8.2 Different groups of variables divided to chronic low back pain

If we consider each individual perspective, it could provide two different types of responses. The first was pursuing a net improvement of treatment effect, which would be necessary to clarify factors that define the person, such as age, sex, body mass index, and so on. chasing in a group intervention, a personalized treatment as closely as possible. Thus, the main factor in making the subgroups born of the characteristics of each subject.

In turn, as has been observed in recent years have seen an expansion of treatment in chronic diseases múscuoloesqueléticas. Of these, the most common of all is the low back, creating groups and specific methods of treatment for this condition. Regardless of whether the agency offers these services is public or private, both seeking to increase efficiency and, therefore, a better balance between cost - effectiveness. This view could prompt more commercial thinking about seeking treatment depersonalization of economic performance just the same, however, studies which demonstrate the optimal frequency of low back pain intervention can help better use of space resources and temporary available, and may favor the increased supply and therefore the number of patients treated and satisfied with the service received.

8.3 Evidence of increased effect: Studies published

In recent years there have been several published studies that attempted to answer this question considering different variables as a criterion for differentiating lumbálgicos groups receiving treatment. The main subdivisions were made based on body mass index, based on the environment where treatment was performed at the age of people who perform it.

He has watched a speech delivered in groups where the criteria of subdivision was the body mass index[113], evolved similar patients in different intervention groups, it seems that this variable does not affect to the evolution of the patient may suffer in terms of symptomatic improvement of low back pain. These results are contradictory to a study that is under review, according to which, people who are obese are not only more likely to suffer back pain, but the treatment effect is inversely proportional to the rate of mass body present.

On the other hand, it has been shown how optimizing available resources are two key aspects to be considered, the number of sessions per week and the medium in which the intervention. This has been shown how a person performing two sessions of physical therapy to improve symptoms of low back pain evolves faster than those who performed only one session per week[87,114]. However, among those who engaged in twice-weekly and three symptomatic evolution could be comparable. This could be in line with the show already in 2007 brought the American College of Sports Medicine from the recommendations of which does not speak of sessions a week, but a cumulative total exercise per week based on the intensity. In paragraph 5 is much deeper in this argument.

Another aspect that has been taken into account when classifying interventions is one in which the environment is considered where the intervention. It has been observed how the subject performs a physical therapy intervention completely dry or a part of the exercise in the water, get a similar evolution in both media. This allows it to be the patient who chooses what kind of environment you prefer when making your own protocol for intervention. However, it has watched a physiotherapy intervention which will supplement water running protocol, the patient experiences an increase in symptom improvement when performing this protocol with respect to when it does.

TREATMENT		ACUTE LBP	SUB-ACUTE LBP	CHRONIC LBP
PHYSICAL THERAPY	Interferential therapy	X	X	X
	Laser therapy	X	X	X
	Lumbar supports	X	X	X
	Shortwave diathermy	X	X	X
	Therapeutic ultrasound	X	X	X
	Thermotherapy	X	X	X
	Traction	X	X	X
	Transcutaneous electrical nerve stimulation (TENS)	X	X	X
Exercise therapy		X	√	√
Bed rest		X	√	√
Active lifestile		√	√	√
Manual therapy	Manipulation/mobilisation	√	√	√
	Massage	X	X	X
Back schools		X	√	√
Minimal contact/brief educational interventions to promote self-care		√	√	√
Cognitive-behavioural treatment methods		√	√	√
Multidisciplinary treatment		X	√	√
Antidepressants		√	√	√
Muscle relaxants		√	√	√
NSAIDs		√	√	√
Capsaicin		√	√	√
Paracetamol		√	√	√
Epidural steroids		X	X	X
Percutaneous electrical nerve stimulation (PENS)			√	√
Acupuncture		X	X	X
Neuroreflexotherapy			√	√

Table 1. Appropriateness of treatment based on pathology

Chronic NLBP	Acute NLBP
Brief. Ed. Interv. Prom. SelfC. = Aerobic Exerc. TENS=Placebo Brief educational interventions to promote self-care. = Usual physiotherapy. Therapeutic Exercise = Gnarl Physiotherapy. TE = Other Exercise TE > General Practice MT = GP	Paracetamol < mefenemic acid Paracetamol = NSAIDs NSAIDs > Placebo NSAIDs = Muscle relaxants NSAIDs = opioid analgesics NSAIDS > non-drug treatments Muscle relaxants > Placebo Spinal Mobilization > Placebo Spinal Mobilization = Therapeutic Exercise Spinal Mobilization = Analgesic
Brief. Ed. Interv. Prom. SelfC. = GP. Back School = Exercise Back School = Manual Therapy. Back School = Brief. Ed. Interv. Prom. SelfC MT > Placebo MT MT = Usual physiotherapy. MT = Back School TE > Passive Interventions MT + GP > GP	Paracetamol = Aspirin Bed rest < Placebo Remain Active > Bed Rest TE > Placebo TE > Bed Rest TE > Brief. Ed. Interv. Prom. SelfC Flexion Exercise > Extension Exercise Paracetamol= indomethacin Spinal Manipulation > Massage TE > Massage Multidisciplinary Treatment > GP Behavioral Treatment > GP
Laser therapy ≠ Placebo Ultrasound ≠ Placebo Massage > Placebo Massage > Acupuncture Massage > Relax therapy Massage = MT TE ≠ Multidisciplinary program Aerobic Exercise > Flexion exercise Diathermia = Placebo Individual Exercise. > Generic exercise Aerobic Exercise = Strength Exercise 2 = 4 Weekly sessions	Back School = Physical Therapy Back School < General Exercise Brief. Ed. Interv. Prom. SelfC > GP Back School = McKenzie exercises
Interferential = Placebo	

LEVEL A	LEVEL B	LEVEL C	LEVEL D

Table 2. Low back pain evidence after revision

9. References

[1] Bigos S, Bowyer O, Braen G et al. Acute low back problems in adults. Clinical practice guideline no. 14. AHCPR publication no. 95-0642. Rockville, MD: Agency for Health Care Policy and Research, Public Health Service, U.S. Department of health and Human Services. December 1994. [USA]

[2] Van Tulder MW, Furlan A, Bouter LM, Bombardier C and the Editorial Board of the Cochrane Back Review Group. Updated Method Guidelines for Systematic Reviews in the Cochrane Collaboration Back Review Group. Spine 2003; 28: 1290-9.

[3] Royal College of General Practitioners. Clinical Guidelines for the Management of Acute Low Back Pain. London, Royal College of General Practitioners, 1996 and 1999. [UK].

[4] Evans G, Richards S. Low back pain: an evaluation of therapeutic interventions. Bristol: Health Care Evaluation Unit, University of Bristol, 1996.

[5] Hagen KB, Hilde G, Jamtvedt G, Winnem M. Bed rest for acute low back pain and sciatica (Cochrane Review) In: The Cochrane Library, Issue 4, 2000. Oxford: Update Software.

[6] Koes BW, van den Hoogen HMM. Efficacy of bed rest and orthoses of low back pain. A review of randomized clinical trials. Eur J Phys Med Rehabil 1994; 4: 86-93.

[7] Van Tulder MW, Koes BW, Bouter LM. Conservative treatment of acute and chronic nonspecific low back pain: a systematic review of randomized controlled trials of the most common interventions. Spine 1997; 22: 2128-56.

[8] Waddell G, Feder G, Lewis M. Systematic reviews of bed rest and advice to stay active for acute low back pain. Br J Gen Pract 1997; 47: 647-52.

[9] Hilde G, Hagen KB, Jamtvedt G, Winnem M. Advice to stay active as a single treatment for low back pain and sciatica (Cochrane Review). In: The Cochrane Library, Issue 1, 2004. Chichester, UK: John Wiley & Sons, Ltd.

[10] Hagen EM, Eriksen HR, Ursin H. Does early intervention with a light mobilization program reduce long-term sick leave for low back pain? Spine 2000; 25: 1973-6.

[11] Rozenberg S, Delval C, Rezvani Y, et al. Bed rest or normal activity for patients with acute low back pain: a randomized controlled trial. Spine 2002; 27: 1487-93.

[12] Malmivaara A, Kotilainen E, Laasonen E, Poussa M, Rasmussen M, Clinical Practice Guidelines: diseases of the low back. (Finnish, available in English) The Finnish Medical Association Duodecim 1999. [Finland]

[13] Faas A, Chavannes AW, Koes BW, Van den Hoogen JMM, Mens JMA, Smeele IJM, Romeijnders ACM, Van der Laan JR. Clinical practice guidelines for low back pain. (Dutch, available in English). Huisarts Wet 1996;39:18-31. [the Netherlands]

[14] Bekkering GE, van Tulder MW, Hendriks HJM, Oostendorp RAB, Koes BW, Ostelo RWJG, Thomassen J. Dutch physiotherapy guideline for low back pain. (KNGF richtlijn lage rugpijn) Ned Tijdschr Fysiother 2001;111 (Suppl. 3): 1-24. [the Netherlands]

[15] Nasjonalt ryggnettverk – Formidlingsenheten. Akutte korsryggsmerter. Tverrfaglige, kliniske retningslinjer. Oslo, 2002: Nasjonalt ryggnettverk. [Norway]

[16] Van Tulder MW, Malmivaara A, Esmail R, Koes BW. Exercise therapy for nonspecific low back pain (Cochrane Review). In: The Cochrane Library, Issue 4, 2000. Oxford: Update Software.

[17] Van Tulder MW, Scholten RJPM, Koes BW, Deyo RA. Non-steroidal anti-inflammatory drugs (NSAIDs) for nonspecific low back pain (Cochrane Review). In: The Cochrane Library, Issue 4, 2000. Oxford: Update Software.

[18] Pohjalainen T, Jekunen A, Autio L, Vuorela H. Treatment of acute low back pain with the COX-2-selective anti-inflammatory drug Nimesulide: results of a randomized, double-blind comparative trial versus ibuprofen. Spine 2000; 25: 1579-85.

[19] Van Tulder MW, Touray T, Furlan AD, Solway S, Bouter LM. Muscle relaxants for nonspecific low back pain (Cochrane Review). In: The Cochrane Library, Issue 1, 2004. Chichester, UK: John Wiley & Sons, Ltd.

[20] Van Tulder MW, Koes BW, Bouter LM. Conservative treatment of acute and chronic nonspecific low back pain: a systematic review of randomized controlled trials of the most common interventions. Spine 1997; 22: 2128-56.

[21] Henry D, Lim LLY, Rodriguez LAG, et al. Variability in risk of gastrointestinal complications with individual nonsteroidal anti-inflammatory drugs: results of a collaborative meta-analysis. Br Med J 1996; 312: 1563-6

[22] van Tulder M, Becker A, Bekkering T, Breen A, del Real MT, Hutchinson A, Koes B, Laerum E, Malmivaara A; COST B13 Working Group on Guidelines for the Management of Acute Low Back Pain in Primary Care. Chapter 3. European guidelines for the management of acute nonspecific low back pain in primary care. Eur Spine J. 2006 Mar;15 Suppl 2:S169-91.

[23] Keel P, Perini Ch, Schutz-Petitjean D, et al Chronicisation des douleurs du dos: problematique, issues. Rapport final du Programme National de Recherche No 26B. Bale: Editions EULAR 1996. [Switzerland].

[24] Keel P, Weber M, Roux E, et al. Kreuzschmerzen: Hintergründe, prävention, behandlung. Basisdokumentation. Verbindung der Schweizer Ärzte (FMH), Bern, 1998. [Switzerland]

[25] Araki S, Kawamura O, Mataka T, et al. RCT ni yoru kyusei yotsu-sho ni taisuru shishin-gun to gishin-gun no tiryou koka [Randomized controlled trial comparing manual acupuncture and sham acupuncture for acute low back pain]. J Japan Soc Acupuncture Moxibustion 2001; 51: 382.

[26] Van Tulder MW, Ostelo RWJG, Vlaeyen JWS, Linton SJ, Morley SJ, Assendelft WJJ. Behavioural treatment for chronic low back pain (Cochrane Review). In: The Cochrane Library, Issue 4, 2000. Oxford: Update Software.

[27] Melloh M, Aebli N, Elfering A, Röder C, Zweig T, Barz T, Herbison P, Hendrick P, Bajracharya S, Stout K, Theis JC. Development of a screening tool predicting the transition from acute to chronic low back pain for patients in a GP setting: protocol of a multinational prospective cohort study.BMC Musculoskelet Disord. 2008 Dec 19;9:167.

[28] Dillingham T. Evaluation and management of low backpain: and overview. State of the Art Reviews 1995;9(3):559-74.

[29] Leboeuf-Yde C, Lauritsen J, Lauritsen T. Why has the search for causes of low backpain largely been nonconclusive? Spine 1997;22(8):877–81.

[30] Dankaerts W, O'Sullivan PB, Burnett AF, Straker LM. The use of a mechanism-based classification system to evaluate and direct management of a patient with non-specific chronic low back pain and motor control impairment--a case report. Man Ther. 2007 May;12(2):181-91.

[31] Dankaerts W, O'Sullivan P. The validity of O'Sullivan's classification system (CS) for a sub-group of NS-CLBP with motor control impairment (MCI): overview of a series of studies and review of the literature. Man Ther. 2011 Feb;16(1):9-14.

[32] O'Sullivan P. Diagnosis and classification of chronic low back pain disorders: maladaptive movement and motor control impairments as underlying mechanism. Man Ther. 2005 Nov;10(4):242-55.

[33] Carragee EJ, Hannibal M (2004) Diagnostic evaluation of low back pain. Orthop Clin North Am, 35(1): 7-16.

[34] Kendall NAS, Linton SJ, Main CJ (1997) Guide to assessing psychosocial yellow flags in acute low back pain: risk factors for long-term disability and work loss., Accident Rehabilitation & Compensation Insurance Corporation of New Zealand and the National Health Committee.: Wellington.

[35] Airaksinen O, Brox JI, Cedraschi C, Hildebrandt J, Klaber-Moffett J, Kovacs F, Mannion AF, Reis S, Staal JB, Ursin H, Zanoli G; COST B13 Working Group on Guidelines for Chronic Low Back Pain.Chapter 4. European guidelines for the management of chronic nonspecific low back pain. Eur Spine J. 2006 Mar;15 Suppl 2:S192-300.

[36] Chou R, Qaseem A, Snow V, Casey D, Cross JT Jr, Shekelle P, Owens DK; Clinical Efficacy Assessment Subcommittee of the American College of Physicians; American College of Physicians; American Pain Society Low Back Pain Guidelines Panel. Diagnosis and treatment of low back pain: a joint clinical practice guideline from the American College of Physicians and the American Pain Society Ann Intern Med. 2007 Oct 2;147(7):478-91

[37] Todd NV. Cauda equina syndrome: the timing of surgery probably does influence outcome. Br J Neurosurg. 2005;19:301-6; discussion 307-8.

[38] Tsiodras S, Falagas ME. Clinical assessment and medical treatment of spine infections. Clin Orthop Relat Res. 2006;444:38-50.

[39] Loblaw DA, Perry J, Chambers A, Laperriere NJ. Systematic review of the diagnosis and management of malignant extradural spinal cord compression: the Cancer Care Ontario Practice Guidelines Initiative's Neuro-Oncology Disease Site Group. J Clin Oncol. 2005;23:2028-37.

[40] Bigos SJ, Bowyer OR, Braen GR, al. e (1994) Clinical Practice Guidelines. Vol. 14, Public Health Service Edition., US Department of Health an Human Services.

[41] Hides JA, Jull GA, Richardson CA. Long-term effects of specific stabilizing exercises for first-episode low back pain. Spine. 2001;26:E243-248.

[42] Hides JA, Stokes MJ, Saide M, Jull GA, Cooper DH. Evidence of lumbar multifidus muscle wasting ipsilateral to symptoms in patients with acute/subacute low back pain. Spine.

[43] Kiesel KB, Uhl TL, Underwood FB, Rodd DW, Nitz AJ. Measurement of lumbar multifidus muscle contraction with rehabilitative ultrasound imaging. Man Ther. 2007;12:161-166.

[44] Kristjansson E. Reliability of ultrasonography for the cervical multifidus muscle in asymptomatic and symptomatic subjects. Man Ther. 2004;9:83-88.

[45] Lee JP, Tseng WY, Shau YW, Wang CL, Wang HK, Wang SF. Measurement of segmental cervical multifidus contraction by ultrasonography in asymptomatic adults. Man Ther. 2006 Sep 18; [Epub ahead of print].

[46] Rankin G, Stokes M, Newham DJ. Size and shape of the posterior neck muscles measured by ultrasound imaging: normal values in males and females of different ages. Man Ther. 2005;10:108-115.

[47] Stokes M, Rankin G, Newham DJ. Ultrasound imaging of lumbar multifidus muscle: normal reference ranges for measurements and practical guidance on the technique. Man Ther. 2005;10:116-126.

[48] Strobel K, Hodler J, Meyer DC, Pfirrmann CW, Pirkl C, Zanetti M. Fatty atrophy of supraspinatus and infraspinatus muscles: accuracy of US. Radiology. 2005;237:584-589.

[49] Teyhen DS, Gill NW, Whittaker JL, Henry SM, Hides JA, Hodges P. Rehabilitative ultrasound imaging of the abdominal muscles. J Orthop Sports Phys Ther. 2007 Aug;37(8):450-66.

[50] Stokes M, Hides J, Elliott J, Kiesel K, Hodges P. Rehabilitative ultrasound imaging of the posterior paraspinal muscles. J Orthop Sports Phys Ther. 2007 Oct;37(10):581-95.

[51] Whittaker JL, Teyhen DS, Elliott JM, Cook K, Langevin HM, Dahl HH, Stokes M. Rehabilitative ultrasound imaging: understanding the technology and its applications. J Orthop Sports Phys Ther. 2007 Aug;37(8):434-49.

[52] Kiesel KB, Uhl T, Underwood FB, Nitz AJ. Rehabilitative ultrasound measurement of select trunk muscle activation during induced pain. Man Ther. 2008 May;13(2):132-8.

[53] Sacket DL, Strauss SE, Richardson WS, Rosenberg W, Haynes RB.). Medicina basada en la evidencia. cómo practicar y enseñar la MBE (2ª ed) Ed Harcourt. 2001

[54] Sackett DL, Richarson WS, Rosenberg W, Hynes RB. Evidence-based medicine: How to practice and teach EBM. London: Churchill-livingstone. 1997

[55] Herbert RD, Jamtvedt G, Mead J, Birger K. Practical evidence-based physiotherapy Ed. Butterworth-Heinemann. 2005

[56] Herbert RD. How to estimate treatment effects from reports of clinical trials. I: Continuous outcomes. Aus J Pyhsio, 2000 (46), 229-235.

[57] CEBP. Center Evidence-based Physiotherapy Tutorial: Reading clinical trials in physiotherapy. Tutorial: Reading clinical trials in physiotherapy. Retrieved 23/12, 2011, from http://www.pedro.fhs.usyd.edu.au/CEBP/index_cebp.html

[58] Oxman AD, Guyatt GH. Validation of an index of the quality of review articles. J Clin Epidemiol, 1991. 44(11): 1271-8.

[59] Hurley DA, Minder PM, McDonough SM, Walsh DM, Moore AP, Baxter DG. Interferential therapy electrode placement technique in acute low back pain: a preliminary investigation. Arch Phys Med Rehabil, 2001. 82(4): 485-93.

[60] Werners R, Pynsent PB, Bulstrode CJ. Randomized trial comparing interferential therapy with motorized lumbar traction and massage in the management of low back pain in a primary care setting. Spine, 1999. 24(15): 1579-84.

[61] Basford JR, Sheffield CG, Harmsen WS. Laser therapy: a randomized, controlled trial of the effects of low-intensity Nd:YAG laser irradiation on musculoskeletal back pain. Arch Phys Med Rehabil, 1999: 80(6): 647-52.

[62] Bjordal JM, Couppe C, Chow RT, Tuner J, Ljunggren EA. A systematic review of low level laser therapy with location-specific doses for pain from chronic joint disorders. Aust J Physiother. 2003, 49(2): 107-16.

[63] Jellema P, van Tulder MW, van Poppel MN, Nachemson AL, Bouter LM. Lumbar supports for prevention and treatment of low back pain: a systematic review within the framework of the Cochrane Back Review Group. Spine. 2001 26(4): 377-86.

[64] van Duijvenbode I, Jellema P, van Poppel MNM, van Tulder MW. Lumbar supports for prevention and treatment of low back pain. Cochrane Datbase of Sytematic Reviews, issue 2 2008. Chichester: John Wiley & Sons Ltd; 2008.

[65] Sweetman BJ, Heinrich I, Anderson JAD (1993) A randomized controlled trial of exercises, short wave diathermy, and traction for low back pain, with evidence of diagnosis-related response to treatment. Journal-of-Orthopaedic-Rheumatology, 6: 159-66.

[66] Philadelphia (2001) Philadelphia Panel evidence-based clinical practice guidelines on selected rehabilitation interventions for low back pain. Phys Ther, 81(10): 1641-74.

[67] van der Heijden GJ, Beurskens AJ, Koes BW, Assendelft WJ, de Vet HC, Bouter LM (1995) The efficacy of traction for back and neck pain: a systematic, blinded review of randomized clinical trial methods. Phys Ther, 75(2): 93-104.

[68] van den Hoogen HM, Koes BW, van Eijk JT, Bouter LM (1995) On the accuracy of history, physical examination, and erythrocyte sedimentation rate in diagnosing low back pain in general practice. A criteria-based review of the literature. Spine, 20(3): 318-27.

[69] Brosseau L, Milne S, Robinson V, Marchand S, Shea B, Wells G, Tugwell P (2002) Efficacy of the transcutaneous electrical nerve stimulation for the treatment of chronic low back pain: a meta-analysis. Spine, 27(6): 596-603.

[70] Milne S, Welch V, Brosseau L, Saginur M, Shea B, Tugwell P, Wells G (2001) Transcutaneous electrical nerve stimulation (TENS) for chronic low back pain. Cochrane Database Syst Rev, (2): CD003008.

[71] Hsieh RL, Lee WC (2002) One-shot percutaneous electrical nerve stimulation vs. transcutaneous electrical nerve stimulation for low back pain: comparison of therapeutic effects. Am J Phys Med Rehabil, 81(11): 838-43.

[72] Yokoyama M, Sun X, Oku S, Taga N, Sato K, Mizobuchi S, Takahashi T, Morita K (2004) Comparison of percutaneous electrical nerve stimulation with transcutaneous electrical nerve stimulation for long-term pain relief in patients with chronic low back pain. Anesth Analg, 98(6): 1552-6.

[73] UK BEAM Trial Team. Brealey S, Coulton S, Farrin A, Morton V, Torgerson D, Burton AK, Garratt A, Harvey E, Letley L, Martin J, Vickers M, Whyte K, Manca A, Klaber Moffett J, Russell I, Underwood M, Williams M (2004a) United Kingdom back pain

exercise and manipulation (UK BEAM) randomised trial: Cost-effectiveness of physical treatments for back pain in primary care. British Medical Journal, 329(7479):1381

[74] Licciardone JC, Stoll ST, Fulda KG, Russo DP, Siu J, Winn W, Swift J, Jr. (2003) Osteopathic manipulative treatment for chronic low back pain: a randomized controlled trial. Spine, 28(13): 1355-62.

[75] Furlan AD, Brosseau L, Imamura M, Irvin E (2002) Massage for low-back pain: a systematic review within the framework of the Cochrane Collaboration Back Review Group. Spine, 27(17): 1896-910.

[76] Hernandez-Reif M, Field T, Krasnegor J, Theakston H (2001) Lower back pain is reduced and range of motion increased after massage therapy. Int J Neurosci, 106(3-4): 131-45.

[77] Walach H, Guthlin C, Konig M (2003) Efficacy of massage therapy in chronic pain: a pragmatic randomized trial. J Altern Complement Med, 9(6): 837-46.

[78] Hsieh LL, Kuo CH, Yen MF, Chen TH (2004) A randomized controlled clinical trial for low back pain treated by acupressure and physical therapy. Prev Med, 39(1): 168-76.

[79] van Tulder MW, Koes B (2003) Low back pain and sciatica: chronic. Clin Evid, (9).

[80] van Tulder MW, Malmivaara A, Esmail R, al. e (2003)Exercise therapy for low back pain., The Cochrane Library: Oxford.

[81] Staal JB, Hlobil H, Twisk JW, Smid T, Koke AJ, van Mechelen W (2004) Graded activity for low back pain in occupational health care: a randomized, controlled trial. Ann Intern Med, 140(2): 77-84.

[82] Gur A, Karakoc M, Cevik R, Nas K, Sarac AJ (2003) Efficacy of low power laser therapy and exercise on pain and functions in chronic low back pain. Lasers Surg Med, 32(3): 233-8.

[83] Jousset N, Fanello S, Bontoux L, Dubus V, Billabert C, Vielle B, Roquelaure Y, Penneau-Fontbonne D, Richard I (2004) Effects of functional restoration versus 3 hours per week physical therapy: a randomized controlled study. Spine, 29(5): 487- 93; discussion 94.

[84] Assendelft WJ, Morton SC, Yu EI, Suttorp MJ, Shekelle PG (2004) Spinal manipulative therapy for low-back pain (Cochrane Review). In: The Cochrane Library, Issue 3. John Wiley & Sons, Ltd.: Chichester, UK.

[85] Low Back Pain: Early Management of Persistent Non-specific Low Back Pain [Internet]. National Collaborating Centre for Primary Care (UK). London: Royal College of General Practitioners (UK); 2009 May.

[86] Haskell WL, Lee IM, Pate RR, et al. Physical activity and public health: updated recommendation for adults from the American College of Sports Medicine and the American Heart Association. Med Sci Sports Exerc. 2007. Aug;39(8);1423-34.

[87] Sato D, Kaneda K, Wakabayashi H, Nomura T. Comparison two-year effects of once-weekly and twice-weekly water exercise on health-related quality of life of community-dwelling frail elderly people at a day-service facility. Disabil Rehabil. 2009;31;84-93.

[88] Rainville J, Jouve CA, Hartigan C, Martinez E, Hipona M. Comparison of short- and long-term outcomes for aggressive spine rehabilitation delivered two versus three times per week. Spine J. 2002;2;402–407.

[89] Mannion AF, Müntener M, Taimela S, Dvorak J. Comparison of three active therapies for chronic low back pain: results of a randomized clinical trial with one-year follow-up. Rheumatology. 2001; 40 (7):772-778.

[90] Hayden JA, van Tulder MW, Malmivaara A, Koes BW. Exercise therapy for treatment of non-specific low back pain. Cochrane Database of Systematic Reviews, Issue 3 2006. Chichester: John Wiley & Sons Ltd; 2005.

[91] Cuesta-Vargas AI, García-Romero JC, Dediego-Acosta AM, González-Sánchez M, Labajos-Manzanares MT. Clinical effect of deep water running on non-specific low back pain: A randomised trial. SA Journal of Physiotherapy. 2009 VOL 65 n° 3 pp1-8.

[92] Cuesta-Vargas A, Garcia-Romero JC,Kuisma R. Maximum and Resting Heart Rate in Treadmill and Deep-Water Running in Male. International Volleyball Players. International Journal of Aquatic Research and Education, 2009, 3, pp 398-405

[93] Cuesta-Vargas AI, Gonzalez-Sanchez M, Garcıa Romero JC, Labajos-Manzanares MT. Efectividad clınica de un programa de fisioterapia multimodal complementado con carrera acuática de alta intensidad sobre la lumbalgia. Un estudio con evaluación previa en el postest. Fisioterapia; 2010, 32(1): pp 17–24

[94] Storheim K, Brox JI, Holm I, Koller AK, Bo K (2003) Intensive group training versus cognitive intervention in sub-acute low back pain: short-term results of a single-blind randomized controlled trial. J Rehabil Med, 35(3): 132-40.

[95] Karjalainen K, Malmivaara A, Mutanen P, Roine R, Hurri H, Pohjolainen T (2004) Mini-intervention for subacute low back pain: two-year follow-up and modifiers of effectiveness. Spine, 29(10): 1069-76.

[96] Frost H, Lamb SE, Doll HA, Carver PT, Stewart-Brown S (2004) Randomised controlled trial of physiotherapy compared with advice for low back pain. Bmj, 329(7468): 708.

[97] Cherkin DC, Eisenberg D, Sherman KJ, Barlow W, Kaptchuk TJ, Street J, Deyo RA (2001) Randomized trial comparing traditional Chinese medical acupuncture, therapeutic massage, and self-care education for chronic low back pain. Arch Intern Med, 161(8): 1081-8.

[98] Karjalainen K, Malmivaara A, Pohjolainen T, Hurri H, Mutanen P, Rissanen P, Pahkajarvi H, Levon H, Karpoff H, Roine R (2003) Mini-intervention for subacute low back pain: a randomized controlled trial. Spine, 28(6): 533-40; discussion 40-1.

[99] Skinner BF (1953) Science and Human Behaviour. New York: The Macmillan Co.

[100] van Tulder MW, Ostelo RW, Vlaeyen JW, Linton SJ, Morley SJ, Assendelft WJ (2004) Behavioural treatment for chronic low back pain (Cochrane Review). In: The Cochrane Library, Issue 3. John Wiley & Sons, Ltd: Chichester, UK.

[101] Ostelo RWJG, de Vet HC, Vlaeyen J, Kerkhoffs MR, Berfelo WM, Wolters PMJC, van den Brandt PA (2003) Behavioral graded activity following first-time lumbar disc surgery. 1- year results of a randomized clinical trial. Spine, 28: 1757-65.

[102] Spinhoven P, Ter Kuile M, Kole-Snijders AM, Hutten Mansfeld M, Den Ouden DJ, Vlaeyen JW (2004) Catastrophizing and internal pain control as mediators of outcome in the multidisciplinary treatment of chronic low back pain. Eur J Pain, 8(3): 211-9.

[103] Brox JI, Sorensen R, Friis A, Nygaard O, Indahl A, Keller A, Ingebrigtsen T, Eriksen HR, Holm I, Koller AK, Riise R, Reikeras O (2003) Randomized clinical trial of lumbar instrumented fusion and cognitive intervention and exercises in patients with chronic low back pain and disc degeneration. Spine, 28(17): 1913-21.

[104] van den Hout JH, Vlaeyen JW, Heuts PH, Zijlema JH, Wijnen JA (2003) Secondary prevention of work-related disability in nonspecific low back pain: does problem-solving therapy help? A randomized clinical trial. Clin J Pain, 19(2): 87-96.

[105] Critchley DJ, Ratcliffe J, Noonan S, Jones RH et al. Effectiveness and cost-effectiveness of three types of physiotherapy used to reduce chronic low back pain disability: a pragmatic randomized trial with economic evaluation. Spine. 2007; 32 (14):1474-1481.

[106] Haldorsen EM, Grasdal AL, Skouen JS, Risa AE, KronholmK, Ursin H (2002) Is there a right treatment for a particular patient group? Comparison of ordinary treatment, light multidisciplinary treatment, and extensive multidisciplinary treatment for long-term sick-listed employees with musculoskeletal pain. Pain, 95(1-2): 49-63.

[107] Guzman J, Esmail R, Karjalainen K, Malmivaara A, Irvin E, Bombardier C (2001) Multidisciplinary rehabilitation for chronic low back pain: systematic review. BMJ, 322(7301): 1511-6.

[108] Bendix T, Bendix A, Labriola M, Haestrup C, Ebbehoj N (2000) Functional restoration versus outpatient physical training in chronic low back pain: a randomized comparative study. Spine, 25(19): 2494-500.

[109] Schonstein E, Kenny D, Keating J, Koes B, Herbert RD (2003) Physical conditioning programs for workers with back and neck pain: a cochrane systematic review. Spine, 28(19): E391-5.

[110] Friedrich M, Gittler G, Arendasy M, Friedrich KM. Long-term effect of a combined exercise and motivational program on the level of disability of patients with chronic low back pain. Spine. 2005; 30 (9):995-1000.

[111] Kääpä EH, Frantsi K, Sarna S, Malmivaara A. Multidisciplinary group rehabilitation versus individual physiotherapy for chronic nonspecific low back pain: a randomized trial. Spine. 2006; 31 (4):371-376.

[112] Smeets RJEM, Vlaeyen JWS, Hidding A, Kester ADM et al. Chronic low back pain: physical training, graded activity with problem solving training, or both? The one-year post-treatment results of a randomized controlled trial. Pain. 2008; 134 (3):263-276.

[113] Mangwani J, Giles C, Mullins M, et al. Obesity and recovery from lower back pain: a prospective study to investigate the effect of body mass index on recovery from lower back pain. Ann R Coll Surg Engl. 2010;92(1):23-26.

[114] Sato D, Kaneda K, Wakabayashi H, Nomura T. The water exercise improves health-related quality of life of frail elderly people at day service facility. Qual Life Res. 2007;16;1577-85.

11

Exercises in Low Back Pain

Krzysztof Radziszewski
Clinic of Rehabilitation,
Military Hospital in Bydgoszcz,
Department of Clinical Fundamentals of Physiotherapy,
Collegium Medicum in Bydgoszcz, Nicolaus Copernicus University,
Poland

1. Introduction

It is commonly believed that physical exercise plays an important role in the treatment of patients with low back pain (LBP) (Alaranta et al., Bendix et al., 1998; 1994; Halldin et al., 2005; Hicks et al., 2005; Hurwitz et al., 2005; Koopman et al., 2004). A serious problem for LBP sufferers is considerable limitation in the range of movement of the trunk and pelvis, often accompanied by shortening of the hamstring tendons and limitation of flexion or extension in the coxofemoral joint. Appropriate dosing of physiological exercise not only improves the condition of soft tissues, but also provides for proper stretching of collagen fibres and enhances the nutrition status of articular cartilage. It is important to prescribe customized programmes of exercises which restore and preserve normal activity of the lumbar spine. An appropriate exercise programme ensures the development of a 'muscle corset' of postural muscles which optimises load on intervertebral discs and passive stabilizers of the spine (ligaments, capsules). Programmes should include stretching as well as endurance- and strength-building exercises. The principle to follow is that movements in joints should be performed within painless limits. Of importance during exercise is appropriate mobility of the lumbar spine–pelvis–lower limb complex. It is often necessary to stretch the hip joint flexors and lumbar extensors as well as to strengthen weak and stretched abdominal and gluteal muscles with the aim of eliminating excessive forward tilt of the pelvis and preventing overload in the lumbar segment as well as ensuring an even distribution of load.

The key to improvement is exercise of spinal muscles to enhance segmental stability, which is compromised by degenerative processes in the disc. Regular physical exercise reduces pain and the accompanying symptoms of depression. Reduction in pain is associated with identifying the most comfortable, 'neutral' position and the ability to assume and maintain that position during motor acts.

Numerous reports emphasise that abdominal muscles are the key to achieving optimal spinal performance (Alaranta et al., 1994; Axler et al., 1997). An essential activity serving to ensure proper spinal function is controlling the posture and position of the spine during movements so that pain is avoided and the range of movement is as close to normal as possible. The above goals are achieved by ensuring appropriate daily posture, including proper lordotic curvature of the spine. Strong muscles of the abdominal wall are essential as they prevent hyperlordosis and excessive forward tilt of the pelvis. It is necessary to simultaneously stretch the iliopsoas muscles, which are usually contractured from working conditions. At the same time, stretching exercises should be included in the exercise programme to restore the proper position of the spine.

Regular exercise is necessary for surgically managed patients. Early on following intervertebral disc surgery, exercises are mostly concerned with static motor activity and particular attention is paid to pain relief. The exercises aim to improve body posture by strengthening postural muscles, while simultaneously avoiding excessive mobilization of lumbar segments of the spine. In order to reduce pain and structural overload of lumbar segments, water exercises are recommended in small doses. It is believed that, by activating plasminogen, physical exercise may reduce the risk of development of periradicular scars (Szymanski et al., 1994).

While injury to the intervertebral disc and the resultant low back pain may be due to a variety of causes, the most important of them are believed to include: a stressful lifestyle, incorrect posture, failure to exercise regularly, and physical injury or disease (Biering-Sørensen & Thomsen, 1986). The mechanism of stress-induced BP includes increased tone of the spinal muscles. Good posture depends on adequate flexibility of the hamstring tendons, hip flexors and extensors, and extensor and flexor muscles of the spine, allowing maintenance of proper spinal caurvatures, which is of importance for appropriate loading and function of the spine.

2. Exercises in the acute and subacute phase

The literature brings conflicting data on the efficacy of exercises to strengthen muscles in the treatment of acute low back pain (Davies et al., 1979; Mitchell & Carmen, 1990; Saal, 1990). Some of the inconsistencies stem from methodological shortcomings, randomisation problems or the lack of precise diagnoses in most of these studies (Donchin et al., 1990). In such papers, the advantages of bending exercises in the treatment of various lumbosacral pain syndromes are compared with those of extension exercises. In one study, bending exercises were shown to be useful in patients with pathologies of the posterior segment, such as spondylolysis or spondylolisthesis (Donchin et al., 1990), while other studies demonstrated efficacy of a programme of extension exercises in patients with low back pain of discopathic origin (Delitto et al., 1993; Stankovic & Johnell). The use of unidirectional exercises (only bends or extensions) is principally therapeutic oversimplification, considering the multiplicity of pathophysiological abnormalities found in patients with acute or recurrent low back pain. McKenzie's exercise programme for patients with intervertebral disc pathology concentrates on centralisation of pain rather than on the movements of bending or extending the spine (McKenzie, 1972). However, this programme is introduced only when the positions associated with pain centralisation have been identified (Donelson et al., 1990). Therapeutic exercise is incorporated in more complex rehabilitation programmes. Techniques enabling stabilisation of the lumbar spine in motion can be applied simultaneously to ensure dynamic muscle control and protection against biomechanical loads, such as tensing, compression, twisting and shearing action. Spinal stabilisation involves synergistic activation or co-activation of the trunk and spinal muscles in the middle segment of their range of motion. Loads are increased by movements of the lower and upper limbs in various planes during therapy and, later, during work and everyday activity. The general objectives of such rehabilitation programmes are the alleviation of pain, development of the protective muscular "corset" of the trunk and spine and reduction of the load on intervertebral discs and other elements acting as static stabilisers of the spine (Saal, (1990; Tulder et al., 1997). Therapeutic sessions should be carried out in an active manner and repeated only as many times as is necessary for the patient to understand the idea behind the programme and master the exercise technique for later unsupervised practice at home. The programme should also involve instructions for the patient, who should be advised to maintain a neutral spinal position and dynamic muscular "corset" action during all daily activities associated with work and recreation. If no improvement is noted following six therapeutic sessions, the patient should be re-evaluated and the rehabilitation specialist consulted. The efficacy of such comprehensive rehabilitation programmes is well-documented and they are widely used in the treatment of professional athletes (Davies et al., 1979; Delitto et al., 1993; Stankovic et al., 1990).

In acute and subacute low back pain, kinesiotherapy should start with a set of exercises selected individually for the specific patient. Following an evaluation of the patient's exercise capacity, the type of exercises is selected together with starting positions. A comprehensive clinical evaluation serves to identify muscle groups in need of strengthening and those likely to benefit from a relaxing action. Motor re-education of the spine and the musculoligamentous apparatus is necessary. An evaluation of spinal mobility identifies hyper- and hypomobile segments. The therapeutic objective of working with hypermobile segments is to effect their stabilisation, while locked, hypomobile areas must undergo motor mobilisation in order to attain maximum motor harmony. Kinesiotherapy is usually preceded by appropriate physical therapy and followed by relaxation-inducing procedures. The exercise programme emphasises strengthening the abdominal muscles and the quadratus lumborum with simultaneous abolition of the lumbar lordosis. Attention is also given to strengthening the crural muscles, hip extensors and gluteal muscles. The application of traction along the spinal axis may be beneficial. To this end, chair traction can be applied in Perschl position, gravitational traction, or pulsed traction. The duration of a session is from several minutes to half an hour. Traction relaxes back muscles and broadens intervertebral spaces (Beurskens et al., 1997).

Exercises are applied in three basic starting positions:

- supine position with limbs flexed at the knees and hips,
- squatting position,
- lateral recumbent position.

The choice of a particular starting position is patient-specific.

Early on, exercises with the patient being hung from pulleys are also possible. When the pain has abated, exercises performed against greater resistance can be introduced, as well as group exercises and further instruction on exercises to be performed by the patient without supervision or assistance.

The exercises must not produce or intensify pain. Exercises should be selected so that it is possible to mobilise all joint-muscle-ligament systems that influence spinal function and health.

3. Exercises in the chronic phase

When the symptoms have become chronic, patients practise in small therapeutic groups. Continuous supervision by the physiotherapist is mandatory. An important component of the programme is patient education regarding optimal working conditions during both professional duties and household chores. Lasting good treatment outcomes depend on the patient exercising regularly in the home.

The treatment of back pain is extremely difficult and prolonged. We need to convince the patient that perseverance in systematic kinesiotherapy and maintaining a healthy life style is a must. Low back pain may recur, existing symptoms may exacerbate and new symptoms may develop.

Various criteria are in use for classifying patients as chronic low back pain sufferers. A temporal criterion can be used (symptoms have been present for more than 6 months) or a symptom-based one (despite back pain, the patient is able to carry on daily activity, including professional duties, be it with some limitations from time to time). Rehabilitation programmes for chronic back pain sufferers are also administered to patients after spinal surgery. Chronic low back pain is characterized by lower pain intensity, a constant level of spinal dysfunction and the presence of permanent neurological deficits. In the chronic low back pain phase, patients often appear depressed and anxious. These are important factors affecting patient motivation to carry out therapeutic exercises. Kinesiotherapy in the chronic phase is based on similar principles as treatment in the acute phase. Differences concern the pace of exercises, loads and exercise types. After exercising individually, the patients can soon join a therapeutic group performing group exercises. Individual exercises should be available to patients following spinal surgery or early on during a symptomatic exacerbation. In patients after spinal surgery, the decision to commence kinesiotherapy must be preceded by collecting detailed information about the operative procedure and the presence of any contraindications to rehabilitation.

Exercises to strengthen weakened phasic muscles are introduced when contractured muscles have been relaxed. An effective way to relax contractured postural muscles is to apply post-isometric muscle relaxation. This technique demands co-operation of the therapist and patient, who contributes to the technique of relaxation. The therapist achieves mild extension of the contractured muscle. The patient uses a minimum force to tense the muscle against the resistance afforded by the therapist's hand for approximately 10 seconds. This is followed by a muscle relaxation phase, lasting 2-3 seconds. As resistance subsides, the therapist gently extends the contractured muscle over several seconds. This cycle should be repeated a few times for each contractured muscle. Exercises associated with uncontrolled extension of passive vertebral stabilisers (ligaments, joint capsules) should be avoided as this may impair spinal stability.

Abdominal muscles are to be strengthened mainly via isometric contractions. Isotonic exercises should only be performed in the supine position. Exercises should be simple and easy to learn and carry out. Exercise intensity should match the patient's capabilities at a given time. The move from less demanding to more strenuous exercises should be gradual.

The DBC method (Documentation Based Care) is a form of kinesiotherapy based on mechanotherapy. It is an active therapy for subacute and chronic spinal ailments. The name emphasizes its documentation-based rationale. The approach to evaluating and analysing treatment outcomes is compatible with the principles of evidence-based medicine. The method is based on modern technology and therapeutic exercise to produce the best possible functional and analgesic effect. Treatment programmes are individualised. The equipment used in DBC has been designed to enable spinal therapy with repeated dynamic loading. The aim of the programme is to restore segmental spinal motion, improve neuromuscular control of these movements, increase mobility and improve muscle exercise capacity. Free and assisted exercises are applied. The exercise technique contributes to muscular relaxation and relaxes the tensed spinal burso-ligamentous structures. Exercises involve controlled flexion in the sagittal plane, extension, rotation and flexion, and spinal rotation and retraction. Supplementary exercises include general toning and relaxing exercises and exercises to strengthen the muscle groups that

3.1 Manipulation and mobilisation

Manipulation has been recognised as an effective method in acute low back pain. However, even though some studies have demonstrated the effectiveness of soft tissue manipulation and mobilisation in the treatment of acute low back pain, other studies have not confirmed this effect (Anderson et al., 1972; Koes et al., 1996; Shekelle et al., 1992; Tulder et al., 1997). Contemporary reports are not reliable due to methodological and procedural shortcomings and the use of poorly measurable parameters for evaluating treatment outcomes. Manipulation should initially be applied once weekly in conjunction with physical exercises. Additionally, supplementary exercises for muscles may be applied two or three times a week. Regular scheduled follow-up visits are necessary to monitor changes in symptoms or signs. The treatment needs to have clear objectives. If there is no improvement after 3-4 sessions, manipulation should be discontinued and the patient re-assessed. Manual techniques should be included in initial treatment of acute low back pain to facilitate physical exercises requiring the patient's active participation. Physicians should be aware of contraindications to manipulation, especially that performed under general anaesthesia, which is associated with considerable risk. While patients undergoing manipulation are very much satisfied with this technique, there is no rationale for performing manipulation after acute pain has subsided.

3.2 Posture

An erect posture is the body's position when standing at ease. Posture changes during life under the influence of the external and internal environment. Serious postural deterioration is usually noted in the fourth decade of life, when the spinal curvatures become more accentuated. This is due to a number of factors: slowly progressive loss of muscle bulk of the abdominal muscles and extensors spinae, gaining weight and degeneration of intervertebral discs.

The lumbar intervertebral discs change with the posture in motion and inactivity. Posture determines the intensity and extent of mechanical tensing of intervertebral discs. Compressive forces acting on the lower lumbar discs decrease nearly to nil in the recumbent position, to increase rapidly in the sitting or standing position. The highest rate of increase in disc compression is associated with physical exertion, especially combined with carrying weights in an inappropriate manner. The intensity of compression depends on the force of gravity and the type and character of the movement being performed. Posture, or the alignment of vertebral bodies against each other and the alignment of the spine along the vertical axis, is of considerable importance for the prevention of back pain.

In the standing position, body mass is distributed equally between vertebral bodies and intervertebral discs. If the spine deviates from the vertical plane, a system of levers begins to operate which increases the pressure acting on intervertebral discs several times. The increase in intervertebral disc compression is the result of the lever action and changes in the plane of action of the levers. The compressive forces do not act on the discs and vertebral bodies at a right angle, but at an acute angle. Shearing forces arise and attempt to dislocate the vertebrae. These shearing forces are counteracted by the intervertebral discs, ligaments, articular processes, and muscles that stabilize the spine.

Changes in vertebral alignment during movement of the spine predominantly affect the annulus fibrosus of the intervertebral disc. Forward and lateral bends, straightening, rotations, or any combinations of these movements, stretch and tense annulus fibrosus fibres. The degree of tensing depends on the amplitude of the movement being performed. The nucleus pulposus takes part in all movements. The gel of the nucleus pulposus is intertwined with the fibrous tissue network growing into the annulus fibrosus. Movements of the spine lead to various degrees of tensing of this fibrous network and the annulus fibrosus. Similarly, forces attempting to dislocate vertebrae are transferred onto the fibrous network and the annulus. These forces, whose intensity depends partially on spinal mobility and partially on posture, have a major influence on degenerative processes within the intervertebral disc. Control of these forces is of basic importance for prevention and the treatment of patients with intervertebral disc damage. Protecting the ailing disc from harmful tensing and loading is a preprequisite for the process of fibrous ankylosis of the affected spinal segment that often produces abolition of symptoms. It is not possible to "switch off" all forces and tensions acting on the lumbar spine. These forces can be reduced and so can their harmful effects. An important role in this regard is played by the maintenance of an appropriate posture both at work and at rest. This must be paralleled by strengthening the muscles that stabilize the lumbar spine.

Good posture plays a major role in protecting the lumbar intervertebral discs from mechanical overload. When the lumbar spine is properly stabilized, a strong extensor spinae and abdominal muscles bear the brunt of many forces that would otherwise be acting directly on the spinal ligaments and joints and intervertebral discs. When an intervertebral disc is damaged, the role of good posture is to ensure maximum spinal performance while simultaneously reducing pressures acting on the spine. Controlling spinal movements prevents repetitive overload of the strands of elastic fibres of the annulus fibrosus and the nucleus pulposus.

Any prevention programme for low back pain should be based on several principles:

- the spine should be maintained in a neutral position. Unnecessary bending, straightening or rotation are to be avoided,
- avoid a 'tired' posture where the physiological spinal curves are accentuated. The abdominal muscles, extensor spinae and the gluteal muscles should maintain a constant appropriate tone,
- the spine should be erected vertically when sitting and standing to reduce the likelihood of the development of shearing forces,

- during movement and exertion, the spine should be controlled by muscles to ensure stability and a safe amplitude of movement.

3.3 Pelvic tilt

Posterior inclination of the pelvis when carrying weights and performing exercises is recommended by many textbooks. This habit leads to spinal flexion and, from the very outset, puts a strain on the annulus fibrosus and posterior spinal ligaments, potentially increasing the risk of damage to the intervertebral disc. A neutrally aligned spinal column (i.e. one that is neither in hyper- or hypolordosis) provides for elastic balance and minimises the risk of damage during increased strain on the spine as a result of muscular contractions. A general practical rule to follow is that the normal lumbo-sacral spinal curvatures should be maintained as they shape out in an erect position (McGill,1998).

3.4 The flexibility

Exercises to enhance trunk flexibility should be limited to the movements of flexion and extension without loading. It is not advisable to attempt to attain the extremes of spinal mobility in particular types of damage (Battié et al., 1990; McGill,1998). The outcomes of numerous rehabilitation programmes confirm the importance of achieving trunk stability through exercises with the spine in a neutral position. It is emphasized that ensuring normal mobility in the hip and knee joints is essential.

Appropriate mobility in the hip and knee joints is required for the maintenance of spine-sparing postures. Normal mobility in the hip and knee joints is necessary to protect the spine from excessive movements during daily activity.

3.5 Strength and endurance

The effectiveness of muscle action is determined by "strength" and "endurance", which should be treated as two different components, especially with regard to planning specific exercise programmes. "Strength" refers to the maximum force that a muscle can produce during a single effort to produce torque in a joint. "Endurance" denotes the ability to exert a sustained force over some time. Decreased muscle strength in patients with spinal pathology is a proven fact (McNeill et al., 1980). Several works have suggested that endurance is more important than strength in prevention (McGill, 1998); McNeill et al., 1980). Many injuries occurring during submaximum efforts are associated with decreased endurance of spinal muscles. Patients with spinal pathology need to ensure necessary stabilisation by tensing their abdominal muscles in the erect position, and especially during flexion. While planning exercises, emphasis should be placed on improving endurance by the application of exercises that take longer to complete but generate less loading (Cady et al., 1979; McNeill et al., 1980). An important aspect of the methodology of endurance-building exercises is that such exercises do not involve joint movements, which facilitates activation of the abdominal muscles.

3.6 Abdominal muscles

Increased intraabdominal pressures are used to stabilise and protect the lumbar spine during movements and carrying weights. Intraabdominal pressure can be increased by appropriate exercises for the rectus abdominis and oblique abdominis muscles. Improvement in abdominal muscle strength and tonus enhances the efficacy of the mechanism for transferring loads and mechanical strain from the skeleton to the muscular system by increasing intraabdominal pressure. As a result, some of the forces representing a load on the lower intervertebral discs are transferred to the pelvic floor and the diaphragm. Moreover, improved abdominal muscle strength helps stabilize the spine better. In the lumbar region, the spine is supported posteriorly by the extensor spinae, anterolaterally by the psoas, and anteriorly by intraabdominal pressure, which depends on abdominal muscle tone.

No single exercise will help develop all abdominal muscles. If the goal is to improve muscle strength and endurance, exercises should be prescribed in increased quantities. Trunk curl-ups mainly strengthen the rectus abdominis with little activity from the psoas muscles and the muscles of the abdominal wall (internal and external oblique and transverse abdominal muscle). Raising an erect trunk (sit-ups), with the lower limbs extended or flexed at the knee, increases psoas activity and increases pressure on the lower spine. Leg raising considerably increases muscle activity and pressure on the spine.

Exercises in the lateral recumbent position are a useful type of exercise for low back pain sufferers as they involve the lateral oblique muscles without generating much load on the lumbar region. These exercises also trigger considerable activity of the quadratus lumborum, which is the most important spinal stabiliser. At the beginning of rehabilitation, exercises for abdominal muscles should involve elevating a curled-up trunk and isometric exercises in the lateral recumbent position with support at the knee and the flexed elbow (Axler & McGill, 1997; Hurwitz et al., 2005).

3.7 Quadratus lumborum muscle

It has been questioned whether the psoas muscle is indeed an important stabiliser of the spine. The activity of the psoas muscles is mostly seen during hip flexion. During flexion and axial loading of the lumbar spine, it is the quadratus lumborum that exhibits greater activity. This suggests an important role for the quadratus lumborum in stabilising the lumbar spine. Strengthening the quadratus lumborum muscle and increasing spinal stability can be achieved with exercises in horizontal lateral support (McGill et al., 1996).

3.8 Extensor spinae

Most exercises for the extensor spinae muscles are associated with considerable load on the spine produced by externally generated pressure and shearing forces.

Exercises involving keeping one leg extended with the body being supported on the hands and the other knee produce little external loading of the spine but simultaneously generate an extension torque, resulting in increased activity of the extensor spinae muscles. Unilateral extensor spinae activity is sufficient. Since the activity of the contralateral extensor spina eis low, the total load on the spine is decreased. Alternate extension of the lower limbs produces alternate engagement of the extensors spinae (Hurwitz et al., 2005).

3.9 Aerobic exercises

Numerous studies have revealed that low back pain sufferers demonstrate reduced aerobic capacity. The importance of aerobic exercise in reducing the incidence of pathology of the lower spine (Cady et al., 1979) and in the treatment of patients with low back pain is well documented (Nutter, 1988).

Some studies raise the causality question as low back pain often affects professional athletes, who have excellent aerobic capacity. Casazza et al. reviewed the available literature on the role of aerobic training and improving cardiovascular performance. They found that it is not clear whether it is low back pain that leads to decreased exercise capacity or whether reduced exercise capacity contributes to the development of low back pain. The authors noted that low back pain has lower intensity in patients with normal exercise capacity and they are convinced that there is a rationale for including aerobic exercise in the rehabilitation programme (Casazza et al, 1998). Videman et al. revealed the presence of more advanced degenerative changes and disc protrusion in weight-lifters and footballers compared to runners (Videman, 1976).

Improved aerobic capacity may increase perfusion and oxygen supply to all tissues, including muscles, vertebrae and spinal ligaments. Aerobic exercise may reduce the influence of mental factors on low back pain by improving mood, diminishing depression and increasing pain tolerance (Anshel & Russell, 1994). It is theoretically possible that such exercises increase the body's ability to lyse scar tissue via the action of tissue plasminogen activator (Szymanski & Pate, 1994). Improvement of aerobic capacity should be combined with a rehabilitation programme aiming to restore normal mobility of the lumbosacral spine, strengthen trunk muscles and restore normal body mechanics. Limiting rehabilitation to aerobic exercise would not be sufficient. It is important to avoid situations that reduce exercise capacity. This principle can be implemented at the very start of treatment by reducing the length of the period of bed rest and immobilisation. Patients with decreased overall exercise capacity should be instructed about the basics of aerobic exercise and evaluation of target exercise intensity by measuring the heart rate or assessing subjective fatigue.

3.10 Regular physical exercise

Particular importance is ascribed to exercising regularly (Ben Salah Frih et al., 2009). Temporary, emergency rehabilitation of patients with disc herniation at L4-L5 does not prevent disease progression. Failure to exercise regularly affects patients' physical performance and results in inability to work and perform self-care in more than 22% of patients within 2 years (Friedrich, 2005). The results of Laursen's observations confirm that regular rehabilitation is indispensable in conservative therapy (Laursen & Fugl, 1995). Observations show that exercise intensity does not have a significant effect on long-term outcomes of rehabilitation of patients with LBP (Mellin et al, 1993). During the immediate post-operative period, programmes of intensive exercises produce better outcomes. (Friedrich et al., 2005; Ostelo et al., 2003).

It is also often emphasised that regular physical exercise has a favourable effect on surgical outcomes in intervertebral disc herniation. The discopathic patient should not wait for a miracle cure to relieve the dysfunction and suffering completely and permanently but should start to participate actively in the treatment process. Intensive exercise from the 4th - 6th week after surgery onwards significantly improves the functional status of patients and reduces the time needed to return to work. A programme of motor rehabilitation introduced at a later stage does not produce such favourable therapeutic effects (Ostelo et al., 2003).

Kjellby argues that repeat surgery is less common in patients engaged in rehabilitation programmes (Kjellby-Wendt et al., 2002).

Patients with acute and subacute low back pain perform exercises most regularly. A study by the present author found that the proportion of those patients exercising and the amount of time devoted to exercise weekly increased with the duration of the disease. Within 6 months following the onset of back pain, 51.4% of patients performed spinal exercises regularly, of whom only 15.4% exercised for 2 hours a week. In long-term follow-up (5 years after onset), 53.6% of respondents reported exercising regularly, 17.9% of whom exercised for more than 2 hours a week.

OUTCOME MEASURE	TIME PER WEEK		
	LESS THAN 1 HUOR	1-2 HOURS	MORE THAN 2 HOURS
Pain intesity V-A scale (1-10)	4,51±1,72	4,12±1,26	3,35±2,31
Functional status OLBPDQ (% of normal)	50,8±11,3	52,8±9,6	59,9±8,4
Occupational activity, F-EORS scale (% of normal)	63,1±21,0	57,7±11,1	59,8±21.3
Depresion index, S-RDS scale	0,61±0,12	0,56±0,10	0,48±0,14

Table 1. Treatment outcomes according to the time alloted to exercise per week

Surgically managed patients appreciated the importance of regular exercise the most during immediate and short-term follow-up. In this period, about 60% of patients reported performing therapeutic exercises, with most, however, exercising for one hour per week. At four years post-surgery, the total number of exercising patients had decreased by approximately 4%, while the number of patients exercising for more than 2-3 hours a week had risen by approximately 4%. Physical exercise was performed by 58.8% of men and 50.4% of women. A beneficial effect of exercise on the functional status, pain intensity and mental state was recorded only in the group exercising for more than two hours a week. The study indicated that the use of physical exercise by patients with low back pain is insufficient, with only approximately 20% of patients exercising long enough. Patients definitely prefer passive treatments to alleviate pain (massage, physiotherapy). Exercises of the backbone are performed for a short period, irregularly and usually only when the pain is more intense. Therefore, the exercises cannot wholly fulfil the important preventive and therapeutic role they are attributed (Radziszewski, 2007).

4. Summary

Numerous authors emphasise that a programme of regular motor rehabilitation is the most efficient modality of conservative therapy (Alaranta et al., 1994; Caby et al., 2010; Kjellby-Wendt et al., 2002; Koopman et al., 2004; Sherman et al., 2010). Regular physical exercise is a way to achieve many beneficial effects, such as reduction of pain, strengthening of the spinal muscles, optimisation of the distribution of load on the spinal structures, enhanced stabilization of the motor segments of the spine, improved posture and increased overall physical capacity of the body. The precise mechanism by which exercise alleviates pain has not been fully elucidated, although it may be associated with enhancing the nutrition status of the disc. Physical exercise, by stimulating changes in pressure within the intervertebral disc, may improve the mechanisms of osmosis that underlie disc nutrition.

The methodology of exercise attributes a significant role to strength- and endurance-building exercises. Muscle strength is of key importance for trunk stability. Augmentation of the spinal curvatures may be due to weakening of the paraspinal muscles. Epidemiologic studies have shown that patients with strong muscles less frequently complain of back pain. In healthy people, the extensor muscles of the trunk are stronger by 30% than the flexor muscles. However, it is believed that decreased strength is less important in back pain syndromes than decreased endurance capacity of dorsal and abdominal muscles (Davies et al., 1979; McGill, 1998).

Exercise accelerates repair and substitution processes in the musculoskeletal system and internal organs, and prevents the development of detrimental substitute motor patterns. It also prevents the development of secondary changes in bones, joints, muscles and ligaments and cardiorespiratory complications. The body's overall physical capacity is also improved. The main aim of exercises involving movement is to break the vicious circle of pain by reducing reflex increase in paraspinal muscle tension. Exercise also serves to improve stability of the lumbar spine by increasing intraabdominal pressure and restoring muscle balance, which prevents the recurrence of symptoms. Kinesiotherapy in low back pain should be well chosen and appropriately dosed. The notion of choice applies to exercise duration, the number of repetitions of an exercise and the duration of a series of exercises. The technique of therapeutic exercises is also important.

An exercise programme should begin with cycles of flexion and extension exercises serving to decrease stiffness and relax elastic structures. This will result in decreased load on the spinal joints during further exercises. The next batch of exercises should serve to improve mobility in the hip and knee joints and should be followed by exercises for the main spinal stabilisers, starting from abdominal muscles, with the spine in a neutral position throughout this stage. These, in turn, are followed by an ordered sequence of exercises in lateral support to strengthen the quadratus lumborum and oblique abdominis muscles, and exercises for the extensors spinae. The programme should be individualized with regard to the number of repetitions and duration of individual exercise items. The goals need to be clearly specified. Importantly, exercises should be performed in the pain-free range as much as possible. General fitness exercises should not be omitted from a programme for rehabilitation of low back pain sufferers (Nutter, 1988). A basic objective of the exercise set recommended by us is to restore normal static and dynamic balance and motor patterns. Improvement in motor function and alleviation of pain can often be observed following several months of exercises (Donchin et al., 1990 ; McGill, 1998). Of significance for LBP prevention is compliance with the principles of ergonomics during daily activities.(Zauner-Dungl et al., 2004))

5. Conclusion

The most important types of exercise for preventing low back pain are exercises for abdominal muscles, dorsal muscles, gluteal muscles and quadratus lumborum muscle. The most appropriate exercises should be chosen for individual patients. "Endurance" rather than "strength" should be emphasized during exercise selection (low-load exercises repeated several times). Exercising on a daily basis is the most effective approach.

6. References

Alaranta, H.; Rytökoski, U.; Rissanen, A.; Talo, S.; Rönnemaa, T.; Puukka, P.; Karppi, S.L.;, Videman, T.; Kallio, V. & Slätis, P. (1994). Intensive physical and psychosocial training program for patients with chronic low back pain. A contolled clinical trial. *Spine*, Vol.19, No. 12, (Jan 1994), pp 1339-1349, ISSN 0362-243

Anderson, R.; Meeker, W.C.; Wirick, B.E.; Mootz, R.D.; Kirk, D.H. & Adams, A. (1992). A meta-analysis of clinical trials of spinal manipulation. *Journal Of Manipulative And Physiological Therapeutics*,Vol.15, No. 3, (Mar-Apr 1992), pp. 181-194, ISSN: 0161-4754

Anshel, M.H. & Russell, K.G. (1994). Effect of aerobic and strength training on pain tolerance, pain appraisal and mood of unfit males as a function of pain location. *Journal Of Sports Sciences [J Sports Sci]*, Vol. 12, No. 6. (Dec 1994), pp. 535-547, ISSN: 0264-0414,

Axler, C.T. & McGill, S.M. (1997). Low back loads over a variety of abdominal exercises: searching for the safest abdominal challenge. *Medicine & Science in Sports & Exercise*, Vol. 29, No. 6, (Juan 1997), pp. 804-811, ISSN: 0195-9131

Battié, M.C.; Bigos, S.J.; Fisher, L.D.; Spengler, D.M.; Hansson, T.H.; Nachemson, A.L. & Wortley, M.D. (1976). The role of spinal flexibility in back pain complaints within industry. A prospective study. *Spine*, Vol. 15, No. 8, (Aug 1990), pp. 768-773

Ben Salah Frih Z., Fendri Y., Jellad A., Boudoukhane S. & Rejeb N. (2009). Efficacy and treatment compliance of a home-based rehabilitation programme for chronic low back pain: a randomizes study. *Annals Of Physical And Rehabilitation Medicine*, Vol. 52, No. 6, (Jul 2009), pp. 485-496,)ISSN: 1877-0665

Bendix, A.E.; Bendix, T.; Haestrup, C. & Busch E. (1998). A prospective, randomized 5-year follow-up study of functional restoration in chronic low back pain patients. *European Spine Journal:Eur Spine J*, Vol. 7, No. 2, (Feb 1998), pp. 111-119, ISSN 0940-6719

Beurskens, A.J.; de Vet, H.C.; Köke, A.J.; Regtop, W.; van der Heijden, G.J.; Lindeman, E. & Knipschild, P.G. (1997). Efficacy of traction for nonspecific low back pain: 12-week and 6-month results of a randomized clinical trial. *Spine*, Vol. 22, No. 23, (Dec 1997), pp. 2756-2762, ISSN: 0362-2436

Biering-Sørensen, F. & Thomsen, C. (1986). Medical, social and occupational history as risk indicators for low-back trouble in a general population. *Spine*, Vol. 11, No. 7, (Sep 1986), pp. 720-725, ISSN: 0362-2436

Caby I., Vanvelcenaher J., Letombe A. & Pelayo P. (2010). Evaluating the efficacy of an intensive, dynamic and multidisciplinary spine-specific functional restoration program in patients with chronic low back pain with or without surgery. *Annals Of Physical And Rehabilitation Medicine*, Vol. 53, No. 10, (Dec 2010), pp. 621-631, ISSN: 1877-0665

Cady, .LD.; Bischoff, D.P.; O'Connell, E.R.; Thomas, P.C. & Allan.,J.H. (1979). Strength and fitness and subsequent back injuries in firefighters. *Journal Of Occupational Medicine*, Vol. 21, No. 4, (Apr 1979), pp. 269-272, ISSN: 0096-1736

Casazza, B.A.; Young, J.L. & Herring, S.A. (1998). The role of exercise in the prevention and management of acute low back pain. *Occupational Medicine*, Vol. 13, No. 1, (Jan-Mar 1998), pp. 47-60, ISSN: 0885-114X

Davies, J.E.; Gibson, T. & Tester ,L. (1979). The value of exercises in the treatment of low back pain. *Rheumatology And Rehabilitation,* Vol. 18, No. 4, (Nov 1979), pp. 243-247, ISSN: 0300-3396

Delitto,A.; Cibulka, M.T.; Erhard, R.E.; Bowling, R.W. & Tenhula, J.A. (1993). Evidence for use of an extension-mobilization category in acute low back pain syndrome: a prescriptive validation pilot study. *Physical Therapy,* Vol. 73, No. 4, (Apr 1993), pp. 216-222, ISSN: 0031-9023

Donchin, M. Woolf, O. Kaplan, L. & Floman, Y. (1990). Secondary prevention of low-back pain: a clinical trial. *Spine ,* Vol. 15, No. 12, (Dec 1990), pp. 1317-1320, ISSN: 0362-2436

Donelson, R.; Silva, G. & Murphy, K. (1990). Centralization phenomenon: its usefulness in evaluating and treating referred pain. *Spine,* Vol. 15. No. 3, (Mar 1990), pp. 211-213, ISSN: 0362-2436

Friedrich, M.; Gittler, G.; Arendasy, M. & Friedrich, K.M. (2005). Long-term effect of a combined exercise and motivational program on the level of disability of patients with chronic low back pain. *Spine,* Vol. 30, No. 9, (May 2005), pp. 995-1000, ISSN 1528-1159

Halldin, K.; Zoëga, B.; Kärrholm, J.; Lind, B.I.; & Nyberg, P. (2005). Is increased segmental motion early after lumbar discectomy related to poor clinical outcome 5 years later? *International Orthopaedics,* Vol. 29, No.4, (Aug 2005), pp. 260-264, ISSN 0341-2695

Hicks, G.E.; Fritz, J.M.; Delitto, A. & McGill, S.M. (2005).Preliminary development of a clinical prediction rule for determining which patients with low back pain will respond to a stabilization exercise program. *Archives Of Physical Medicine And Rehabilitation,* Vol. 86, No. 9, (Sept 2005), pp. 1753-1762, ISSN 0003-9993

Hurwitz, E.L.; Morgenstern, H. & Chiao, C. (2005). Effects of recreational physical activity and back exercises on low back pain and psychological distress: findings from the UCLA Low Back Pain Study. *American Journal Of Public Health,* Vol. 95, No. 10, (Oct 2005), pp. 1817-1824, ISSN: 0090-0036

Kjellby-Wendt, G.; Carlsson, S.G. & Styf, . (2002). Results of early active rehabilitation 5-7 years after surgical treatment for lumbar disc herniation. *Journal Of Spinal Disorders & Techniques,* Vol. 15, No 5, (Oct 2002), pp. 404-409, ISSN 1536-0652

Koes,B.W.; Assendelft, W.J.; van der Heijden, G.J. & Bouter, L.M. (1996). Spinal manipulation for low back pain: an update systematic review of randomized clinical trials. *Spine,* Vol.21, No. 24, (Dec 1996), pp. 2860-2871, ISSN: 0362-2436

Koopman, F.S.; Edelaar, M.; Slikker, R.; Reynders, K.; van der Woude, L.H. & Hoozemans, M.J. (2004). Effectiveness of multidisciplinary occupational training program for chronic low back pain: a prospective cohort study. *American Journal Of Physical Medicine & Rehabilitation,* Vol. 83, No. 2, (Feb 2004), pp. 94-103, ISSN 0894-9115

Laursen, S.O. & Fugl, I.R. (1995). Outcome of treatment of chronic low back pain in inpatients. Effect of individual physiotherapy including intensive dynamic training in inpatients with chronic low back trouble evaluated by means of low back pain rating scale. *Danish Medical Bulletin,* Vol. 42, No. 3, (Jun 1995), pp. 290-29, ISSN 0907-8916

McGill, S.; Juker, D. & Kropf P. (1996). Appropriately placed surface EMG electrodes reflect deep muscle activity (psoas, quadrates lumborum, abdominal wall) in the lumbar spine. *Journal Of Biomechanics,* Vol. 29, No. 11, (Nov 1996), pp. 1503-1507, ISSN: 0021-9290

McGill, S.M. (1998). Low back exercises: evidence for improving exercise regimens. *Physical Therapy,* Vol. 78, No. 7, (Jul 1998), pp. 754-765, ISSN: 0031-9023

McKenzie, R.A. (1972). Chiropractic treatment. *The New Zealand Medical Journal,* Vol. 75, No. 477, (Feb 1972), pp. 119, ISSN: 0028-8446

McNeill, T.; Warwick, D.; Andersson, G. & Schultz, A. (1980). Trunk strengths in attempted flexion, extension and lateral bending in healthy subjects and patients with low-back disorders. *Spine*, Vol. 5, No. 6, (Nov-Dec 1980), pp. 529-538, ISSN: 0362-2436

Mannion, A.F.; Müntener, M.; Taimela, S. & Dvorak, J. (2001). Comparison of three active therapies for chronic low back pain: results of a randomized clinical trial with one-year follow-up. *Rheumatology*, Vol. 40, No. 7, (Jul 2001), pp. 772-778, ISSN: 1462-0324

Mellin, G.; Härkäpää, K,; Vanharanta, H.; Hupli, M.; Heinonen. R. & Järvikoski, A. (1993). Outcome of multimodal treatment including intensive physical training of patients with chronic low back pain. *Spine*, Vol. 18, No. 7, (Jun 1993), pp. 825-829, ISSN 0362-2436

Mitchell, R.I. & Carmen, G.M. (1990). Results of a multicenter trial using an intensive active exercise program for the treatment of acute soft tissue and back injuries. *Spine*, Vol. 15, No. 6, (Jun 1990), pp. 514-521, ISSN 0362-2436

Nutter, P. (1988). Aerobic exercise in treatment and prevention of low back pain. *Occupational Medicine*, Vol. 3, No. 1, (Jan-Mar 1988), pp. 137-145, ISSN: 0885-114X

Ostelo, R.W.; de Vet, H.C.; Waddell, G.; Kerckhoffs, M.R.; Leffers, P. & van Tulder, M. (2003). Rehabilitation following first-time lumbar disc surgery: a systematic review within the framework of the cochrane collaboration. (2003). *Spine*, Vol. 28, No. 3, (Feb 2003), pp. 209-218, ISSN 1528-1159

Radziszewski, K.R. (2007). Physical exercise in the treatment of patients with lumbar discopathy. *Ortopedia Traumatologia Rehabilitacja*, Vol. 9, No. 1. (Jan-Feb 2007), pp. 98-106, ISSN 1509-3492

Saal,J.A. (1990). Dynamic muscular stabilization in the nonoperative treatment of lumbar pain syndromes. *Danish Medical Bulletin*, Vol. 19, No. 8, (Aug 1990), pp. 691-700, ISSN: 0094-6591

Shekelle, P.G.; Adams, A.H.; Chassin, M.R.; Hurwitz, E.L.& Brook, R.H. (1992). Spinal manipulation for low-back pain. *Annals Of Internal Medicine*, Vol. 117, No 7, (Oct 1992), pp. 590-598, ISSN: 0003-4819

Sherman K.J., Cherkin D.C., Cook A.J., Hawkes R.J., Deyo R.A., Wellman R. & Khalsa P.S. (2010). Comparison of yoga versus stretching for chronic low back pain: protocol for the Yoga Exercise Self-care (YES) trial. *Trials*, Vol. 11, No. 36, (Mar 2010), pp. 36, ISSN: 1745-6215

Stankovic, R. & Johnell, O. (1990). Conservative treatment of acute low-back pain: a prospective randomized trial: McKenzie method of treatment versus patient education in "mini back school". *Spine*, Vol. 15, No. 2, (Feb 1990), pp. 120-123, ISSN: 0362-2436

Szymanski, L.M. & Pate, R.R. (1994). Effects of exercise intensity, duration, and time of day on fibrinolytic activity in physically active men. *Medicine And Science In Sports Exercise*, Vol. 26, No. 9, (Sep 1994), pp. 1102-1108, ISSN: 0195-9131

Videman, T.; Sarna, S.; Battié, M.C.; Koskinen, S.; Gill, K.; Paananen, H. & Gibbons, L. (1976). The long-term effects of physical loading and exercise lifestyles on back-related symptoms, disability, and spinal pathology among men. *Spine*, Vol. 20, No. 6, (Mar 1995), pp 699-709, ISSN: 0362-2436

Zauner-Dungl A. (2004). Is Qi Gong suitable for the prevention of low back pain? *Wiener Medizinische Wochenschrift*, Vol. 154, No. 23,24, (Dec 2004), pp. 564-567, ISSN: 0043-5341

12

Yoga as a Treatment for Low Back Pain: A Review of the Literature

Erik J. Groessl[1,2], Marisa Sklar[3] and Douglas Chang[1,2]
[1]*VA San Diego Healthcare System,*
[2]*University of California San Diego,*
[3]*SDSU/UCSD Joint Doctoral Program in Clinical Psychology,*
USA

1. Introduction

Chronic low back pain (CLBP) affects millions of people worldwide. In addition to chronic pain, CLBP is associated with increased disability and psychological symptoms, and reduced health-related quality of life (HRQOL). There are many treatment options for chronic low back pain, although no single therapy stands out as being the most effective. In the past 10 years, yoga interventions have been studied as an additional approach for treating CLBP. The objective of this chapter is to provide an introduction to yoga as a treatment for CLBP before reviewing the published literature to date supporting the efficacy of yoga for CLBP. Two large randomized controlled trials (RCTs) published late in 2011 provide the most conclusive evidence to date in this area. With few exceptions, previous studies and the recent RCTs indicate that yoga can reduce pain and disability, can be practiced safely, and is well received by participants. Some studies also indicate that yoga can reduce pain medication use and improve psychological symptoms, but these effects are currently not as well established. We summarize these results, discuss their implications, and examine caveats and limitations of the current research evidence. Finally, we provide suggestions for future avenues of research.

2. Chronic low back pain

Back pain is the second most common reason for physician visits and approximately 25% of the US population report having had back pain that lasted all day in the prior 3 months. (Deyo, Mirza, & Martin, 2006) It is estimated that 90% of all acute back pain episodes resolve within 4 weeks, (Anderson, 1997) up to a third of those who sought treatment for their back pain reported persistent pain one year later, (Von Korff & Saunders, 1996) with 20% also reporting limitations of activity. It was estimated that back pain-related health care costs were about $26 billion in 1998 and that the health care costs of back pain patients are 60% higher than those without back pain. (Luo, Pietrobon, Sun, Liu, & Hey, 2004)

Low back pain is the most common type of back pain and is a prevalent condition that afflicts about 70% of people in developing countries at some point in their lifetime. (Anderson, 1997) The incidence of low back pain is greatest in persons of young adult and middle age, with 74% of all health visits for low back pain made by persons between the ages of 18 and 64 years. (AAOS, 2008) Additionally, in this group, low back pain is often associated by reduced ability to work or inability to work at all. The total economic impact (health care costs plus socioeconomic costs) has therefore been estimated at over $100 billion each year. (AAOS, 2008) In the past, chronic low back pain was defined as low back pain lasting 12 weeks or more, but current guidelines now primarily differentiate between acute low back pain lasting less than 4 weeks and chronic, subacute low back pain lasting greater than 4 weeks. (Chou et al., 2007) This distinction coincides with the data cited above showing most back pain resolves on its own within 4 weeks.

Chronic low back pain results in more than just pain and discomfort. Persons with chronic low back pain also experience a variety of other symptoms and functional limitations. These include increased psychological symptoms such as depression, (Currie & Wang, 2004; Sullivan, Reesor, Mikail, & Fisher, 1992) anxiety, (Manchikanti, Pampati, Beyer, Damron, & Barnhill, 2002; Thompson, Bower, & Tyrer, 2007) increased disability, (Guo, Tanaka, Halperin, & Cameron, 1999) and reduced health-related quality of life (HRQOL). (Burstrom, Johannesson, & Diderichsen, 2001; Kosinski et al., 2005) Low back pain has a major impact on workforce productivity, with millions of workdays (Guo et al., 1999) (costing billions of dollars) lost for employees with back pain each year in the US. Research on disability and lost productivity among people with low back pain indicates that psychological factors are independently associated with lost productivity, increased disability, (Schiphorst Preuper et al., 2007) and increased healthcare utilization. (Keeley et al., 2008) Using formal diagnostic criteria, results of a 2004 research study found that 20% of persons with chronic back pain had major depression while only 6% of pain-free individuals were classified this way. (Currie & Wang, 2004) Higher rates of depression among individuals with low back pain have been found previously in many other studies, (Manchikanti et al., 2002; Sullivan et al., 1992) along with elevated rates of other disorders such as anxiety and somatoform disorder. (Manchikanti et al., 2002) Although the causal relationship between psychological symptoms and CLBP is complex, research evidence indicates that psychological symptoms often improve in low back pain patients after exercise interventions, even if the interventions were not specifically designed to affect the psychological symptoms. (Roche et al., 2007) Conversely, placebo or sham treatments for low back pain have not resulted in significant changes in psychological symptoms. (Thompson et al., 2007)

Current treatments for chronic low back pain

Treatment recommendations for low back pain have been updated in 2007 and begin with an effort to categorize patients into three groups: Nonspecific low back pain, low back pain with radiating leg pain, and low back pain from a specific cause (e.g. fracture, malignancy, infection, cauda equine syndrome, or ankylosing spondylitis). (Chou et al., 2007) The majority of chronic low back pain cases (85%) are nonspecific and are not linked to specific physical abnormalities. (van Tulder, Assendelft, Koes, & Bouter, 1997) When a treating physician deems low back pain to be non-specific, health care providers are strongly recommended to begin treatment by providing patients with evidence-based information and to also encourage them to stay active and perform self-care activities. Self-care or self-management activities are strongly recommended because they are inexpensive and are almost as effective as other non-pharmacological options. Another front-line option for patients with nonspecific chronic back pain is medication. (Chou & Huffman, 2007a; Chou et al., 2007) Patients that do not improve after treatment with self-care activities and/or medications are good candidates for non-pharmacological treatments. Non-pharmacological treatments include physical treatments (i.e. heat, ice, ultrasound, massage therapy), spinal manipulation, and forms of injection therapy. (Chou & Huffman, 2007b) Other studies have examined interventions such as exercise therapy, yoga, back schools, acupuncture, psychological therapies, laser treatment, lumbar supports, traction, and transcutaneous electrical nerve stimulation.

Non-pharmacological treatments

Non-pharmacological treatments are diverse, and vary considerably in the quality and amount of evidence supporting them and in the effect sizes they produce [14]. Despite varying evidence of their effectiveness, non-pharmacologic treatment options are widely recommended, especially by primary care physicians when their patients have not improved. (Di Iorio, Henley, & Doughty, 2000; Freburger, Carey, & Holmes, 2005) Ratings of the level of evidence for non-pharmacological treatments in recent guidelines are as follows: "good" scientific evidence was available for spinal manipulation (moderate effects), multidisciplinary approaches (moderate effects), exercise (small to moderate effects), and some psychological interventions (moderate effects), exercise (small to moderate effects), and some psychological interventions (moderate effects); (Chou & Huffman, 2007b) a "fair" level of evidence was found for yoga (moderate effects), acupuncture (moderate effects), functional restoration (moderate effects), back schools (small effects), and continuous traction (not effective); and finally, effects were not rated for the seven other therapies for which evidence was judged as "Poor". Overall, the recommendations suggest that several non-pharmacological treatments are moderately effective, but none stand out as exceptionally beneficial. Thus, the characteristics, preferences and resources of individual patients, the cost and risk of the interventions, and consideration of the disease's natural history itself become important factors in treatment decision-making for chronic low back pain. For instance, some patients are at greater risk for developing addictions when treated with narcotic pain medications, making non-pharmacological treatments a more appealing choice.

Medical procedures

Injectional therapy to treat back conditions has become increasingly popular. Some injections (e.g. trigger point injections, acupuncture, prolotherapy) can be considered one of the many sundry non-pharmacological treatments. Other injections (e.g. epidural steroid injections, facet injections, medial branch blocks, radiofrequency ablation) are performed more frequently for spinal conditions and deserve specific discussion. The utilization rates for injectional therapies has risen about 250% between 1994 and 2001. (Chou, Atlas, Stanos, & Rosenquist, 2009) However, the evidence for these therapies is controversial. There are few well designed studies that support their usage and many studies with limitations that show either benefit or no benefit.

The best evidence supports the use of epidural steroid injections in the treatment of radicular pain. Bush et al. (Bush, Cowan, Katz, & Gishen, 1992) followed 165 patients with lumbar radicular pain for one year. The patients were given ~3 lumbar epidural steroid injections (using a caudal approach). 14% of the patients opted for surgical decompression, the rest had a satisfactory clinical recovery, with 94% reduction in visual analog scale pain and partial to complete resolution of disk herniations and disk bulges. Riew et al. followed

55 patients for five years with lumbar radicular pain who had initially opted for surgery. (Riew et al., 2006) The patients were offered lumbar epidural steroid injection therapy (using a transforaminal approach) prior to the planned surgery. After two years, 29 of the patients avoided surgery. After five years, 21 of the 29 patients were identified and re-evaluated. Four of the 21 patients had opted for surgical treatment, while 17 continued to avoid surgery. These 17 had significantly decreased neurological symptoms and pain.

Facet joint injections and medial branch blocks have been proposed to treat axial (non-radiating) low back pain. While there is good research to support their usage in cervical spine pain, the evidence to treat lumbar pain is more limited. (Chou et al., 2009) In one study, 95 patients were followed for 6 months following a beneficial response to anesthetic injections into the lumbar facet joints of subjects with back pain. (Carette et al., 1991) The patients were randomized for another treatment with cortisone versus saline. Variable treatment responses were observed. There was no additional benefit of steroid over saline after the initial anesthetic injection.

Lastly, surgical treatment of non-specific low back pain has not been shown to be reliably successful. (Zigler et al., 2007) Depending on the outcome measure or surgery utilized, "success" rates for surgery for low back pain only range from 40% - 65%.

3. Yoga

The word "yoga" means union, and refers to the goal of uniting individual human spirit or will with divine spirit or the True Self. (Bhaktivedanta Swami Prabhupada, 1997; Stiles, 2000) Classical yoga (Raja Yoga) is an ancient discipline that was first formally described by Patanjali around 200 BC in the Yoga Sutras. It has roots in Hindu religion and philosophy (Stiles, 2000) and was designed to create harmony of mind and body, and aid in achieving enlightenment or oneness with God. Although yoga has at times been misunderstood in the West as primarily "stretching", the postures or poses ('asanas'), comprise just one of eight components of a broader discipline of comprehensive physical, mental, and spiritual health and balance for individuals. However, many types of yoga do not include or do not emphasize stretching or postures, and are not considered Hatha yoga. (Sivananda, 1999; Yogananda, 1998) Modern Hatha yoga usually includes other classical yoga components such as breathing exercises ('pranayama'), concentration (pratyhara), and mindfulness/meditation (dhyana). (Iyengar, 1979) Thus, a typical Hatha yoga program consists of an instructor leading a group of students or practitioners through a series of yoga postures while performing deep breathing exercises for. Most classes last 60-90 minutes, and the instructor demonstrates the correct posture for practitioners, and provides verbal suggestions that encourage practitioners focus their attention or concentrate on deep breathing, postural alignment, on bodily sensations produced by the asanas. Depending on their training and often the class setting, instructors often encourage students to embrace positive cognitions or attitudes towards the world and themselves. This usually occurs at the beginning or end of the session and the instructors model these attitudes as well. Some yoga instructional centers provide a more complete social and spiritual community in which the additional components of classical yoga are also practiced.

There are many different types of Hatha yoga (Ashtanga, Anusara, Viniyoga, Bikram, etc). These styles or schools of Hatha yoga differ on variables such as pace, or the amount of time spent in each pose, the extent to which deep breathing is emphasized, level of emphasis on proper bodily alignment, room temperature, spiritual emphasis, meditation time, and the overall intensity and difficulty of the poses. Hundreds or possibly thousands of postures and variations have been developed over time, each one designed to stretch, strengthen, or engage specific areas of the body. When modified, Hatha yoga can be practiced by almost anyone, not just the healthy and flexible. This can be achieved by the use of props which enables people of all ages and ability levels (physical and mental) to perform poses that achieve benefit. (Iyengar, 1979) Yoga can be tailored to people with various physical or psychological limitations and can range from gentle to strenuous, with some types of yoga providing a cardiovascular workout, and others focused on relaxation and a calm mind. To be improve physical and mental health, the practice of yoga is usually performed at least once per week (twice is recommended), with increasing frequency of practice either at home or in a class, and gradual practice of more advanced postures as conditioning improves and strength increases. (Stiles, 2000)

The popularity of yoga has grown tremendously in recent years. Data from the National Center for Complementary and Alternative Medicine (NCCAM) show that the usage of complementary and alternative medicine (CAM) treatments for all conditions is on the rise in the US. Back pain is the most common condition for which CAM treatments are sought. Yoga was the 5th most commonly used CAM treatment and its use increased significantly between 2002 and 2007. Yoga was used by 6.1% of all US adults and 2.1% of all children in the use in 2007.

Broader effectiveness of yoga therapies

Although there are many studies claiming yoga can be an effective treatment for improving a wide variety of conditions (musculoskeletal problems, (Greendale, McDivit, Carpenter, Seeger, & Huang, 2002) cardiopulmonary function, (Raub, 2002) lipid and carbohydrate metabolism, (Bera & Rajapurkar, 1993) sleep problems, (Harinath et al., 2004) anxiety and depression, (Waelde, Thompson, & Gallagher-Thompson, 2004)) study quality has been lacking, with a clear need for larger randomized, controlled trials (RCTs). (Luskin et al., 2000) The limitations of most previous yoga studies include being non-randomized, a lack of validated outcome measures, a lack of data on dose response, and little examination of the underlying mechanisms. In addition, the yoga interventions being studied are often not well described. Yoga is multi-dimensional, so it is important to describe all of the components of each yoga intervention in order to compare across interventions and better understand which components are best for different disease populations. More recently, some larger, higher quality randomized studies have been conducted in areas including depression, (Sharma, Das, Mondal, Goswampi, & Gandhi, 2005) stress and anxiety, (Granath, Ingvarsson, von Thiele, & Lundberg, 2006; Smith, Hancock, Blake-Mortimer, & Eckert, 2007) HIV, (Brazier, Mulkins, & Verhoef, 2006) irritable bowel syndrome, (Kuttner et al., 2006) and chronic low back pain. (Sherman et al., 2011; Tilbrook et al., 2011) With very few exceptions, these more recent trials indicate that yoga has demonstrable beneficial effects, is rarely harmful, and is well received by participants with a wide variety of health problems. The psychological benefits of yoga are almost as well established as the physical benefits, as suggested by studies on stress, anxiety, and depression.

In summary, chronic low back pain affects millions of people on a daily basis, and while there are many treatment options, none stand out as being highly effective. Yoga is a promising inexpensive alternative for treating CLBP with few anticipated side effects. It has moderate effectiveness and the next section reviews the published literature in more detail, including two large RCTs that were recently published.

4. Literature review: Yoga for chronic low back pain

The impact of yoga on physical functioning and disability

Almost all studies of yoga intervention for treating chronic low back pain measure physical functioning/disability as a primary outcome. It is viewed as a more reliable and objective measure of CLBP because it is often either measured by actual physiological performance, or by questionnaires with items that are tied to specific behaviors. Pain severity is typically an internal experience and more subjective. Virtually all studies measuring functioning/disability have demonstrated beneficial effects of yoga among adults with CLBP. (See Table 1) In 2004, Galantino et al. conducted a small randomized controlled trial to assess the impact of Hatha yoga on chronic low back pain. (Galantino et al., 2004) Participants were randomized to either the yoga group, consisting of twice-weekly, 60-minute, yoga classes for 6 weeks, or a wait-list control. Outcomes related to physical functioning included flexibility as assessed with the forward reach and sit and reach tests, and disability as assessed with the Oswestry Disability Index. Results of this study demonstrated non-significant trends towards improved balance and flexibility and decreased disability for the yoga group. However, sample size and participant attrition weakened this study's power, demonstrating the need for larger studies assessing the impact of yoga on chronic low back pain. Additionally, the 6-week yoga program is shorter than the 10-12 week programs that are most frequently studied.

Williams et al. conducted a randomized controlled trial to assess the impact of Iyengar yoga therapy in participants with non-specific chronic low back pain. (K. A. Williams et al., 2005) The study compared a standardized yoga intervention to an educational control group. Both the intervention group and the control group programs were 16 weeks long. Both groups received 16 weekly newsletters on back care, and two lectures of occupational/physical therapy education regarding chronic low back pain with instructional handouts. The yoga intervention consisted of one 90-minute class each week for 16 weeks at a community yoga studio, and participants were encouraged to practice yoga at home for 30-min, 5 days a week. Study results revealed less functional disability in the yoga group than in the control group at the post-treatment assessment.

The efficacy of a week-long intensive residential yoga program on disability caused by pain and spinal flexibility in patients with chronic low back pain was studied by Tekur et al. (Tekur, Singphow, Nagendra, & Raghuram, 2008) Eighty participants who were previously admitted to a health home in Bangalore, India were randomized to yoga and control groups. The yoga group followed a daily routine of meditation, yogic physical practices, yogic hymns, lectures on yogic lifestyle, yogic breathing, deep relaxation, counseling, and meditation with yogic chants. The control group followed a daily routine of exercise, non-yogic safe breathing exercises and lectures on causes of back pain, stress and chronic low back pain, and benefits of physical exercises. Control participants also watched video shows

Table 1. Continued

First author, (year)	Study Design	*n; setting*	Yoga Intervention	Comparison Intervention	Relevant Outcomes	Main Results
Galantino (2004)	RCT	*22*	2x-weekly 60-min classes, 6 weeks	Waitlist control	Forward reach; Sit and reach; Oswestry Disability Index,	Non-significant trends towards improved flexibility and balance, decreased disability for the yoga group. Limited sample size.
Williams (2005)	RCT Pilot	*60*	Weekly 90-min classes, 16 weeks,	Information-only	Pain Disability Index	Yoga group had significantly greater reductions in functional disability than the control group.
Tekur (2008); (2010)	RCT	*80*; India	Week-long, all-day intensive yoga training, subsequent self- practice.	Week-long daily non-yoga exercise and lectures	Oswestry Disability Questionnaire; Spinal flexion, physiological movements	Yoga group showed greater decrease in disability, and greater increase in spinal flexion, spinal extension, and left lateral flexion, and leg raising than the control group.
Telles (2009)	RCT	*291*; India	60 days of yoga practice, 60-min	Waitlist control	Cornell Musculoskeletal Discomfort Questionnaire; Hand grip strength; Low back and hamstring flexibility	Improvements in low back flexibility, hamstring flexibility, and handgrip strength for in the yoga group.
Saper (2009)	RCT Pilot	*30*; ethnic minorities	Weekly 75-min classes, 12 weeks	Wait-list usual care	Roland-Morris Disability Questionnaire	No significant differences in disability outcomes. Limited by sample size.
Williams (2009)	RCT	*90*	2x-weekly, 90-min classes, 24 weeks	Waitlist usual care	Oswestry Disability Questionnaire,	Greater reductions in functional disability and pain intensity in the yoga group. Depression was significantly lower in the yoga group. No difference in medication use.

First author, (year)	Study Design	*n; setting*	Yoga Intervention	Comparison Intervention	Relevant Outcomes	Main Results
Cox (2010)	RCT Pilot	*20*	Weekly 75-min classes, 12 weeks	Usual care	Roland-Morris Disability Scale	No significant differences in function/ disability but not adequately powered to detect them. Established methodological issues to inform a full-scale trial.
Evans (2010)	Non-random between groups	*53;* self-selected treatment groups	Weekly 120-min classes, 6 weeks	2x weekly physical therapy, 45-60-min	Roland Morris Disability Questionnaire	No significant group differences in treatment effect on disability at 6 weeks.
Ülger (2011)	Single group, Pre-post	*27;* Female	2x-weekly 60-min classes, 4 weeks	n/a	Static balance; Gait parameters	Improvements on all gait and static balance parameters after the intervention. Limited by sample size and single group design.
Sherman (2011)	RCT	*228*	Weekly 75-min classes, 12 weeks	Weekly 75-min stretching classes, 12 weeks, Self-care book	Roland-Morris Disability Scale	Greater reductions in back-related dysfunction for yoga group when compared to self-care. Similar effects of yoga on function/ disability for yoga and stretching groups.
Tilbrook (2011)	RCT	*313;* England	Weekly 75-min classes, 12 weeks	Usual care	Roland-Morris Disability Scale;	Greater improvements for yoga group in back-function at 3, 6, and 12 month follow-up when compared with usual care.

Table 1. Studies that examined the effect of yoga on functioning/ disability.

on animals, plants, nature, etc. Outcomes included spinal mobility, as measured using a dialtype goniometer, and the Oswestry Disability Index. Results showed a significant difference between groups in disability, with the yoga group experiencing a greater decrease in disability than the control group. Spinal flexion, spinal extension, and left lateral flexion, increased in both groups, with the yoga group showing a greater increase in flexibility than the control group. Greater improvements were also found in straight leg raises for right and left legs for yoga group. (Tekur, Chametcha, Hongasandra, & Raghuram, 2010).

In 2009, Telles et al. presented results of a randomized control trial examining the effect of yoga on musculoskeletal discomfort and motor functions in professional computer users in India (n = 291). (Telles, Dash, & Naveen, 2009) Employees who used a computer for at least 6 hours each day, 5 days a week were randomized into a yoga intervention, or waitlist control. The yoga group participated in an hour of yoga practice each day, 5 days per week. Employees in the wait-list control spent the hour in a recreation center. Both groups were assessed at baseline and after 60 days on hand grip strength, tapping speed, and low back and hamstring flexibility. The yoga group demonstrated significant increases in handgrip strength for both hands and significant improvements in low back and hamstring flexibility. Results also demonstrated group differences in changes in tapping speed following the 60 days.

Williams et al. published additional results on the effectiveness of Iyengar yoga on chronic low back pain in 2009. (Williams et al., 2009) In this study, a total of 90 participants were randomized to the yoga intervention (n = 43) and wait-list control (n = 47) groups. The yoga intervention consisted of biweekly, 90-minute, Iyengar yoga classes over a 24 week period. Yoga participants were also asked to practice 30 minutes of yoga at home on non-class days, and were given props, a DVD, and an Iyengar yoga instruction manual. Participants in the control group continued their standard medical care, and were offered the yoga classes 6 months after the conclusion of the study. Individuals randomized to the yoga group showed greater improvements in functional disability than those randomized to the control group. Differences between the yoga and control groups were even stronger when limiting analyses to "completers" (30 individuals who completed the yoga intervention per protocol and 43 individuals not lost to follow-up in the waitlist control). Williams et al. (2009) report several limitations to their study, including reliance only on self-report measures, minimal disability among one-third of the participants, and the yoga group received greater attention and group support than did individuals from the control group.

In 2010, Cox et al. led a small randomized controlled pilot study (n=20) with the goal of informing a larger multicenter trial on the effectiveness of yoga for chronic low back pain. (Cox et al., 2010) The study compared 12 weekly, 75-minute, yoga back classes with usual care. As part of the study, a yoga manual was developed for yoga practitioners and their students. Outcomes including the Roland-Morris Disability Scale were assessed at baseline, 4 and 12 weeks following randomization. No significant effects were found, as the pilot study was not powered to detect differences. The study did provide useful data for the larger study on feasibility of recruitment, attendance, and retention.

In 2010, Evans et al. studied the predictors of outcomes in individuals who self-selected yoga or physical therapy to treat chronic low back pain. (Evans et al., 2010) Specifically, yoga participants (n = 27) were recruited from a series of five 6-week, once weekly, yoga classes offered through a hospital based complementary and alternative medicine clinic.

Physical therapy participants (n = 26) were recruited from 1 private and 1 hospital-based outpatient physical therapy clinic. Participants completed a clinical and demographic questionnaire at baseline and again after 6 weeks of treatment. Results suggested no significant group differences in treatment effect on disability at 6 weeks. However, their results indicated that self-efficacy was the most important predictor of disability and health status at 6 weeks for both groups. Additionally, the authors found a group by self-efficacy interaction upon predicting disability at 6 weeks. Specifically, self-efficacy was a stronger predictor of disability at 6 weeks for the physical therapy group. Because participants self-selected into the yoga or physical therapy group, a significant limitation of this study rests in fact self-selection bias may explain the differences in outcomes between the groups.

In 2011, Ülger and Yağli studied the effects of yoga on balance and gait in women (n = 27) with musculoskeletal disorders including low back pain and osteoarthritis. (Ülger and Yağli, 2011) The effect of 8 sessions of yoga treatment was assessed on gait (gait cycle, walking speed, maximum walking distance, step length, and ambulation index) and balance evaluations. Results suggested participants' gait parameters improved statistically following the 8 week yoga intervention. Additionally, improvements were also observed in the balance parameters. Although the authors conclude yoga has positive effects on physical problems such as gait and balance, significant limitations to this study include the absence of a control group/intervention, and small sample size. It is thus difficult to attribute the improvements in gait/balance to their yoga intervention.

Two larger randomized trials have recently been published in 2011 regarding yoga on chronic low back pain. Sherman et al. compared three different approaches designed to decrease the negative effects of back pain on participants' (n = 228) lives. (Sherman et al., 2011) Specifically, a series of yoga classes were compared to stretching exercises and to a self-care book. Yoga and stretching series consisted of twelve standardized, weekly 75-minute classes. Interviews were conducted at baseline and at 6, 12, and 26 weeks after randomization. Results suggested similar effects for yoga and stretching in individuals with low back pain. Back-related dysfunction declined over time in all groups, with the yoga group and stretching group reporting superior function than the self-care group at follow up assessments. At 12 weeks, the yoga group was significantly less bothered by symptoms than the self-care group. Both the yoga and stretching groups were more likely to rate their back pain as improved at all follow-up times, and were more likely to report being very satisfied with their care. Consequently, Sherman et al. suggest that yoga's benefits are largely attributable to the physical benefits of stretching and strengthening the muscles and not to its mental components.

In another study, Tillbrook et al. compared the effectiveness of yoga and usual care for chronic or recurrent low back pain using patients (n = 313) from 13 non-National Health Service premises in England, using long-term follow-up methods. (Tilbrook et al., 2011) The yoga intervention consisted of twelve 75-minute classes (1 class per week). Yoga participants were given a student manual, a mat, a relaxation compact disc which featured four narrated guided relaxations, and home practice sheets delivered at four intervals. Yoga participants were encouraged to use the compact disc, and to practice yoga for 30-minutes daily or to practice at least 2 times per week. All participants received a back pain education booklet and usual care. Additionally, fidelity assessments were used to ensure fidelity to the standardized treatment. Outcomes were measured before randomization, at baseline, and at 3, 6, and 12 months follow-up. Results suggested the yoga group had significantly greater improvements than the usual care group in back-function at 3, 6, and 12 month follow-up. The authors conclude that a 12 week yoga intervention leads to greater improvements in back function than usual care treatment for up to 12 months.

The impact of yoga on pain

A number of studies, including many of the studies discussed above, also demonstrate the effectiveness of yoga in reducing pain in individuals with chronic low back pain. For example, in addition to studying yoga's effect on functional disability, Williams et al. (2005) also assessed clinical levels of pain, pain-related fears of movement, and pain attitudes. Their results suggested that in addition to the yoga group having less functional disability at post treatment, the yoga group demonstrated two times greater reductions in pain, than the control group.

Beginning in 2005, military veterans who began attending a clinical yoga program at a large VA medical center in California completed a battery of health questionnaires before and after attending a 10-week yoga program. Baseline data and 10-week follow-up data were available for 33 participants as of August 2007. Statistically significant improvements were found for pain between baseline and 10-weeks. Among the various indicators of the amount of yoga practiced, correlations indicated that actual attendance was significantly correlated with decreased pain. These effects were found despite the fact that some participants did not attend regularly and the sessions were only offered once per week. Participants were encouraged to practice yoga postures at home and self-reports of the frequency of home practice were also associated with improvements in back pain. Further analyses with an expanded sample (n = 53) from the same study indicate that women improved more than men in the yoga program after controlling for baseline differences. Female participants had significantly greater improvements than male participants for "average" pain levels. No differences were found between men and women for pain "at its worst"or a total pain score. Women and men did not differ on attendance or home practice.

Saper et al. (2009) also found greater decreases in pain scores for yoga participants than the control group from baseline to 12 weeks. The yoga group participants also reported larger global improvements in back pain at week 12 than control group participants. Results from this pilot study also provide support for the feasibility of recruiting, retaining, and treating a sample of predominantly minority adults for a 12 week yoga intervention. However, a number of limitations exist for this study. The small sample size limited their statistical power, there was substantial attrition to long-term follow-up in the yoga group, and many non-study treatments including yoga were used by the control group, making it difficult to draw conclusions from their 26-week data.

As discussed above, Telles et al. presented results of a randomized control trial examining the effect of yoga on musculoskeletal discomfort and motor functions in professional computer users (n = 291). (Telles, Dash, & Naveen, 2009) At the end of 60 days, they found greater decreases in the degree of interference due to musculoskeletal discomfort in the yoga group. Limitations noted by the authors include a high attrition rate from the follow-up assessment in both groups, but attrition rates did not differ between the groups. Of the 57 individuals who dropped out from the yoga group, only 6 did so because they preferred to use the 60-minute period for a recreational activity of their choosing. A second limitation of the intervention they studied was the high level of commitment required to sustain a 5-day/week, 60-minute, yoga practice on working days.

The 2009 study by Williams et al. discussed earlier also demonstrated the effectiveness of Iyengar yoga on improving pain for individuals with chronic low back pain. (K. Williams et al., 2009) Individuals randomized to the yoga group showed greater improvements in pain intensity than those randomized to the control group. Differences between the yoga and control groups were even stronger when limiting analyses to "completers" (30 individuals who completed the yoga intervention per protocol and 43 individuals not lost to follow-up in the waitlist control).

The Cox et al. study in 2010 measured pain-related outcomes using the Aberdeen Back Pain Scale and pain efficacy. At the 4-week follow-up, the yoga group reported greater decreases in pain. At both follow-up points, a non-significant trend in the yoga group showing an improvement in pain self-efficacy over the usual care group was observed. The results of the large RCT published by the same research group found no significant differences in pain severity at any assessment periods. They did find greater improvements in pain self-efficacy for the yoga group at 3 & 6 month follow-ups than those randomized to usual care.

In 2010, Evans et al. studied back pain bothersomeness, and back pain self-efficacy, in individuals who self-selected yoga or physical therapy to treat chronic low back pain. Results suggested no significant group differences in treatment effect on pain at 6 weeks. Their results also indicated that self-efficacy was the most important predictor of pain and health status at 6 weeks for both groups. Finally, Sherman et al. measured pain "bothersomeness" instead of pain severity because of the more subjective nature of reporting pain severity. Results indicate that the yoga group had significantlygreater reductions in pain "bothersomeness" than the self-care group at 12 weeks. However, they found similar effects of yoga on pain for yoga and stretching groups. Similar to the disability outcomes, both groups had reductions in pain after participating in the interventions.

Medication use

Five of the studies reviewed reported the effectiveness of yoga on reducing the use of medications. The results of Williams (2005) suggest a greater decrease in the use of pain medications than the control group. Saper et al. (2009) also reported on the beneficial effects of yoga on the use of medications. They found that the use of pain medicine differed significantly between the yoga and control groups such that the yoga participants decreased their use of pain medicine while the control group did not change. Opiate analgesic use increased for the control group participants, but decreased to zero for the yoga participants—another statistically significant difference between groups. Williams et al. (2009) found non-significant reductions in pain medication use at 12 and 24 weeks that was comparable in both their yoga group participants, and their control group who continued self-directed standard medical care. However, Williams et al. report a trend for the yoga group to have a higher success rate in decreasing their use of pain medication than at both 12 and 24 weeks follow up than the control group. Subgroup analyses that examined the use of pain medication in participants with moderate disability at baseline indicate that yoga participants with moderate disability showed a significantly greater reduction in pain medication at 12 weeks than their control group counterparts. In 2010, Evans et al. studied pain medication use in individuals who self-selected yoga or physical therapy to treat chronic low back pain. Results suggested that both self-selected groups decreased pain medication use by similar amount (52% and 57% among yoga physical therapy groups, respectively). In the largest study of the impact of yoga on medication use to date, Sherman et al. found greater decreases in medication use in the yoga group when compared to self-care, but no difference between the yoga and stretching groups.

Psychological impacts of yoga

The broader effectiveness of yoga to the psychological well being of participants has been debated. Results from the literature are not yet conclusive regarding whether yoga can improve participants' psychological well being. For example, in 2004, Galantino et al. also assessed the impact of Hatha yoga on depression as assessed with the Beck Depression Inventory. Results of this study demonstrated non-significant trends towards decreased depression for the yoga group. However, sample size and participant attrition weakened this study's power, demonstrating the need for larger studies assessing the impact of yoga on chronic low back pain.

Groessl et al. also reported the influence of yoga on the psychological well being of participants among San Diego veterans. The study found significant improvements in depression as measured with the CES-D 10, and the Mental Health Scale of the SF-12. Among the various indicators of the amount of yoga practiced, correlations indicated that self-reported home practice was significantly correlated with improved outcomes for depression.

Williams et al. (2009) also reported on the impact of Iyengar yoga on the psychological well being of participants with chronic low back pain. Specifically, in reducing depression among individuals with chronic low back pain. Using the Beck Depression Inventory, individuals randomized to the yoga group showed greater improvements in depression than those randomized to the control group. As mentioned above, differences between the yoga and control groups were even stronger when limiting analyses to "completers".

In 2010, Tekur et al. (Tekur, Chametcha, Hongasandra, & Raghuram, 2010) presented additional results from their 2008 study. The authors used the WHOQOL Bref psychological subscale to measure the impact of yoga on mental health. They found significantly greater improvements in WHOQOL Bref psychological subscale for the yoga group compared with the control group. However, the intervention included many more elements (formal meditation, interactive lectures, spirituality) than the typical Hatha yoga interventions being studied in the other research we have reviewed, and the benefits were documented only at 7 days after baseline.

Two studies by the same research group in the UK measured psychological impact with the Short From 12 Mental Component Scale (SF-12 MCS). The earlier pilot found no significant differences but has little power (n =20) to detect differences. The Tilbrook study was adequately powered but found non-significant trends toward greater improvements among the yoga group at 3- and 6-month assessments.

Other outcomes

A variety of other outcomes were measured across the studies that have been reviewed. Some were very specific to the population being studied such as hand tapping speed for computer programmers. Other measures such as health-related quality of life were measured in a number of studies and are not study specific.

Safety of yoga

It is important to address the concern that yoga could potentially be harmful to those with chronic low back pain. Popular media has tapped into this concern, often with anecdotal stories of dangers and injury, but little data. Like other exercise activity, the risks of injury from improperly performing yoga postures likely vary depending on how, where, and with whom the yoga is practiced. The initial practice of yoga under the direction of experienced yoga instructors is preferable to simply reading a book or following a video at home, and many of the programs being studied have been modified specifically for people with the condition of chronic low back pain. For optimal safety, people with either acute or chronic health conditions should consult their physician before starting a yoga program.

Data from research studies with experienced yoga instructors have shown occasional adverse events. The 2005 Sherman et al. study reported no serious adverse events. Of 36 patients assigned to the yoga group, one patient discontinued yoga because it precipitated migraines. Similarly, of 35 patients in the exercise group, one individual in the exercise group discontinued the intervention because of a back strain. Data from the Williams et al. study in 2005 show one serious adverse event among 30 patients randomized to yoga. This patient had symptomatic osteoarthritis and herniated a disc during the study. However, the event was reviewed by a medical panel and it was determined that the event was not caused by practicing yoga in this study. A larger, more recent study by Sherman et al. found equal numbers of mild to moderate adverse events in the yoga and stretching interventions, with temporary increases in back pain the leading cause. One serious adverse event, a herniated disc occurred among the 87 yoga participants. The other recent large RCT by Tilbrook et al. found 1 serious adverse event and 12 nonserious events among 156 yoga participants, all related to increased back pain. The more general review of nonpharmacological treatments for chronic low back pain concluded that these interventions seldom cause harm, but better studies and better reporting are needed (Chou & Huffman, 2007b).

5. Discussion

Chronic low back pain is an extremely prevalent condition that results in a great deal of lost productivity, disability, discomfort, and reduced quality of life for those afflicted. CLBP patients have higher health care costs in both the short-term and long-term.

Current treatments for CLBP are variable in the quality of evidence supporting them and in their overall levels of effectiveness. Medication management works for some patients but others require stronger narcotic agents which heighten the risk of addiction. None of the non-pharmacologic treatments stand out as clearly superior. With the exception of exercise and yoga, most of the treatments with solid supporting evidence and at least moderately sized effects are performed in a one-on-one provider setting or require expensive equipment. Thus, treatment modalities such as spinal manipulation, physical therapy, acupuncture, etc. may be more expensive than yoga or exercise interventions that can be delivered in group format, or once learned, can be self-administered at home. Actual data and cost analyses on yoga interventions for chronic low back pain are needed.

Our review of the current literature indicates that yoga has reduced disability and improved daily functioning in most studies when compared with usual care, or information alone. Most studies use one of two well-validated measures of functioning/disability, and some studies also included physiological measures such as grip strength and flexibility (See Table

1). The two most informative studies have been published in recent months and have not been included in previous reviews. Each of these recent studies found that yoga improved function more than usual care or self-care. The Sherman et al. study employed a three group design, and thus, provided important "comparative effectiveness" data by comparing yoga to an exercise program led by physical therapists. It is notable that was not statistically superior to this exercise intervention. The only other study that used a comparison group of proven efficacy was Evans et al who also found no significant differences on function/disability. Thus, we conclude that yoga may not be superior to other non-pharmacological interventions with moderate effects sizes. However, attendance and satisfaction rates were higher among the yoga group in the Sherman study, indicating that it may be a more attractive intervention to many individuals.

With the exception of a few smaller studies, yoga interventions have been shown to reduce pain severity or the "bothersomeness" of pain, when compared with usual care, or information alone (See Table 2). In looking at the recent RCTs, the Sherman study found that yoga patients were less bothered by low back pain than self-care patients, while the Tilbrook study found no significant differences in back pain severity. The Tilbrook finding is a bit surprising, even though self-reported pain severity is different than pain bothersomeness. Sherman et al. specifically chose to measure pain bothersomeness because self-reported pain severity may be harder to measure reliably across various groups. It is also possible that the design of the Tilbrook study (13 different private practices across the UK) may have affected the results obtained. This may have resulted in greater heterogeneity among the instructors, intervention, or participants, and it is unclear whether the statistical analysis accounted for clustering with the 13 cohorts.

Our review also suggests that yoga can reduce reliance on pain medication when compared with usual or self-care. However, only a few studies have published results on these outcomes so conclusions remain more tentative (See Table 3). With the exception of the Williams at el study, very little information is provided on how medication was measured. Measuring medication use poses its own challenges, with self-reported interview data often differing from medical record information or pill counts. Future research should consider other methods for measuring medication usage including the use of medical record information when possible.

Depression and other indicators of the impact of yoga on psychological outcomes were assessed in a small number of studies (See Table 4). Significant effects were found in a few of the smaller studies, but only non-significant trends were found for the SF-12 MCS in the full-scale trial in which they were measured. The Sherman study did not publish data on psychological variables in their initial manuscript but these results may be forthcoming. Given the cognitive and relaxation components of yoga, along with the higher rates of depression among individuals with chronic low back pain, further research in this area is very important.

We also reviewed the safety of yoga for some of the larger randomized controlled trials. Data from the largest and most recent trials suggests that two serious adverse events occurred among a combined total of 243 participants. These events were related to increased back pain, one being a herniated disc. Another 10% of these yoga participants experienced non-serious adverse events that were almost exclusively increases in back pain. Thus, participating in yoga interventions by persons with chronic low back pain is not without risk, but the vast majority of participants had no problems and experienced considerable benefit for a chronic debilitating condition.

First author, (year)	Study Design	*n*	Yoga Intervention	Comparison Intervention	Relevant Outcomes	Main Results
Williams (2005)	RCT Pilot	*60*	Weekly 90-min classes, 16 weeks,	Information-only	Pain (PDI, SF-MPQ, PPI, VAS); Pain-related fears (TSK); Pain attitudes (SOPA);	Yoga group had two times greater reductions in pain.
Groessl (2008)	Single group, Pre-post	*49;* Veterans	Weekly 60-min classes, 10 weeks	n/a	Bodily Pain Index	Significantly less pain 10 weeks after starting the program. Frequency of home practice was associated with less pain. Limited by sample size, single group design.
Saper (2009)	RCT Pilot	*30;* Ethnic Minority	Weekly 75-min classes, 12 weeks	Wait-list usual care	Numerical rating scale (0=no pain to 10=worst possible pain)	Yoga group has greater decreases in pain.
Telles (2009)	RCT	*291;* Bangalore, India	60-min yoga sessions, 5 days/week for 60 days	Waitlist control	Cornell Musculoskeletal Discomfort Questionnaire	Greater decrease in frequency and level of musculoskeletal discomfort for whole body and both hands.
Cox (2010)	RCT Pilot	*20*	Weekly 75-min classes, 12 weeks	Usual care	Aberdeen Back Pain Scale; pain self-efficacy	No significant differences in pain but not adequately powered to detect them.
Evans (2010)	Non-random between groups	*53;* self-selected into treatment groups	Weekly 120-min classes, 6 weeks,	2x-weekly physical therapy, 45-60-min	Back pain bothersomeness; Back Pain Self-Efficacy Scale;	No significant group differences for pain at 6 weeks.
Sherman (2011)	RCT	*228*	Weekly 75-min classes, 12 weeks	Weekly 75-min stretching classes, 12 weeks, Self-care book	Pain bothersomeness	Yoga group significantly less bothered by pain than the self-care group at 12 weeks. Similar effects of yoga on pain for yoga and stretching groups.
Tilbrook (2011)	RCT	*313;* England	Weekly 75-min classes, 12 weeks	Usual care	Aberdeen Back Pain Scale; Pain Self-Efficacy	No significant differences in pain severity. Greater improvements in the yoga group in pain self-efficacy at 3 & 6 month follow-ups.

Table 2. Studies that examined the effect of yoga on pain.

First author, (year)	Study Design	*n*	Yoga Intervention	Comparison Intervention	Relevant Outcomes	Main Results
Williams (2005)	RCT Pilot	60	Weekly yoga classes for 16 weeks, 90-min	Weekly newsletters, 2 lectures, and handouts on chronic low back pain	Pain medication use	Yoga group had a greater decrease in the use of pain medications than the control group.
Saper (2009)	RCT Pilot	30; Ethnic Minority	Weekly Hatha yoga classes for 12 weeks, 75-min	Waitlist usual care	Analgesic and opiate medication use	Yoga group reported less analgesic use and less opiate use than the usual care group.
Williams (2009)	RCT	90	24 weeks of twice-weekly 90-min yoga classes	Waitlist usual care	Pain medication use	No difference in medication use.
Evans (2010)	Non-random between groups	53; self-selected into treatment groups	Weekly yoga classes for 6 weeks, 120-min	Twice-weekly individualized physical therapy sessions, 45-60-min	Pain medication use;	No significant group differences in the use of pain medications.
Sherman (2011)	RCT	228	Weekly yoga classes for 12 weeks, 75-min	Weekly stretching classes for 12 weeks, 75 min; Self-care book	Back pain-related medication use.	Greater decreases in medication use in the yoga group when compared to self-care. Similar changes in medication use for yoga and stretching groups.

Table 3. Studies that examined the effect of yoga on medication use.

First author, (year)	Study Design	*n*	Yoga Intervention	Comparison Intervention	Primary Outcomes	Main Results
Galantino (2004)	RCT	*22*	2x-weekly 60-min classes, 6 weeks	Waitlist control	Beck Depression Inventory	Non-significant trends toward decreased depression for the yoga group. Limited sample size and dropout rate contribute to non-significance.
Groessl (2008)	Single group, Pre-post	*49*; Veterans	Weekly 60-min classes, 10 weeks	n/a	CESD-10; SF-12 mental health	Significant decreases in depression and SF-12 MCS scores. Frequency of home practice was associated with improved outcomes.
Williams (2009)	RCT	*90*	24 weeks of twice-weekly 90-min yoga classes	Waitlist usual care	Beck Depression Inventory	Greater decreases in depression in the yoga group.
Cox (2010)	RCT Pilot	*20*	Weekly 75-min classes, 12 weeks	Usual care	SF-12 mental health	No significant differences in pain but not adequately powered to detect them.
Tekur (2008); (2010)	RCT	*80*; India	Week-long, all-day intensive yoga training, self- practice.	Week-long daily non-yoga exercise and lectures	WHOQOL Bref psychological subscale	Greater improvements in WHOQOL Bref psychological subscale for yoga group.
Tilbrook (2011)	RCT	*313*; England	Weekly 75-min classes, 12 weeks	Usual care	SF-12 mental health	Non-significant trends toward decreased SF-12 MCS for the yoga group.

Table 4. Studies that examined the effect of yoga on psychological health.

Overall, our results are similar to and confirmatory of those published in a review article in 2011. This prior review was useful, but was released before the results of the two largest randomized controlled trials that have been published to date. Thus, we believed it was important to add these studies to the body of existing literature. We conclude that yoga interventions impact multiple outcomes that are important to the health and well-being of people afflicted with chronic low back pain. Recent, high quality evidence suggests that yoga provides comparable effects to, and is more appealing than, formal stretching and strengthening programs led by physical therapists. The recent data suggest that it would behoove health care organizations and the members they serve, to have yoga as an available health service option at little or no cost.

6. References

Anderson, G. B. J. "The Epidemiology of Spinal Disorders." In *The Adult Spine: Principles and Practice.*, edited by JW Frymoyer, 93-141. New York: Raven Press, 1997.

Barnes, P. M., E. Powell-Griner, K. McFann, and R. L. Nahin. "Complementary and Alternative Medicine Use among Adults: United States, 2002." *Adv Data*, no. 343 (2004): 1-19.

Barnes, P. M., B. Bloom, and R. L. Nahin. "Complementary and Alternative Medicine Use among Adults and Children: United States, 2007." *Natl Health Stat Report* 10, no. 12 (2009): 1-23.

Broad, W. J. "How Yoga Can Wreck Your Body." *New York Times*, January 5, 2012 2012.

Choo, P. W., C. S. Rand, T. S. Inui, M. L. Lee, E. Cain, M. Cordeiro-Breault, C. Canning, and R. Platt. "Validation of Patient Reports, Automated Pharmacy Records, and Pill Counts with Electronic Monitoring of Adherence to Antihypertensive Therapy." *Med Care* 37, no. 9 (1999): 846-57.

Chou, R., A. Qaseem, V. Snow, D. Casey, J. T. Cross, Jr., P. Shekelle, and D. K. Owens. "Diagnosis and Treatment of Low Back Pain: A Joint Clinical Practice Guideline from the American College of Physicians and the American Pain Society." Ann Intern Med 147, no. 7 (2007): 478-91.

Chou, R., and L. H. Huffman. "Medications for Acute and Chronic Low Back Pain: A Review of the Evidence for an American Pain Society/American College of Physicians Clinical Practice Guideline." *Ann Intern Med* 147, no. 7 (2007): 505-14.

Chou, R., and L. H. Huffman . "Nonpharmacologic Therapies for Acute and Chronic Low Back Pain: A Review of the Evidence for an Aps/American College of Physicians Clinical Practice Guideline." *Ann Intern Med* 147, no. 7 (2007): 492-504.

Cox, H., H. Tilbrook, J. Aplin, A. Semlyen, D. Torgerson, A. Trewhela, and I. Watt. "A Randomised Controlled Trial of Yoga for the Treatment of Chronic Low Back Pain: Results of a Pilot Study." *Complement Ther Clin Pract* 16, no. 4 (2010): 187-93.

Currie, S. R., and J. Wang. "Chronic Back Pain and Major Depression in the General Canadian Population." *Pain* 107, no. 1-2 (2004): 54-60.

Deyo, R. A., S. K. Mirza, and B. I. Martin. "Back Pain Prevalence and Visit Rates: Estimates from U.S. National Surveys, 2002." *Spine* 31, no. 23 (2006): 2724-7.

Evans, D. D., M. Carter, R. Panico, L. Kimble, J. T. Morlock, and M. J. Spears. "Characteristics and Predictors of Short-Term Outcomes in Individuals Self-Selecting Yoga or Physical Therapy for Treatment of Chronic Low Back Pain." *Pm R* 2, no.11 (2010): 1006-15.

Galantino, M. L., T. M. Bzdewka, J. L. Eissler-Russo, M. L. Holbrook, E. P. Mogck, P. Geigle, and J. T. Farrar. "The Impact of Modified Hatha Yoga on Chronic Low Back Pain: A Pilot Study." Altern Ther Health Med 10, no. 2 (2004): 56-9.

Groessl, E. J., T. G. Ganiats, and A. J. Sarkin. "Sociodemographic Differences in Quality of Life in Rheumatoid Arthritis." *Pharmacoeconomics* 24, no. 2 (2006): 109-21.

Groessl, E. J., K. R. Weingart, K. Aschbacher, L. Pada, and S. Baxi. "Yoga for Veterans with Chronic Low-Back Pain." *J Altern Complement Med* 14, no. 9 (2008): 1123-29.

Groessl, E.J., K. R. Weingart, N. Johnson, and S. Baxi. "The Benefits of Yoga for Women Veterans with Chronic Low Back Pain." *J Altern Complement Med* (in press).

Johnson, Andrew, and Richards Marged. "Celebrity Power Yoga: The New Craze from over There Causing Bad Karma over Here." *The Independent. (U. K.)* , Sunday, 30 January 2005.

Liu, H., C. E. Golin, L. G. Miller, R. D. Hays, C. K. Beck, S. Sanandaji, J. Christian, T. Maldonado, D. Duran, A. H. Kaplan, and N. S. Wenger. "A Comparison Study of Multiple Measures of Adherence to Hiv Protease Inhibitors." *Ann Intern Med* 134, no. 10 (2001): 968-77.

Luo, X., R. Pietrobon, S. X. Sun, G. G. Liu, and L. Hey. "Estimates and Patterns of Direct Health Care Expenditures among Individuals with Back Pain in the United States." *Spine* 29, no. 1 (2004): 79-86.

Posadzki, P., and E. Ernst. "Yoga for Low Back Pain: A Systematic Review of Randomized Clinical Trials." *Clin Rheumatol* 30, no. 9 (2011): 1257-62.

Saper, R. B., K. J. Sherman, D. Cullum-Dugan, R. B. Davis, R. S. Phillips, and L. Culpepper. "Yoga for Chronic Low Back Pain in a Predominantly Minority Population: A Pilot Randomized Controlled Trial." Altern Ther Health Med 15, no. 6 (2009): 18-27.

Sherman, K. J., D. C. Cherkin, J. Erro, D. L. Miglioretti, and R. A. Deyo. "Comparing Yoga, Exercise, and a Self-Care Book for Chronic Low Back Pain: A Randomized, Controlled Trial." *Ann Intern Med* 143, no. 12 (2005): 849-56.

Sherman, K. J., D. C. Cherkin, R. D. Wellman, A. J. Cook, R. J. Hawkes, K. Delaney, and R. A. Deyo. "A Randomized Trial Comparing Yoga, Stretching, and a Self-Care Book for Chronic Low Back Pain." *Arch Intern Med* (2011).

Sullivan, M. J., K. Reesor, S. Mikail, and R. Fisher. "The Treatment of Depression in Chronic Low Back Pain: Review and Recommendations." *Pain* 50, no. 1 (1992): 5-13.

Tekur, P., S. Chametcha, R. N. Hongasandra, and N. Raghuram. "Effect of Yoga on Quality of Life of Clbp Patients: A Randomized Control Study." Int J Yoga 3, no. 1 (2010): 10-7.

Tekur, P., C. Singphow, H. R. Nagendra, and N. Raghuram. "Effect of Short-Term Intensive Yoga Program on Pain, Functional Disability and Spinal Flexibility in Chronic Low Back Pain: A Randomized Control Study." J Altern Complement Med 14, no. 6 (2008): 637-44.

Telles, S., M. Dash, and K. V. Naveen. "Effect of Yoga on Musculoskeletal Discomfort and Motor Functions in Professional Computer Users." *Work* 33, no. 3 (2009): 297-306.

Tilbrook, H. E., H. Cox, C. E. Hewitt, A. R. Kang'ombe, L. H. Chuang, S. Jayakody, J. D. Aplin, A. Semlyen, A. Trewhela, I. Watt, and D. J. Torgerson. "Yoga for Chronic Low Back Pain: A Randomized Trial." *Ann Intern Med* 155, no. 9 (2011): 569-78.

Ülger, Ö., and N. V. Yağli. "Effects of Yoga on Balance and Gait Properties in Women with Musculoskeletal Problems: A Pilot Study." Complement Ther Clin Pract 17, no. 1 (2011): 13-5.

Williams, K. A., J. Petronis, D. Smith, D. Goodrich, J. Wu, N. Ravi, E. J. Doyle, Jr., R. Gregory Juckett, M. Munoz Kolar, R. Gross, and L. Steinberg. "Effect of Iyengar Yoga Therapy for Chronic Low Back Pain." *Pain* 115, no. 1-2 (2005): 107-17.

Williams, K., C. Abildso, L. Steinberg, E. Doyle, B. Epstein, D. Smith, G. Hobbs, R. Gross, G. Kelley, and L. Cooper. "Evaluation of the Effectiveness and Efficacy of Iyengar Yoga Therapy on Chronic Low Back Pain." *Spine (Phila Pa 1976)* 34, no. 19 (2009): 2066-76.

13

Stabilization Exercise for the Management of Low Back Pain

A. Luque-Suárez, E. Díaz-Mohedo,
I. Medina-Porqueres and T. Ponce-García
Physiotherapy Department, Malaga University, Spain

1. Introduction

Lumbopelvic stabilization model

The lumbopelvic stabilization model is an active approach to low back pain, as proposed by Waddel (Waddel et al., 1997), based on a motor control exercises program. The main aim of this program is to reestablish the impairment or deficit in motor control around the neutral zone of the spinal motion segment by restoring the normal function of the local stabilizer muscles.

Stabilization exercise program has become the most popular treatment method in spinal rehabilitation since it has shown its effectiveness in some aspects related to pain and disability. However, some studies have reported that specific exercise program reduces pain and disability in chronic but not in acute low back pain, although it can be helpful in the treatment of acute low back pain by reducing recurrence rate (Ferreira et al., 2006).

Studies comparing Stability programs and others

Despite stabilization exercises have become a major focus in spinal rehabilitation as well as in prophylactic care such as sports injury prevention (Zazulak et al., 2008), the therapeutic evidences in terms of postural control variables have not been well documented. Some randomized controlled trials have comprehensively reported the effects of core stability exercises versus conventional physiotherapy treatment regimes on pain characteristics, recurrence and disability scores in chronic low back pain patients emphasizing patient centered outcomes (Dankaerts et al., 2006; Liddle et al., 2007). These studies have addressed the need of homogenous chronic low back pain group for better clinical outcomes. Evaluating postural control parameters such as centre of pressure displacements, moments and forces following interventions, particularly stability exercises, may provide insight into how this surrogate outcomes are mediated by different subgroups or heterogeneous chronic low back pain patients and identifying subgroups of chronic low back pain patients who are most likely to benefit after particular intervention (Muthukrishnan et al., 2010).

The core stability exercises cannot be superior to conventional physiotherapy exercises in terms of reducing pain and disability. However, core stability exercise demonstrates significant improvements in: distribution of ground reaction forces, use of optimized postural adjustments in the direction of perturbation, 20% absolute risk reduction of flare-up during intervention and 40% absolute risk reduction for resolution of back pain after core instability exercises (Muthukrishnan et al., 2010).

Core stability exercise is an evolving process, and refinement of the clinical rehabilitation strategies is ongoing. Further work is required, however, to refine and validate the approach, particularly with reference to contemporary understanding of the neurobiology of chronic pain (Hodges, 2003).

Related to the comparison between Pilates method and stabilization programs, Pilates method did not improve functionality and pain in patients who have low back pain when compared with control and lumbar stabilization exercise groups (Pereira et al., 2011).

To contrast the efficacy of two exercise programs, segmental stabilization and strengthening of abdominal and trunk muscles, on pain, functional disability, and activation of the transversus abdominis (TrA) muscle, in individuals with chronic low back pain. Both techniques lessened pain and reduced disability. Segmental stabilization is superior to superficial strengthening for all variables. Superficial strengthening does not improve TrA activation capacity (Franca et al., 2011).

Comparing traditional exercise program and core stabilization program one group of Soldiers (N = 2616) between 18 and 35 years of age were randomized to receive a traditional exercise program (TEP) with sit-ups or Core Stabilization exercise program (CSEP). CSEP did not have a detrimental impact on sit-up performance or overall fitness scores or pass rates. There was a small but significantly greater increase in sit-up pass rate in the CSEP (5.6%) versus the TEP group (3.9%) (Childs et al., 2009).

Who is suitable for getting benefits from a stabilization program?

This sort of program has shown to produce short-term improvements in global impression of recovery and activity for people with chronic low back pain, maintaining the results after 6 and 12 months (Costa et al., 2009), as well as be superior to minimal intervention at long term follow-up (Macedo et al., 2009; Kriese, 2010). Improvements in pain intensity and functional disability were also demonstrated in groups of patients with low back pain suffering from a spondylolisis or a spondylolisthesis (O'Sullivan, 2000) and a significant decrease of symptoms in people with hypermobility (Fritz et al., 2005).

However, before approaching this model, for better understanding the theory basis some of the crucial terms will be described.

Neutral Position

"The posture of the spine in which the overall internal stresses in the spinal column and muscular effort to hold the posture are minimal" (Panjabi, 1992b)

Neutral Zone

"That part of the physiological intervertebral motion, measured from the neutral position, within which the spinal motion is produced with a minimal internal resistance. It is the zone of high flexibility or laxity" (Panjabi, 1992b).

Spinal instability. Panjabi's Hypotheses

Can be defined as "a significant decrease in the capacity of the stabilizing system of the spine to maintain the intervertebral neutral zones within the physiological limits so that there is no neurological dysfunction, no major deformity, and no incapacitating pain" (Panjabi, 1992b). Therefore, an unstable spinal segment might not be able to maintain the correct vertebral alignment. The excessive movement in an unstable spine may either stretch or compress pain sensitive structures, leading to inflammation (Panjabi, 1992a).

It is also necessary to differentiate between instability and hypermobility because in both cases the range of motion is greater than normal. The main difference is that hypermobility might be asymptomatic, however, instability exits when dysfunctions, which can induce pain while performing active physiological movements (Paris, 1985).

1.1 The stabilization system of the spine

Panjabi conceptualized the basis of the stabilization system of the spine, subdividing it into three different subsystems: the active subsystem, the passive subsystem and the control subsystem.

The Passive subsystem consists on the ligamentous system and does not generate or produce itself any motion at the spine. It produces reactive forces by the end of the ranges of motion but its prime assignment is to work as a signals transducer to the neural subsystem and to send any sense of vertebral position or motion, especially those produced by the vicinity of the neutral zone (Panjabi, 1992a).

The Active subsystem is composed of muscles and tendons which generate forces to supply the stability to the spine (Panjabi, 1992a). Poor postural control can leave the spine vulnerable to injury by placing excessive stress on the body tissues (Kendall et al., 1993). In the lumbar spine, the trunk muscles protect spinal tissues from excessive motion. To do this, however, the muscle surrounding the trunk must be able to co-contract isometrically when appropriate (Richardson, 1990). The synergistic interaction between various trunk muscles is complex: some muscles act as primary movers to create the gross movements of the trunk, whereas others function as stabilizers (fixators) and neutralizers to support the spinal structures and control unwanted movements. Rehabilitation through active lumbar stabilization not only deals with the torque- producing capacity of muscles, as it is true for many traditional programs, but also seeks to enable a person to unconsciously and consistently coordinate an optimal pattern of muscle activity (Jull&Richardson, 1994a).

The Neural Control subsystem. Its function is to receive all the sensory feedback from the transducers of the passive system, determine the stability requirements and make the active system to achieve those stability goals. It also has an important role in measuring the forces generated in each muscle through the transducers located inside the tendons (Panjabi, 1992).

In a normal situation, the stabilization system provides the stability required to fulfill the demands of the constantly changing stability provoked by variations in posture and static and dynamic loads. To meet all those needs, the three subsystems must work together in harmony. However, dysfunction of any of these three components might incite a fail in the whole system, leading, over time, to chronic dysfunction and pain (Panjabi, 1992a).

Each of these three interrelated systems has its own role in maintaining the spinal stability. Inert tissues (in particular ligaments) provide passive support; contractile tissues give active support; and neural control centers links the passive and active systems, receives information about the position and direction of the movements and coordinates and control the muscles ability to contract and maintain stability (i.e., to increase stiffness and reduce the size of the neutral zone). This will depend on the speed and accuracy with which the information is relayed. The vital aspects of neural system development are therefore accuracy of movement and speed of reaction. Thus, the stabilization program emphasizes accuracy of movements early on; speed comes later.

Generally speaking, the main strategy of the stabilization model is to reduce the size of the neutral zone by increasing stiffness offered by muscles contraction (Norris, 2008)

Following with the Stabilization model, we are focusing now on the active support system. In this concept we must avoid *muscle imbalance* that occurs when one muscle, the "agonist", is stronger than the opposite, the "antagonist", or when one or the other is abnormally shortened or lengthened.

1.2 Types of muscles

We can categorize muscles into two groups: stabilizers or "postural muscles" and mobilizers or "task muscles" (Janda&Schmid, 1980; Richardson, 1990).

Stabilizers or postural muscles: stabilize a joint and approximate the joint surfaces. Tend to be more deeply placed in the body and are usually monoarticular muscles. Stabilizers can be subdivided into primary and secondary types (Jull&Richardson, 1994). Many of these smaller muscles have and important proprioceptive functions. For example, the intertransversarii muscles of the lumbar spine and the interspinals muscles both have a dense concentration of muscle spindles indicating a significant proprioceptive function (Adams et al., 2002). Intertransversarii muscles and interspinals muscles have demonstrated their influence over low back pain. The secondary stabilizers are the main torque producers, being large monoarticular muscles attaching via extensive aponeurosis.

Despite there is no actual evidence whether pain or motor control impairments come first, Panjabi (1992a) suggested that changes in the active support system might lead to a poor control of the joints and repeated microtrauma and pain. Supporting this idea, many research works have been conducted to explain all those fails in controlling the stability of the spine. According to this, changes in automatic control of TrA have been found in people with low back pain (Ferreira et al., 2004), a delayed onset of its contraction (Hodges&Richardson, 1996) and a loss of its tonic and preadjusting function (Hodges, 1999), what indicates a motor control deficit and is hypothesized to result in inefficient muscular stabilization of the spine (Hodges, 1996, 1999). The activation of the other stabilizer muscles also appears delayed, but to a lesser extent (Hodges, 1999).

On the other hand, there are many research papers about the changes that occur in other stabilizers as a consequence of or associated to chronic low back pain. Some of these changes are: a reduction in the cross-sectional areas of multifidus, psoas, and quadratus lumborum (Kamaz et al., 2007), asymmetric atrophy between both side of the symptomatic level (Hides et al., 2006) and fat infiltrations in multifidus muscles (Kjaer et al., 2006; Mengiardi et al.,

2006). Nevertheless, it has been reported some good results in recovering these changes with a specific stabilization program (Hides et al., 1996; Hides et al., 2008).

Mobilizers: are superficial and are often biarticular (two-joint) muscles. They can develop angular rotation more effectively than the stabilizers. This group of muscles acts as stabilizers only in conditions of extreme need. When they do, the precision of movement is often lost, creating and observable movement dysfunction.

In table 1 we can see stabilizers and mobilizers characteristics (Norris, 2008).

Stabilizers	Primary stabilizers: • Deep, close to joint • Slow twitch • Usually monoarticular (1joint) • No significant torque • Short fibers Secondary stabilizers: • Intermediate depth • Slow twitch • Usually monoarticular • Primary source of torque • Attachments are multipennate	• Build tension slowly, more fatigue resistant • Better activated at low levels of resistance • More effective in closed chain movement • In muscle imbalance, tend to weaken and lenghten
Mobilizers	• Superficial • Fast twitch • Often biarticular (2 joints) • Secondary source of torque	• Build tension rapidly, fatigue quickly • Better activated at high levels of resistance • More effective in open chain movements • In muscle imbalance, tend to tighten and shorten

Table 1. Stabilizers and mobilizers characteristics.

In this table, stabilizer and mobilizer muscles that affect the low back are presented. Muscles with (*) can work in different ways.

STABILIZERS		MOBILIZERS
Primary	Secondary	
Multifidus	Gluteus maximus	Iliopsoas * Rectus femoris
Transversus abdominis	Quadriceps	Hamstrings
Internal oblique	Iliopsoas *	Tensor fasciae lata
Gluteus medius	Subscapularis	Hip adductors
Vastusmedialis	Infraspinatus	Piriformis
Serratus anterior	Upper trapezius	Rectus abdominis External oblique Quadratus lumborum *
Lower trapezius	Quadratus lumborum *	Erector spinae
Deep neck flexors		Upper trapezius Levator scapulae
		Sternomastoid Scalenes
		Rhomboids Pectoralis minor Pectoralis major

Table 2. Stabilizer and mobilizer muscles that affect the low back

2. Diagnosis in lumbopelvic stabilization model

The main purpose of our diagnosis is to identify the abnormal segmental control of a motion segment. For that assessment, passive intervertebral manual pressures directly applied on the spinous process can be utilized in the search of an excessive or uncontrolled segmental translation. Usually, the application of that force on an affected or unstable segment may provoke pain or reproduce the symptoms. Multifidus muscles atrophy at any level could be another sign to detect a dysfunctional spinal segment. This can be assessed by palpation at both sides of the spinous process of every level and might be either unilateral or bilateral (figure 12).

Referring movement impairment changes in body segment alignment and the degree of segmental control (the ability to move one body segment without moving any others) form the basis of the movement impairment tests.

On the other hand, tightness and weakness in muscle imbalance alters body segment alignment and changes the equilibrium point of a point. If the muscles on one side of a joint are tight and the opposing muscles are lax, the joint will be pull out alignment toward the tight muscle. This alteration in alignment throws weight-bearing stress out a smaller region of the point surface, increasing pressure per unit area. Furthermore, the inert tissues on the shortened (closed) side of the joint will contract over time.

The combination of stiffness (hypoflexibility) in one body segment and laxity (hyperflexibility) in an adjacent segment leads to the development of relative flexibility (White&Sahrmann, 1994).

In contrast, radiologists have tried to determine the intervertebral instability using imaging techniques to assess both normal and abnormal ranges of movements. Most common techniques used to measure those intervertebral ranges of movements are neutral radiographs and functional in both flexion and extension taken in sagittal plane (Alam, 2002; Leone et al, 2007). Some of the measurements taken by many authors in different studies are shown in the table below.

Author	Spinal Level	Translation (mm)	Rotation (degrees)
Hayes et al.	L1-5	2-3	7-13
	L5-S1	3	14
White et al.	L1-5	3	13
	L5-S1	3	20
Froming & Frohman	L1-5	3	9
	L5-S1	3	17
Kanayama et al.	L1-5	4	10

Table 3. The upper limits of motion in a normal spine as seen on functional radiography.

According to White and Panjabi (1978), the radiographic criteria established as spinal instability are the following:

Flexion–extension radiographs

- Sagittal plane translation > 4.5 mm or 15%
- Sagittal plane rotation

15° at L1-2, L2-3, and L3-4

20° at L4-5

25° at L5-S1

Resting radiographs

- Sagittal plane displacement >4.5 mm or 15%
- Relative sagittal plane angulation >22°

Despite this measurements techniques are commonly used in taking care of some spinal pathologies, especially degenerative disorders, are not really relevant in clinical practice when talking about stabilization exercise program and its used as an instability evaluation technique has not been reported in any of the stabilization research papers.

Now some examples of different tests related to tight muscles, lax muscles and movement impaired are presented.

2.1 Tight muscles tests

2.1.1 Thomas test

Goal: to assess the length of the hip flexors.

The patient begins in supine position on the examination table. He/she is told to lift both knees up to his/her chest, keeping his/her back flattened to a point where the sacrum just begins to lift away from the examination table surface, but not further. As he holds on leg close to his chest in order to maintain the pelvic position, the opposite lower limb is gradually extended until it rests on the table. An increase of lumbar lordosis or the impossibility to complete the knee extension (figure 3b) indicates shortened hip flexors (iliopsoas mainly).

The same procedure with the examined leg out of the table (figure 3c) elucidates a shortened rectus femoris. Optimal alignment occurs with the femur horizontal and aligned with the sagittal plane (no abduction) and with the subject's shoulder, hip, and knee more or less in line. A positive test is indicated when the tibia loses their vertical position due to knee extension. The test is negative when the tibia remains vertical.

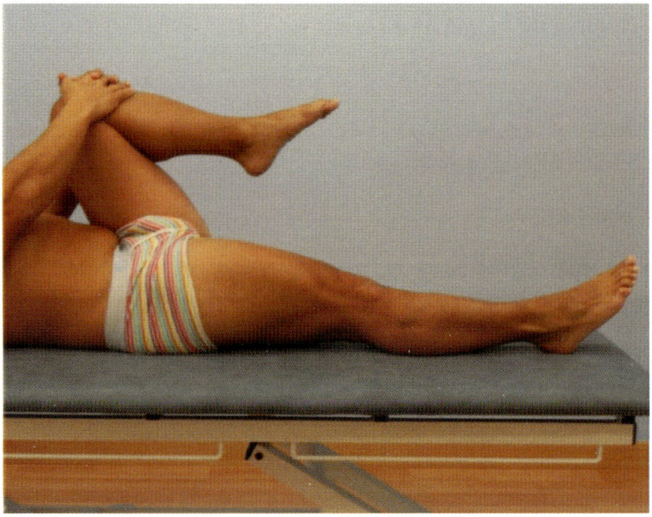

Fig. 3(a). Thomas test (no shortness).

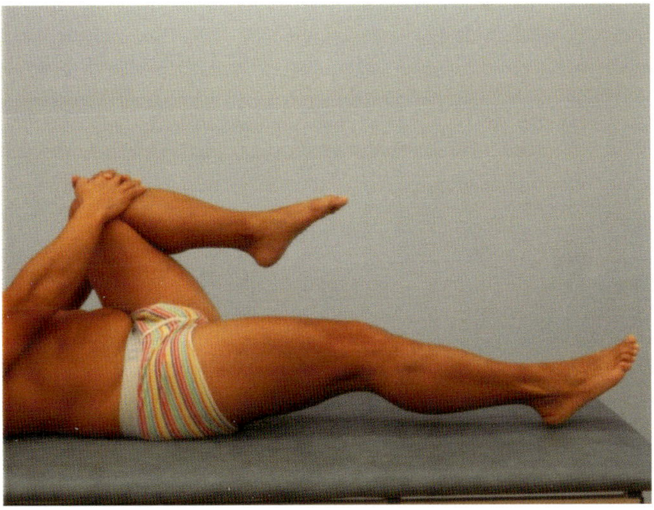

Fig. 3(b) Thomas test (iliopsoas shortened).

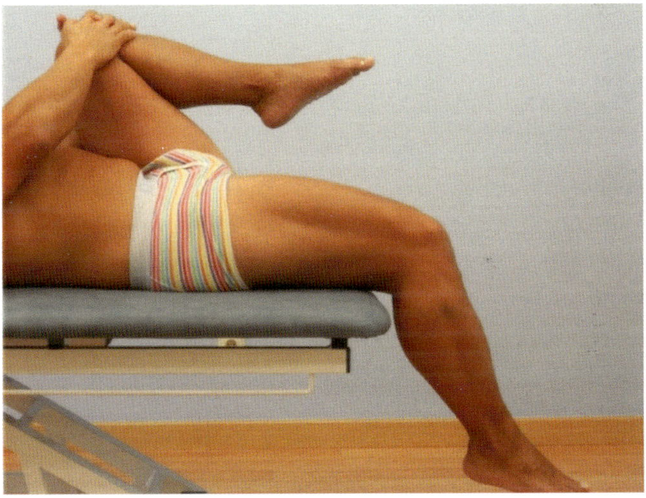

Fig. 3(c). Modified Thomas test (rectus femoris shortened).

2.1.2 Ober Test

Goal: to assess the length of tensor fasciae lata muscle.

The patient adopts a side-lying position with the pelvis in neutral. Contralateral knee is bent in order to improve overall body stability while the examiner stabilizes the pelvis to avoid lateral pelvic dipping. Patient abducts the homolateral leg to 15° above the horizontal and then extends his hip about 15°. While maintaining extension patient is then told to adduct his/her leg. Optimal muscle length would be confirmed if he/she is able to lower the homolateral leg to the level of the table.

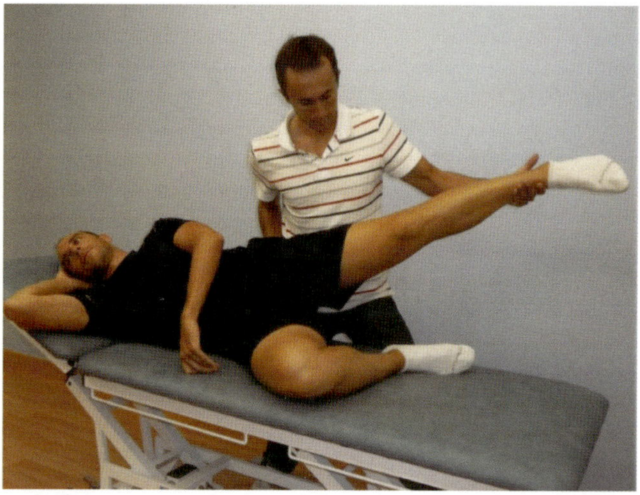

Fig. 4(a). Ober test; started position.

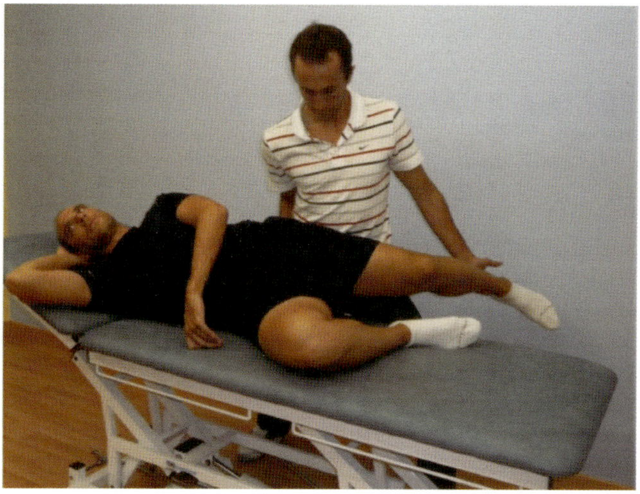

Fig. 4(b). Ober test; ended position.

2.1.3 Straight-leg raise test

Goal: to assess tightness in hamstrings.

The patient lies supine on the examination table, with one leg slightly bent. The patient is told to raise the other leg, keeping it completely straight. The examiner palpates the anterior rim of the pelvis to note the point at which the pelvis begins to posteriorly tilt because of hamstrings tightness. Optimal muscle length will permit degrees of flexion around 60-70°.

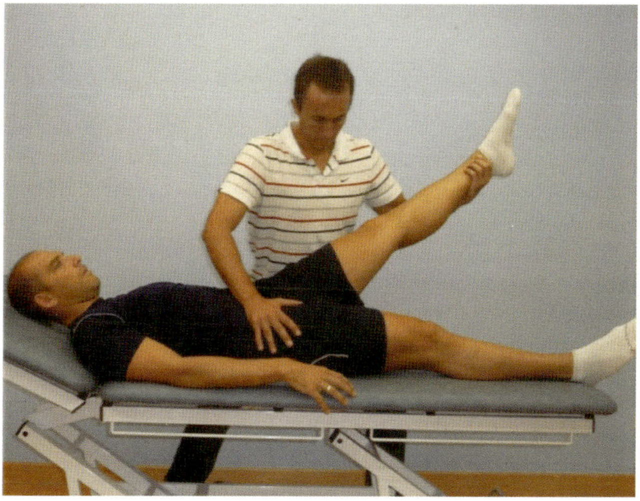

Fig. 5. Straight-leg raise test.

2.2 Lax muscles tests

2.2.1 Assessing muscle balance in the gluteus medius

Goal: to determine if the gluteus medius muscle is capable of holding the hip in full inner-range combined abduction and external rotation.

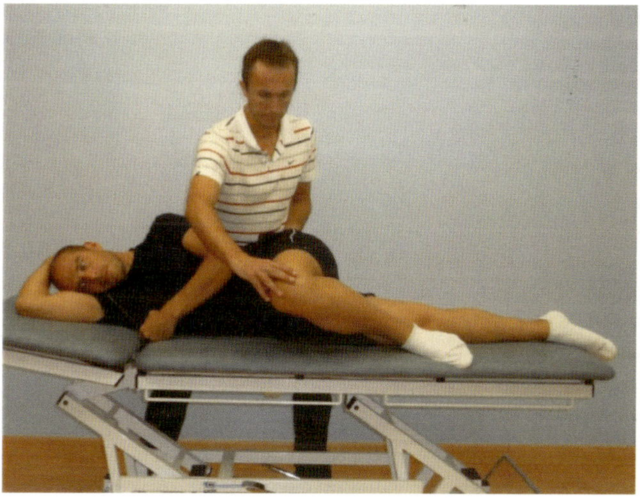

Fig. 6(a). Assessing muscle balance in the gluteus medius; started position.

The action in this test combines hip abduction and slight lateral rotation to emphasize the posterior fibers of the muscle. Patient lies on one side with his knees flexed and feet together. This position will identify where muscle tone is poor. People should rotate their trunk forward until the chest is on the couch and allow the knee to drop over the couch side. From this position they lift the leg as before.

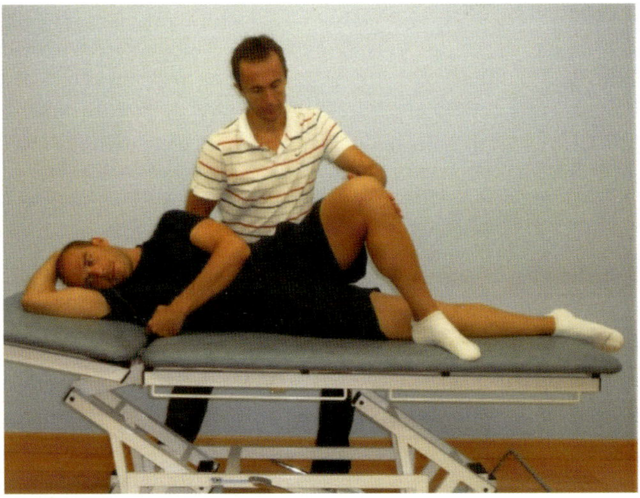

Fig. 6(b). Assessing muscle balance in the gluteus medius; ended position.

2.2.2 Sorensen test (low back fatigue test)

Goal: to determine isometric endurance of trunk extensor muscles.

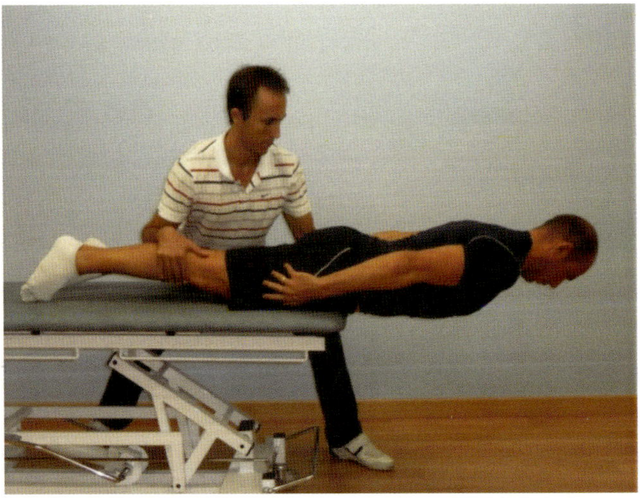

Fig. 7. Sorensen test.

The test consists in measuring the amount of time a person can hold the unsupported upper body in a horizontal prone position with the lower body fixed to the examining table.

Maximum values:

Healthy women: 171 sec. Healthy men: 239 sec.

Low back pain women: 99 sec. Low back pain men: 109 sec.

2.2.3 Prone abdominal hollowing test using pressure biofeedback

Goal: to assess patient's ability to hold the inner range of the deep abdominals.

With the patient lying prone, a pressure biofeedback unit is placed under his/her abdomen with the upper edge of the device's bladder below his navel. The unit is then inflated to 70 mmHg and patient is instructed to perform the abdominal hollowing maneuver. The aim is to reduce the pressure reading on the biofeedback unit by 6 to 10 mmHg and to maintain this contraction for 10 repetitions of 10 sec. each while breathing normally.

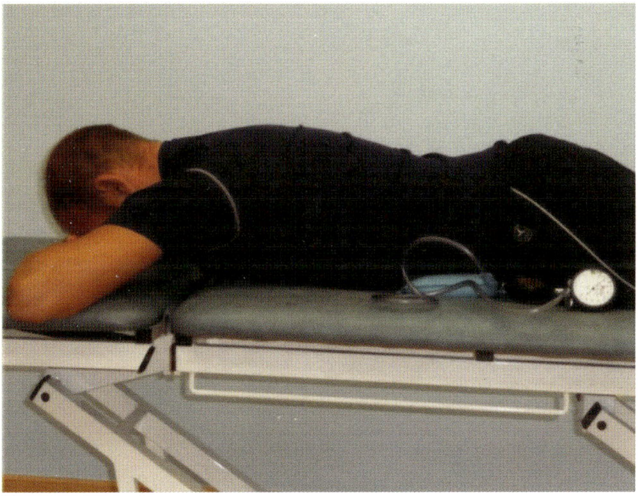

Fig. 8. Prone abdominal hollowing test using pressure biofeedback.

2.3 Movement impaired test

2.3.1 Functional low back movements

Goal: to determine the quality of each movement (flexion, extension, side-bending and rotation).

Patient stands up and is asked to move into flexion, extension, side-bending and rotation. Pelvis and low back is monitored any time in a quantitative and qualitative way.

2.3.2 Kneeling rock-back

Goal: to determine control of the hip relative to the lumbar-pelvic region while kneeling.

Patient is kneeling on a mat on all fours, with his/her hand directly beneath his shoulder and his knee beneath his hip. The test begins with the lumbar spine in a neutral position and then is rocked backward, pulling the hip behind the knees. Examiner should monitor the pelvic tilt angle and lumbar lordosis. Motion should begin at the hip for an optimal segmental control. Once hip flexion passes about 120° (depending on patient´s body proportions), his pelvis should posteriorly tilt and his lumbar spine flatten. Examiner should ensure that he moves slowly, and determine whether the sequence is motion at the hip-pelvis-lumbar spine. Poor segmental control will be present if the pelvic tilts and the lumbar spine flattens at the beginning of the rock-back.

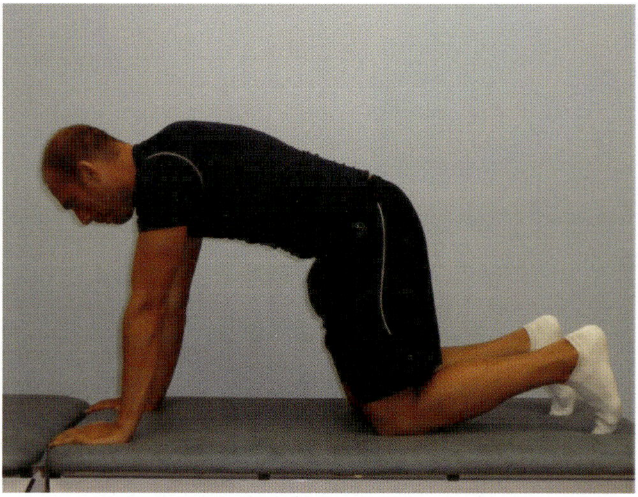

Fig. 9(a). Kneeling rock-back; starting position.

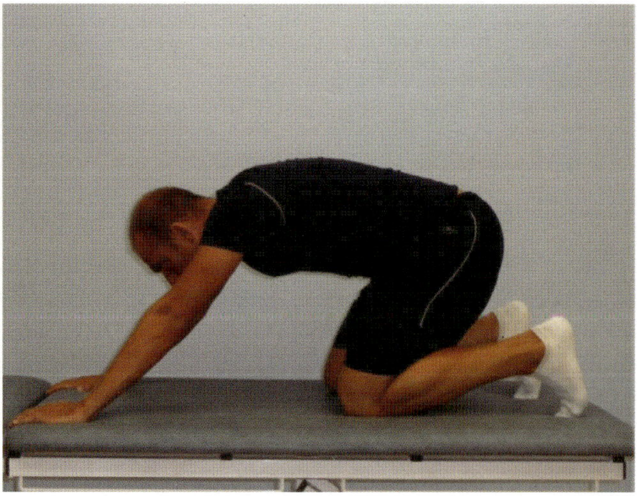

Fig. 9(b). Kneeling rock-back; ended position.

2.3.3 One-leg lift

Goal: to assess lumbar-pelvic control during one-leg lifting.

Patient stands side-on to a wall with one hand on the wall for balance if needed. He/she is instructed to slowly lift one leg, with the knee bent. The leg should reach a comfortable position -usually above hip height- and then lower. The examiner monitors the lumbar-pelvic region from the front and the side. In optimal alignment, the pelvis should remain level horizontally as the patient lifts his leg, and the sequence should be hip motion (flexion) followed by pelvic motion (posterior tilt) followed by lumbar motion -lordosis flattens and then reverses-. Poor control exits when the pelvis drops as the leg is lifted, and the lumbar spine flexes during the early stages of the movement.

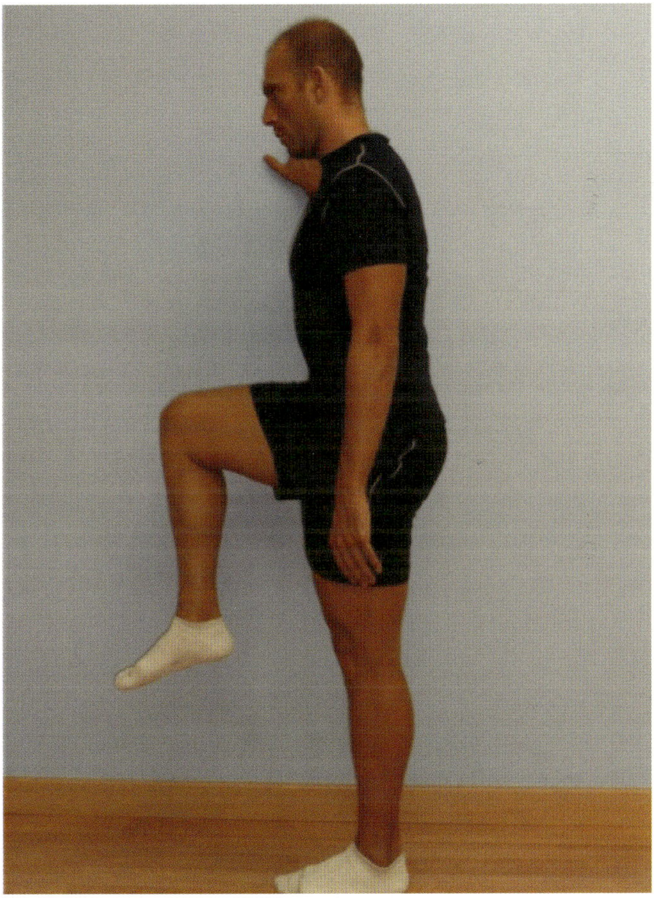

Fig. 10. One-leg lift.

2.3.4 Forward bending

Goal: to determine lumbar-pelvic control in bending.

Patient stands with his/her feet shoulder-width apart, facing the seat of a chair. He/she is instructed to bend forward, to touch the chair seat, and to stand back up again. Optimal control occurs when the patient unlocks his/her knees and anteriorly tilts his pelvis, flexing only slightly at the lumbar spine. Poor control will be present when he locks out and hyperextends the knees; he/she should not tilt his pelvis but instead should flex markedly at the lumbar and thoracic spine.

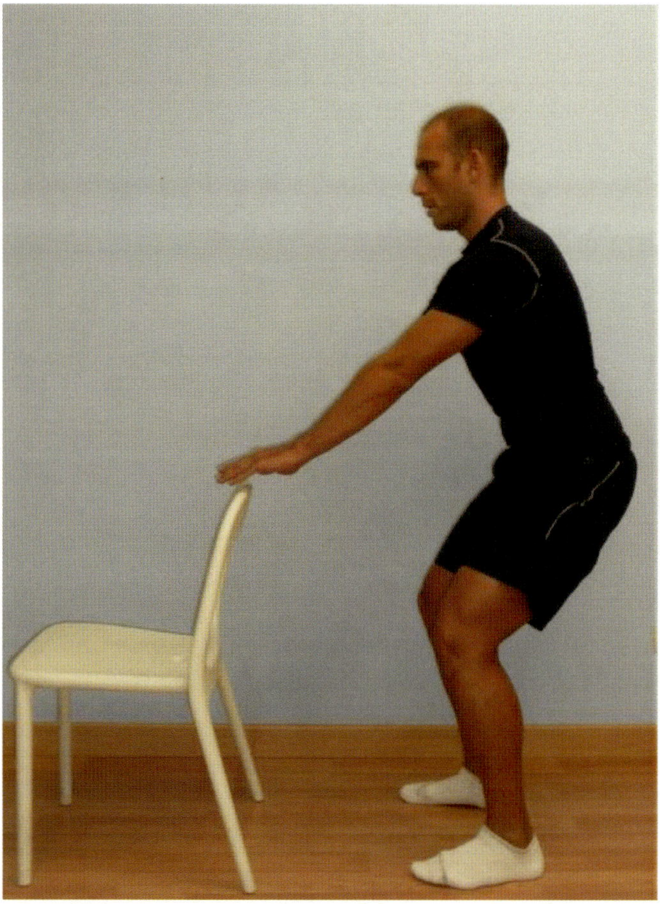

Fig. 11. Forward bending test.

3. Phases of treatment: Lumbopelvic stabilization program

The first consideration before establishing phases of treatment is to determine testing procedures. Many experimental assessment procedures, some of them described before, give essential information about joint protection mechanisms, especially in the lumbopelvic region.

Lumbopelvic stabilization program needs to involve a problem-solving approach, where clinical tests, reflecting the dysfunction mechanisms, are used to decide the best type of treatment approach for an individual client. In order to achieve this, assessments and their related treatments have been simplified by dividing them into progressive stages, where one stage of assessment and treatment is ideally completed prior to proceeding to the next stage. The segmental approach we have devised develops through three stages of segmental control, with each stage exposing the individual patient to increasing challenges to his/her joint protection mechanisms (Richardson et al., 2004).

- Segmental control over primary stabilizers (mainly TrA, deep multifidus, pelvic floor and diaphragm)
- Exercises in closed chain, with low velocity and low load
- Exercises in open chain, with high velocity and load

3.1 Phase 1

Key: Segmental control over primary stabilizers.

We refer to re-establishing directly the simultaneous contraction of the deep muscle synergy independently of the secondary stabilizers and mobilizers. This simultaneous contraction of the synergy, independent of the global muscles, should occur with the postural cue to "draw in the abdominal wall". The weight of the body is minimized in order to allow the patient to focus on this specific skill involved in joint protection.

Training local segmental control involves activating and facilitating the local muscle system, while using techniques (e.g. feedback) to reduce the contribution of the global muscles, most particularly the mobilizers. Instructional cues, body position and various feedback techniques (including palpation, electromyography and real-time ultrasound) are used simultaneously to facilitate the local synergy and inhibit or relax the more active global muscles. The ability to hold this pattern through developing specific muscular control, without addition of any load, may serve also to help to restore kinaesthetic awareness and lumbopelvic position sense, usually found to be impaired in the patient with low back pain.

The precise position of the lumbopelvic region may itself be facilitatory for activation of the local synergy muscles. Recent research has shown that better co-activation of the TrA occurs when the pelvic floor is contracted with the lumbar spine place in a more neutral position (Sapsford et al., 1997b). There is a consensus that local muscles are involved in segmental support and, therefore, contribute to the precise positioning of the lumbosacral curve.

Lumbar multifidus activation

In order to get a suitable activation of lumbar multifidus (LM), a submaximal contraction was elicited with the contralateral arm lift maneuver, while holding a small hand weight, as previously demonstrated to elicit approximately 30% of the maximal voluntary contraction of the LM muscle (Koppenhaver et al., 2011).

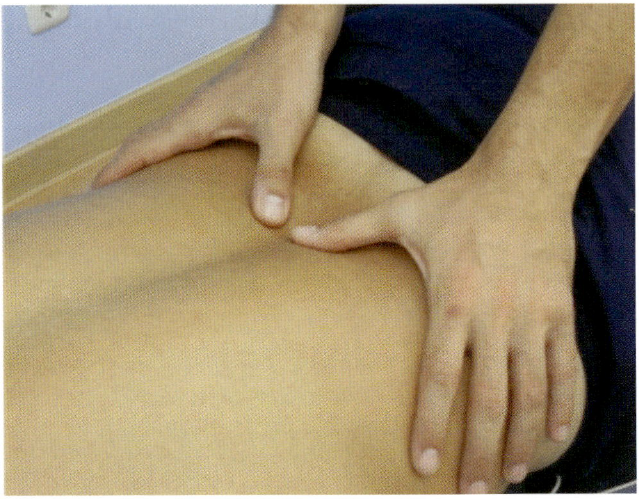

Fig. 12. Activation of multifidus in prone position.

Transversus abdominis activation

In order to get a suitable contraction of TrA, we propose to use the hollowing-in maneuver. Performance of the abdominal hollowing maneuver may be difficult, even in healthy subjects. Contraction of the pelvic floor muscles may promote contraction of the TrA during the abdominal hollowing maneuver. Participants were instructed to "take a relaxed breath in and out, hold the breath out and then draw in your lower abdomen without moving your spine." Alternate cues of "cut off the flow of urine" or "close your rear passage" were sometimes given in an attempt to optimize contraction of the TrA with minimal to no thickening of the internal oblique (IO) muscle (Koppenhaver et al., 2011).

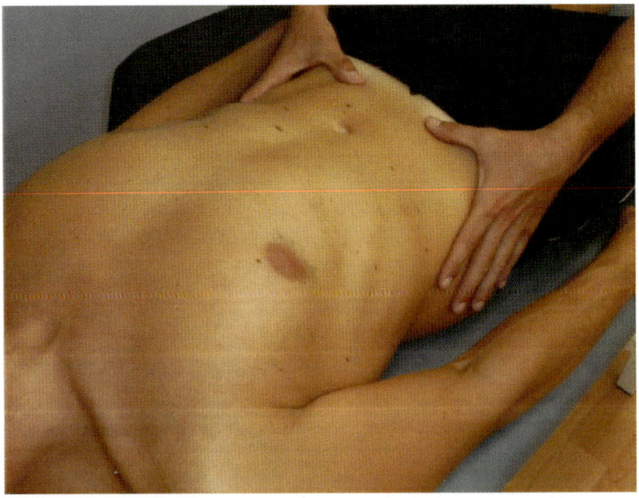

Fig. 13. Abdominal hollowing; activation of transversus abdominis in crook-lying position.

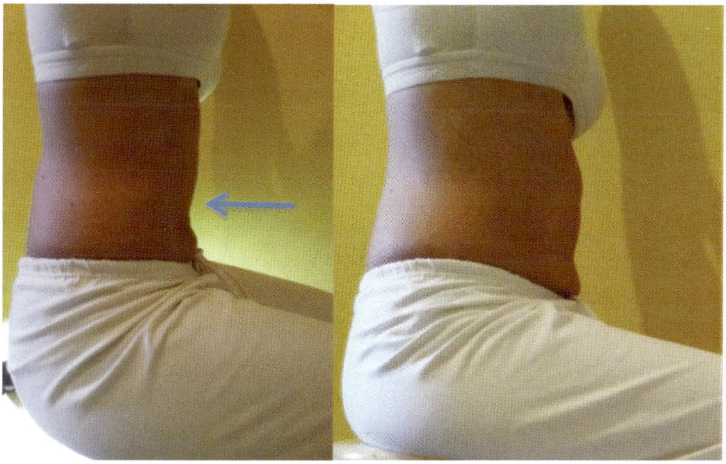

Fig. 14. Abdominal hollowing: activation of transversus abdominis in sitting.

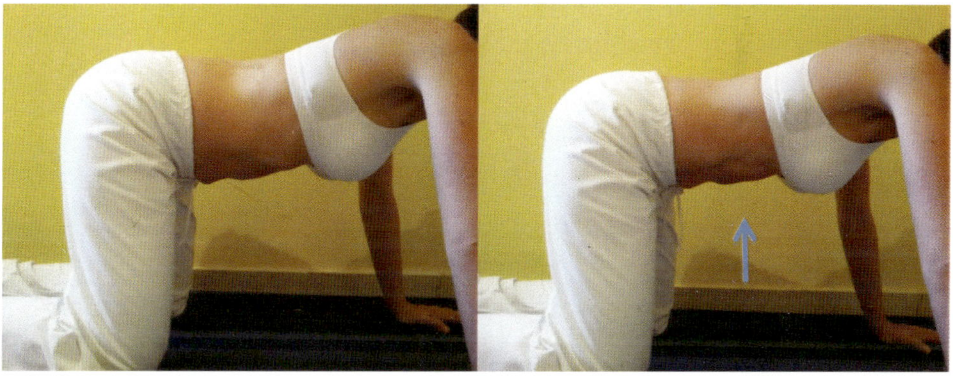

Fig. 15. Abdominal hollowing: activation of transversus abdominis in four point kneeling.

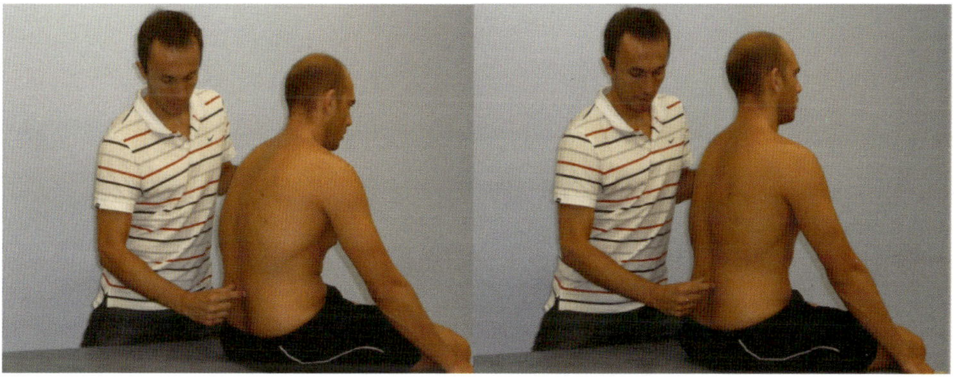

Fig. 16. Activation of multifidus from sitting to lumbar neutral position: looking for neutral position.

3.2 Phase 2

Key: Exercises in closed chain, low velocity and low load.

The purpose is to maintain local muscle synergy contraction, while gradually progressing load cues through the body using weightbearing closed chain exercises. Weightbearing load is added very slowly, ensuring any weightbearing muscle at any kinetic chain segment is activated in order to give effective antigravity support and provide efficient and safe load transfer through the segments of the body. The focus is especially to ensure activation of the local and weightbearing muscles of the lumbar spine and pelvis, and the ability to maintain a static lumbolpelvic posture for weightbearing. These muscles are likely to be dysfunctional in patients with low back pain. In addition, lifestyle factors of many individuals, which could have led to a dysfunction in these muscles, need to be addressed, as they may place them at risk of sustaining further low back injury.

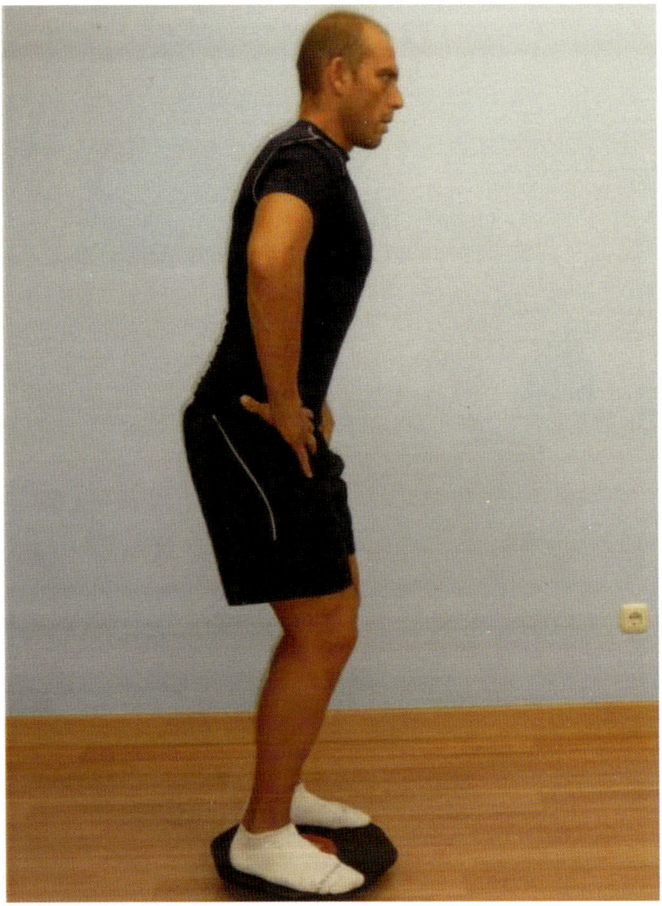

Fig. 17. Stand-up position on unstable surface.

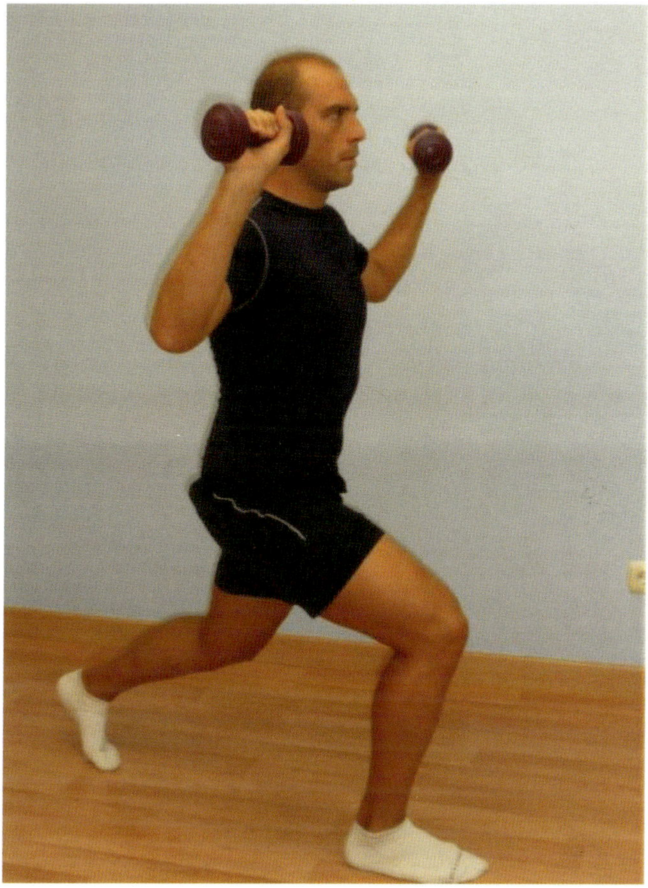

Fig. 18. Closed chain lunge exercises, with the addition of hand weights.

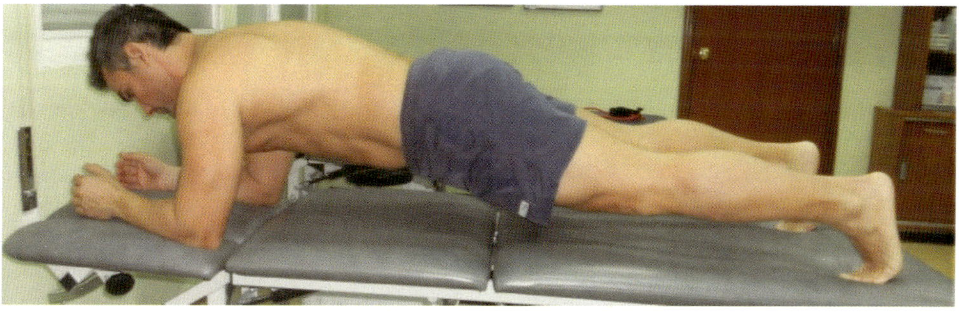

Fig. 19. Bridge in prone position

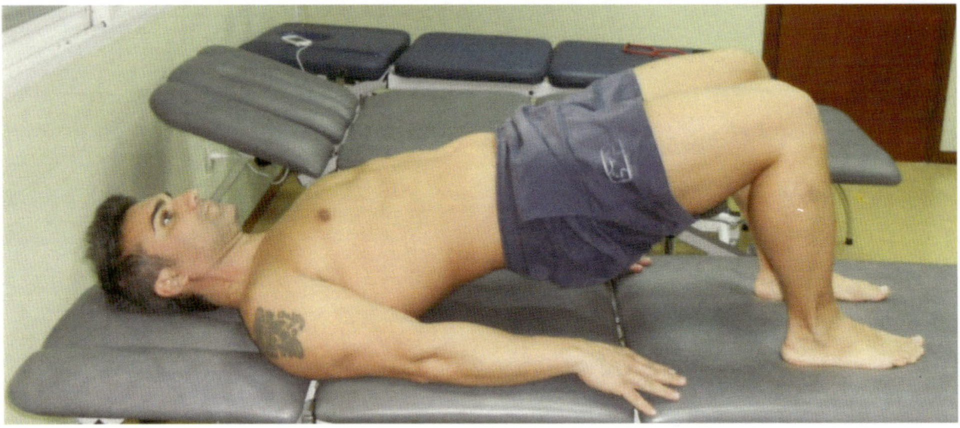

Fig. 20. Bridge in supine position.

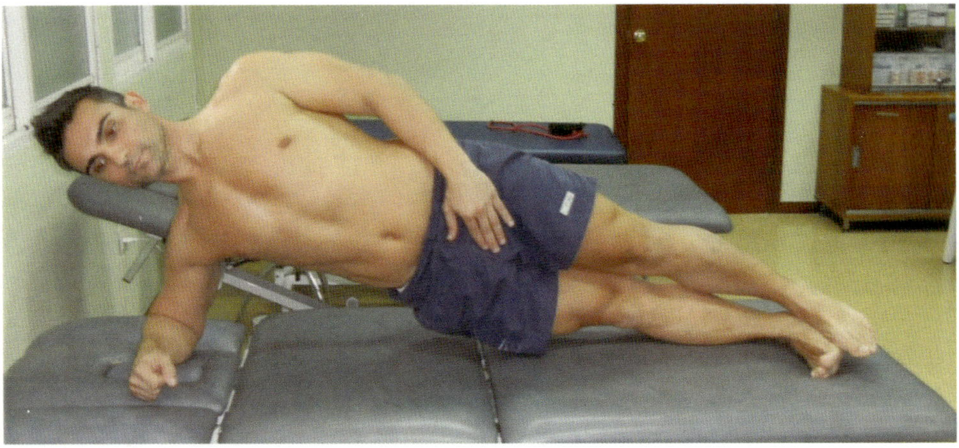

Fig. 21. Lateral bridge.

3.3 Phase 3

Key: Exercises in open chain, high velocity and high load.

The aim is to continue to maintain local segmental control while load is added through open kinetic chain movement of adjacent segments. This final step is to direct progression so that all muscles are integrated into functional movement tasks in a formal way.

This third stage allows any loss of local segmental control during high loaded open chain tasks to be detected, as well as ensuring that there is no compensation by the more active (i.e. non-weightbearing) muscles. In addition, loss of range of asymmetry of joints adjacent to the lumbopelvic region needs to be addressed to ensure that loss of movement range does not interfere with the ability of the individual to maintain lumbopelvic stability during movement.

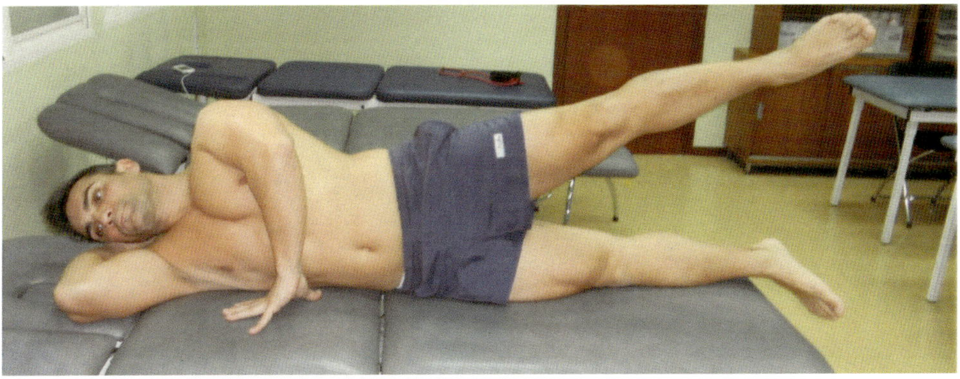

Fig. 22. Lower limb abduction.

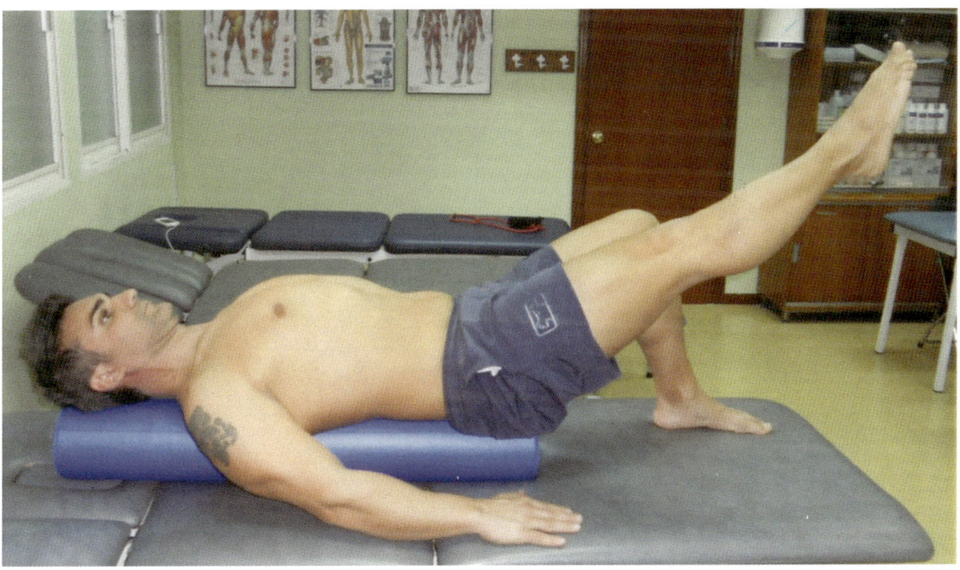

Fig. 23. Knee extension in supine position on roller.

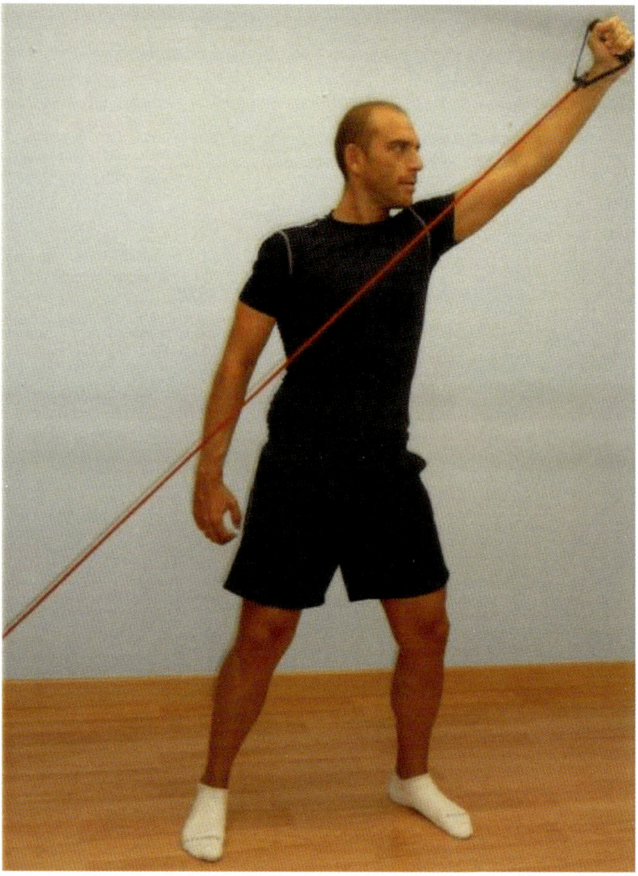

Fig. 24. Open chain exercise of upper limb after co-contraction of transversus abdominis and multifidus.

4. Gym ball and foam roller exercises

4.1 Gym ball

We can obtain good levels of stability using exercise with gym balls (also called stability balls or Swiss balls). These exercises require quite complex movements and will help increase the stability already obtained through previous exercises in this book. They can also strengthen stability muscles that otherwise might not be exercised. It is an inexpensive and effective apparatus for back stability. A 26 in. (65 cm) gym ball provides the optimal sitting position for most people although it can be used 21.6 in. (55) cm and 29.5 in. (75 cm). People should be able to sit on the ball with their femurs horizontal and their hips and knees both at 90° to 100° of flexion, so that their knees are slightly below their hips.

4.1.1 Practical considerations (Norris, 2008)

- Patients should warm up before use them.
- Return to the neutral position when the exercise is complete and keep their abdomens hollowed when stress is imposed on the spine.
- Progression with stability ball exercises: we might start with 8 to 10 repetitions, and then increase to 12 to 15. At first a slow count of 4 to 5 to move into a holding position should be used; hold the designated position for a count of 5, and then use a count of 4 or 5 to move back into the starting position. Patients can progress by adding reps or increasing the holding time.
- Deflate the ball slightly to increase its contact area.
- Begin with simple actions and progress to more complex movements.

4.1.2 Some exercises

- Sitting knee raise on gym ball. Goal: maintain stability in the presence of hip movement on a reduced base of support.

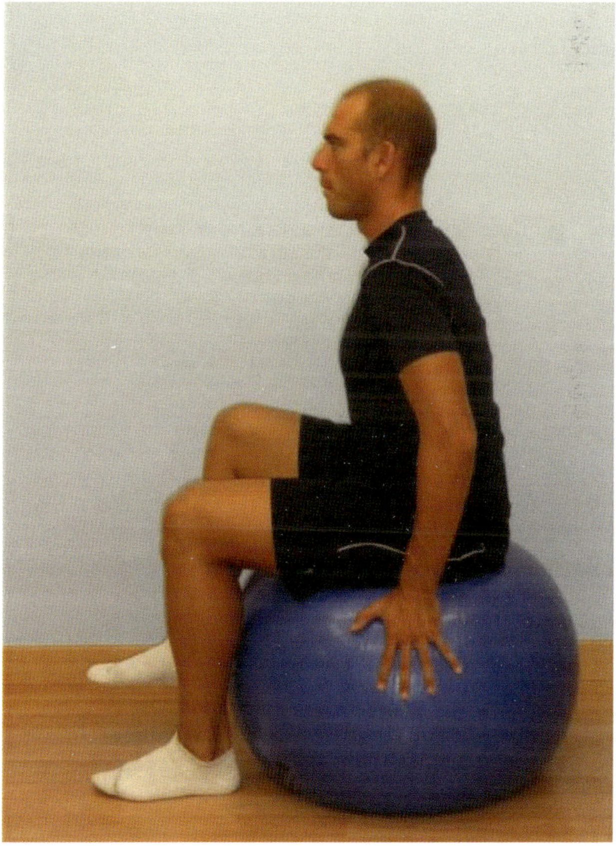

Fig. 25. Sitting knee raise on gym ball.

- Abdominal slide. Goal: control action of the rectus abdominis while moving.

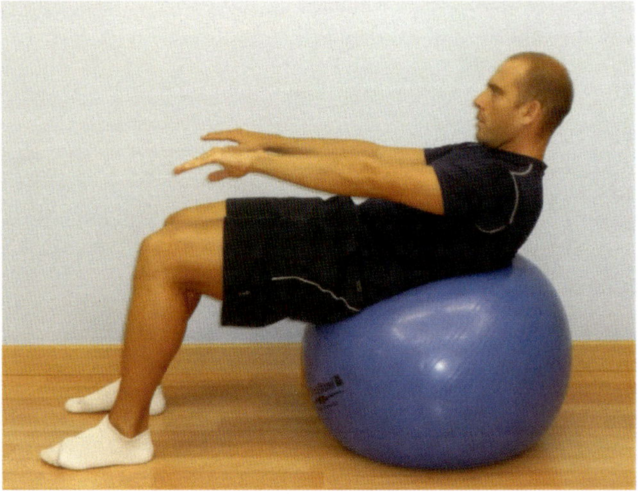

Fig. 26. Abdominal slide.

- Lying trunk curl with leg lift. Goal: strengthen upper and lower abdominals.

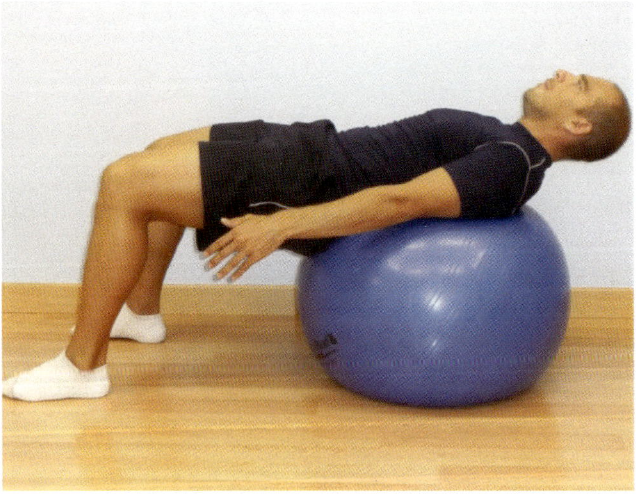

Fig. 27. Lying trunk curl with leg lift.

- Basic superman. Goal: strengthen the spinal and hip extensors.

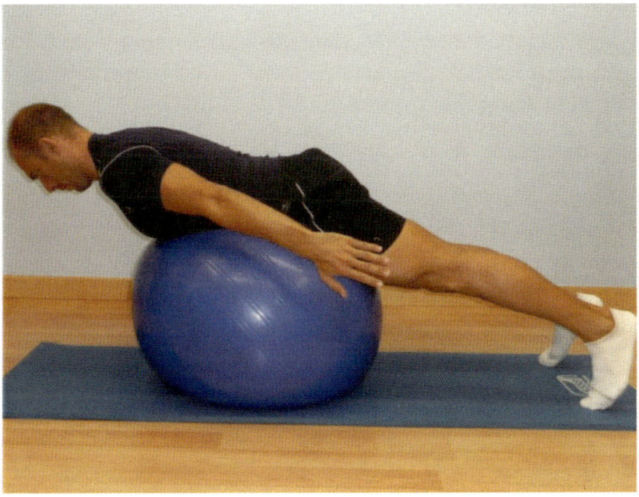

Fig. 28. Basic superman.

- Bridge with therapist pressure. Goal: strengthen hip and trunk stability muscles by challenging stability with continuously variable overload from multiple directions.

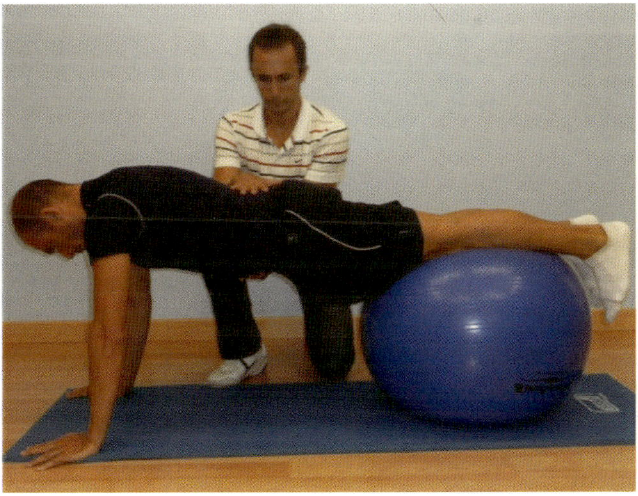

Fig. 29. Bridge with therapist pressure.

4.2 Foam roller

Foam rollers are commonly used within physical therapy for rehabilitation and during exercise classes such as Pilates (Norris, 2008). They are normally 3 ft (1 m) long and either 3 or 6 in. (7.6 or 15.2 cm) in diameter. Rollers may be either full rolls (circles) or half rolls (D-shaped), made of polyurethane or similar materials, which are durable and suitable for weight bearing up to 350 lb (150kg) (figures 23, 30, 31 and 32).

Because the rollers are narrow, their contact area with the floor is quite small, making them ideal as an unstable base of support. Because they are firm but forgiving, they are especially useful for exercises that require direct body contact. Foam rollers have the advantage over wooden wooble boards in this feature.

Each exercise should be performed for 10 repetitions or 5 reps to each side (10 in total) if using single-side movements. Because these are balance exercises, they may be progressed through timing and complexity.

4.2.1 Some exercises

Supine-lying leg lift. Goal: to develop back stability in an unstable lying position.

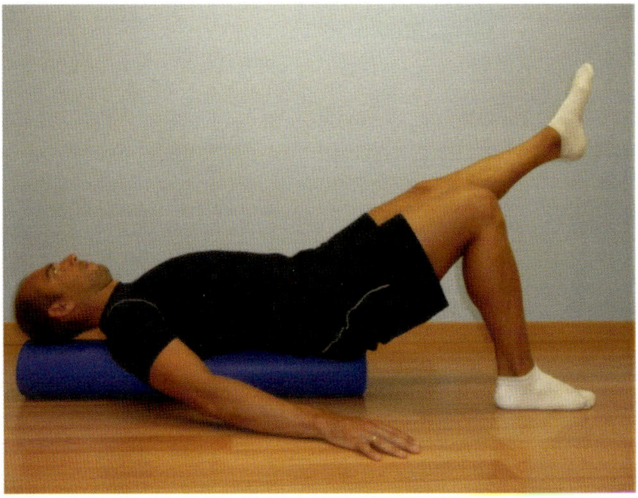

Fig. 30. Supine-lying leg lift.

- Bridge with heel raise on roller. Goal: develop spinal extensor and gluteal muscle endurance on an unstable platform.

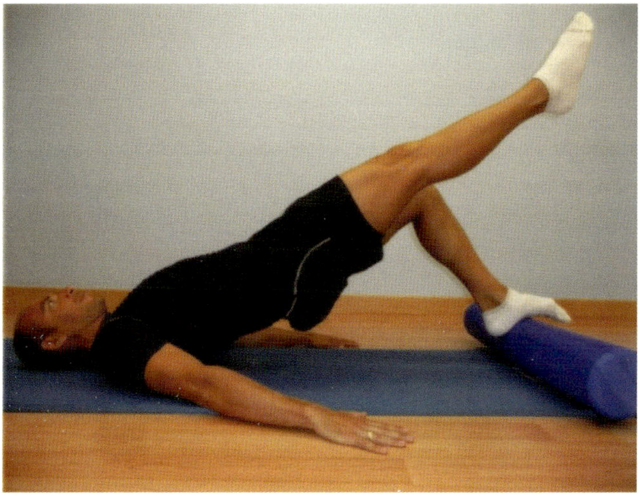

Fig. 31. Bridge with heel raise on roller.

- Prone tuck on roller. Goal: to develop whole trunk strength and range of motion.

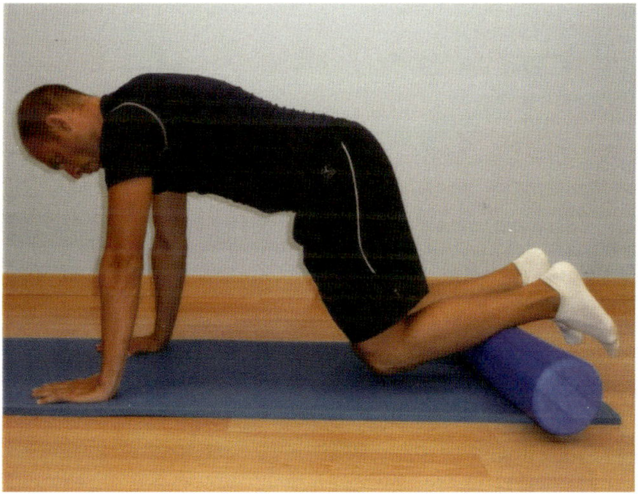

Fig. 32. Prone tuck on roller.

5. Conclusions

Lumbopelvic stabilization approach seems to be useful for the management of low back pain. Based on a solid biomechanical model (Panjabi's hypotheses), it has demonstrated positive effects over pain and return to activity, but it is not clear the optimal type of exercise, duration or number of repetitions, among other variables. Furthermore there is no strong evidence that conclude whether lumbopelvic stabilization programs provide better results than other different methods such as Pilates, Yoga, or Aerobics. Further research focusing on these topics is needed.

6. References

Alam A. Radiological evaluation of lumbar intervertebral instability. Ind J Aerospace Med 2002; 46(2): 48-53.

Adams M, Bogduk N, Burton K, Doland P. The biomechanics of back pain. Edinburgh, UK: Churchill Livingstone; 2002.

Childs JD, Teyhen DS, Benedict TM, Morris JB, Fortenberry AD, McQueen RM, Preston JB, Wright AC, Dugan JL, George SZ. Effects of sit-up training versus core stabilization exercises on sit-up performance. Med Sci Sports Exerc 2009; 41(11): 2072-83.

Costa LOP, Maher CG, Latimer J, et al. Motor control exercise for chronic low back pain: a randomized placebo-controlled trial. Phys Ther 2009; 89: 1275-86.

Dankaerts W, O'Sullivan P, Burnett, A, Straker L. Altered patterns of superficial trunk muscle activation during sitting in nonspecific chronic low back pain patients: importance of subclassification. Spine 2006; 31(17): 2017-23.

Ferreira PH, Ferreira ML, Hodges PW. Changes in recruitment of the abdominal muscles in people with low back pain: ultrasound measurement of muscle activity. Spine 2004; 29(22): 2560-6.

Ferreira PH, Ferreira ML, Maher CG, Herbert RD, Refshauge K. Specific stabilisation exercise for spinal and pelvic pain: a systematic review. Aust J Physiother 2006; 52(2): 79-88.

França FR, Burke TN, Hanada ES, Marques AP. Segmental stabilization and muscular strengthening in chronic low back pain: a comparative study. J Manipulative Physiol Ther 2011; 34(2): 98-106.

Fritz JM, Whitman JM, Childs JD. Lumbar spine segmental mobility assessment: an examination of validity for determining intervention strategies in patients with low back pain. Arch Phys Med Rehabil 2005; 86(9): 1745-52.

Hides J, Gilmore C, Stanton W, Bohlscheid E. Multifidus size and symmetry among chronic LBP and healthy asymptomatic subjects. Man Ther 2008; 13: 43-9.

Hides JA, Stanton WR, MacMahon S, Sims K, Richardson CA. Effect of stabilization training on multifidus muscle cross-sectional area among young elite cricketers with low back pain. J Orthop Sports PhysTher 2008; 38(3): 101-8.

Hodges PW, Richardson CA. Inefficient muscular stabilization of the lumbar spine associated with low back pain. A motor control evaluation of transversus abdominis. Spine 1996; 21(22): 2640-50.

Hodges PW, Richardson CA. Delayed postural contraction of transversus abdominis in low back pain associated with movement of the lower limb. J Spinal Disord 1998; 11: 46-56.

Hodges PW. Is there a role for transversus abdominis in lumbopelvic stability? Man Ther 1999; 4(2): 74-86.

Hodges PW. Core stability exercise in chronic low back pain. Orthop Clin North Am 2003; 34(2): 245-54.

Janda V, Schmid HJA. Muscles as a pathogenic factor in back pain. In: Proceedings of the International of OrthopaedicManupulative Therapists (4th conference, 17-18). Auckland, New Zealand; 1980.

Jull GA, Richardson CA. Active stabilization of the trunk. Course notes. University of Edinburgh, Edinburgh, UK; 1994.

Kamaz M, Kıreşi D, Oğuz H, Emlik D, Levendoğlu F. CT measurement of trunk muscle areas in patients with chronic low back pain. Diagn Interv Radiol 2007; 13: 144-48.

Kankaanpää M, Taimela S, Airaksinen O, Hänninen O.The efficacy of active rehabilitation in chronic low back pain. Effect on pain intensity, self-experienced disability, and lumbar fatigability. Spine 1999; 24(10): 1034-42.

Kendall FP, McCreary EK, Province PG. Muscles. Testing and function, 4ed. Baltimore: Williams&Wilkins; 1993.

Kjaer P, Bendix T, Sorensen JS, Korsholm L, Leboeuf-Yde Ch. Are MRI-defined fat infiltrations in the multifidus muscles associated with low back pain? BMC Medicine 2007; 5:2.

Koppenhaver SL, Fritz JM, Hebert JJ, Kawchuk GN, Childs JD, Parent EC, Gill NW, Teyhen DS. Association between changes in abdominal and lumbar multifidus muscle thickness and clinical improvement after spinal manipulation. J Orthop Sports Phys Ther 2011; 41(6): 389-99.

Kriese M, Clijsen R, Taeymans J, Cabri J. Segmental stabilization in low back pain: a systematic review. Sportverletz Sportschaden 2010; 24(1): 17-25.

Leone A, Guglielmi G, Cassar-Pullicino V, Bonomo L. Lumbar Intervertebral Instability: A Review. Radiology 2007; 245: 62-77.

Liddle SD, Gracey JH, Baxter GD. Advice for the management of low back pain: a systematic review of randomised controlled trials. Man Ther 2007; 12(4): 310-27.

Liebenson C. Rehabilitation of the spine. 2 ed. Baltimore: Williams&Wilkins; 1996.

Macedo LG, Maher CG, Latimer J, McAuley JH. Motor control exercise for persistent, nonspecific low back pain: a systematic review. Phys Ther 2009; 89: 9-25.

Mengiardi B, Schmid MR, Boos N, Pfirrmann C, Brunner F, Elfering A, Hodler J. Fat content of lumbar paraspinal muscles in patients with chronic low back pain and in asymptomatic volunteers: Quantification with MR Spectroscopy. Radiology 2006; 240: 786-92.

Muthukrishnan R, Shenoy SD, Jaspal SS, Nellikunja S, Fernandes S. The differential effects of core stabilization exercise regime and conventional physiotherapy regime on postural control parameters during perturbation in patients with movement and control impairment chronic low back pain. Sports Med Arthrosc Rehabil Ther Technol 2010; 2: 13.

Norris CM. Back Stability. Champaign, IL: Human Kinetics; 2008.

O'Sullivan PB, Phyty GD, Twomey LT, Allison GT. Evaluation of specific stabilizing exercise in the treatment of chronic low back pain with radiologic diagnosis of spondylolysis or spondylolisthesis. Spine 1997; 22(24): 2959-67.

O'Sullivan PB. Lumbar segmental "instability": clinical presentation and specific stabilizing exercise management. Man Ther 2000; 5(1): 2-12.

Panjabi MM, Abumy K, Duranceau J, Oxland T. Spinal stability and intersegmental muscle forces. A biomechanical model. Spine 1989; 14: 194-200.

Panjabi MM. The stabilizing system of the spine. Part I. Function, dysfunction, adaptation, and enhacement. J Spinal Disord 1992; 5: 383-9.

Panjabi MM. The stabilizing system of the spine. Part II. Neutral zone and instability hypothesis. J Spinal Disord 1992; 5(4): 390-7.

Panjabi MM. Clinical spinal instability and low back pain. J Electromyogr Kinesiol 2003; 13: 371–9.

Paris SV. Physical signs of instability. Spine 1985; 10(3): 277-9.

Pereira LM, Obara K, Dias JM, Menacho MO, Guariglia DA, Schiavoni D, Pereira HM, Cardoso JR. Comparing the Pilates method with no exercise or lumbar stabilization for pain and functionality in patients with chronic low back pain: Systematic review and meta-analysis. Clin Rehabil 2011.

Richardson C, Toppenberg R, Jull G. An initial evaluation of eight abdominal exercises for their ability to provide stabilization for the lumbar spine. Aust J Physiother 1990; 36: 6-11.

Richardson CA, Hodges PW, Hides J. Therapeutic Exercise for Lumbopelvic Stabilization: A Motor Control Approach for the Treatment and Prevention of Low Back Pain. 2 ed. Edinburgh: Churchill Livingstone; 2004.

Waddell G, Feder G, Lewis M. Systematic reviews of bed rest and advice to stay active for acute low back pain. Br J General Pract 1997; 47: 647-52.

White AA, Panjabi MM. Clinical biomechanics of the spine. Philadelphia: JB Lippincott; 1978.

White SG, Sahrmann SA. A movement system balance approach to management of musculoskeletal pain. In: Grant R. Physical therapy of the cervical and thoracic spine. New York: Churchill Livingstone; 1994.

Zazulak B, Cholewicki J, Reeves NP. Neuromuscular control of trunk stability: clinical implications for sports injury prevention. J Am Acad Orthop Surg 2008; 16(9): 497-505.

14

Conservative Management for Patients with Sacroiliac Joint Dysfunction

Kyndall Boyle
Appalachian State University
USA

1. Introduction

Conditions involving one or both sacroiliac joints (SIJs) are often referred to as sacroiliac joint pain (SIJP), sacroiliac joint dysfunction (SIJD), or pelvic girdle pain (PGP). SIJP is defined as pain arising from intra-articular structures such as the anterior sacroiliac ligament, posterior sacroiliac ligament, interosseous ligaments, and articular cartilage in the SIJ. SIJD is a state of altered mechanics, either an increase or decrease from the expected normal or the presence of an aberrant motion.[1] It includes pain arising from extra-articular structures that surround the SIJs such as the sacrotuberous, sacrospinous, and/or iliolumbar ligaments. Lastly, PGP is pain experienced between the posterior iliac crest and the gluteal fold, particularly in the vicinity of the SIJs.[2] SIJP and SIJD are therefore considered subgroups of PGP. [2]

The prevalence of sacroiliac joint pain has been reported between 13-30%.[3, 4] Specifically 13% of individuals with low back pain have pain arising from the SIJ as evidenced by relief of their pain after an intra-articular anesthetic block.[3] Thirty percent of all patients seen in out-patient clinics have pain arising from the SIJs,[4] 25% of pregnant women have PGP, and 7% of post partum women have "serious" PGP.[5]

2. Diagnosis

2.1 Subjective data

Making a clinical diagnosis of a patient with certainty that pain is originating from the SIJs is challenging.[1] Reliability and validity of many special tests (particularly motion palpation tests) are poor[6, 7], and the existence of a Gold standard test is controversial.[4, 8] Subjective history specifics, location of pain/symptoms, and special tests called provocation testing are helpful and important in this endeavor. Patients who complain of pain when they arise after long term sitting present a classic sign of pain from the SIJs.[9] It is also common for patients to point directly over their left (L) and/or right (R) SIJs (posterior superior iliac spine (PSIS) region). This is referred to as Fortin's Finger Test.[10] A complaint of *unilateral* pain (on one side only) rather than bilateral pain is also considered more likely to be coming from an SIJ.[9] Another classic sign indicative of SIJ pain referral is the absence of lumbar pain above L5.[9] Pain perceived over one or both PSIS/SIJs and just lateral and/or inferior, in the buttock, is also a strong indicator of SIJP.[11] This area is called Fortin's Area and was discovered and defined as three centimeters lateral to the PSIS/SIJ and ten centimeters caudal to the PSIS/SIJ, based on a study in which the SIJs were injected with a contrast medium (arthrography) to stimulate pain, and then the area of referred pain was mapped.[11]

3. Special tests

3.1 Load transfer

A myriad of special tests have been discussed in the literature, including a load transfer test[12], many provocation tests designed to provoke pain in one or both SIJs, and motion palpation tests designed to assess asymmetry in SIJ motion and/or hyper- or hypomobility of the SIJs. The Active Straight Leg Raise Test (ASLR) assesses the ability of the patient to effectively transfer load between their lower limbs and trunk.[12] This test can be used to help rule in pain arising from the SIJ(s) but is not limited to the SIJs. The ASLR test can also be used to assess many conditions involving the trunk and pelvis. The test is done with the patient lying supine. The clinician then asks the patient to raise their leg 5 cm off the supporting surface (plinth) (Figure 1) and determines how much effort was required on a scale of 0-5 (0=No effort, 5=Max effort).[13] If the patient has optimal ability to effectively transfer load during the test, the leg will rise up effortlessly without any pelvic movement. The clinician observes for movement during the test and watches for compensatory movement resulting from instability. Examples of aberrant motion may include drawing the rib cage inward from over activation of the external obliques, flaring the lower ribs out from over activation of the internal obliques or thoracic extension from over activation of the

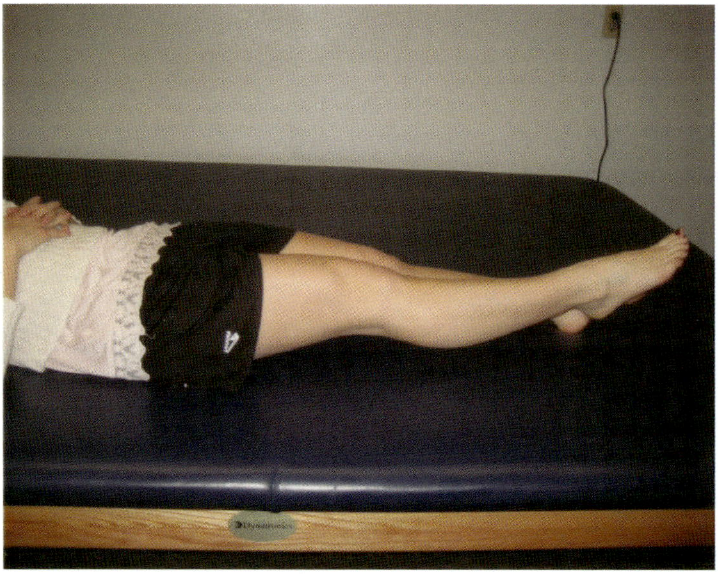

Fig. 1. Active Straight Leg Raise (ASLR) (step one)

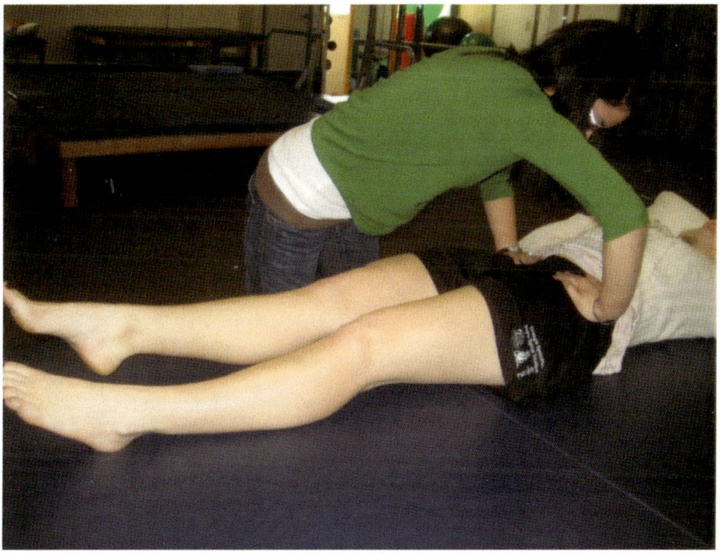

Fig. 2. Active Straight leg Raise (ASLR) with manual compression
Copyright © Kyndy Boyle 2010, used with permission

erector spinae. The abdomen may also bulge, potentially indicating that the patient is holding their breath during the test to compensate for poor load transfer.[13] The clinician then repeats the test while applying manual pelvic compression in the area of compensatory motion (Figure 2). The clinician asks the patient if the heaviness or effort of lifting their leg has decreased. The test is positive if effort or heaviness is lessened or abolished with manual compression. A positive test indicates the need for greater stability around the SIJ, also called force closure, which will be discussed later in this chapter.

3.2 Pain provocation tests

Pain provocation tests (PPTs) such as Resisted Abduction, Patrick's Sign, Distraction, Gaenslen's, and Sacral Thrust have shown adequate reliability, sensitivity, and specificity, especially when performed as a cluster.[8 14, 15] PPTs are limited by the difficulty they present for the clinician to identify whether intra-articular or peri-articular structures are stressed by the tests. The possibility of false negatives due to physical properties of the tissues constitutes another limitation and may require PPTs to be held up to two minutes to avoid.[16] From my observation over 21 years, they are seldomly held for that length of time in the clinic. Three or more positive PPTs appear to provide the highest discriminatory power, with a sensitivity of .85 and a specificity of .76.[8] A few individual PPTs are recommended: The Thigh Thrust Test, also called the Posterior Shear Test, and the Compression Test.[8] The Thigh Thrust/Posterior Shear Test has a reported sensitivity of .81 and specificity of .66 (Figure 3). The Compression Test has a reported sensitivity of .63 and specificity of .69 (Figure 4).

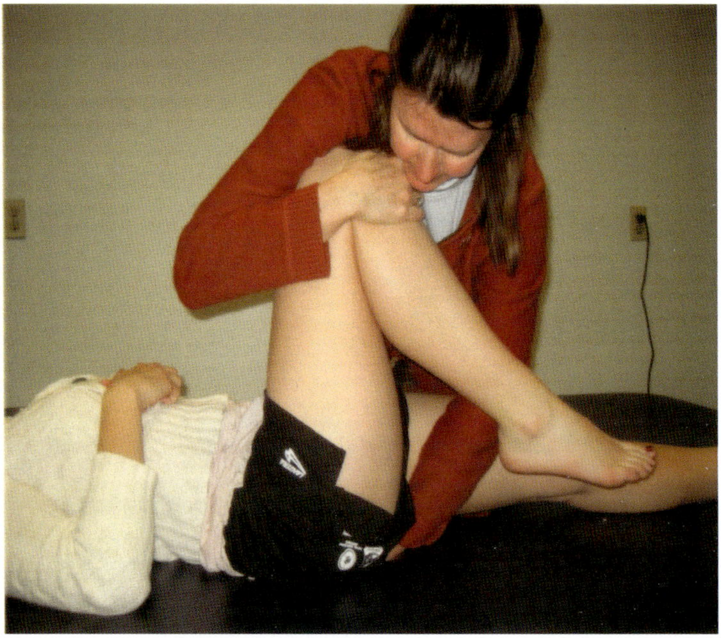

Fig. 3. Posterior Shear Test (Pain Provocation)
Copyright © Kyndy Boyle 2010, used with permission

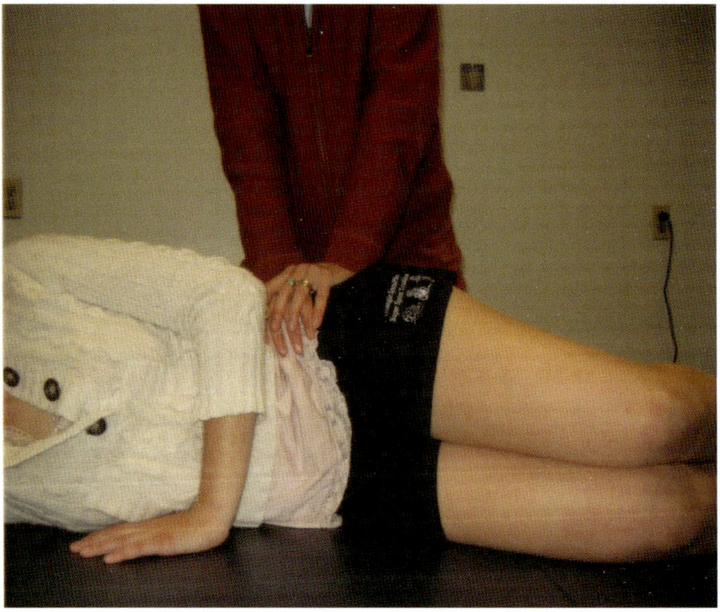

Fig. 4. Compression Test (Pain Provocation)
Copyright © Kyndy Boyle 2010, used with permission

3.3 Motion palpation tests

Motion palpation tests such as the Standing Flexion Test, Prone Knee Flexion Test, Supine Long Sitting Test, Sitting PSIS, and Heel-bank Test are not recommended for diagnosing patients with SIJP or SIJD.[6, 7, 17] Movement of the SIJ(s) cannot be reliably assessed by manual palpation, especially in weight bearing. The reliability, reported as Kappas between 0.19-0.37, is too low for clinical use.

Two opinions exist as to whether there is a gold standard for diagnosis of SIJP/SIJD. One opinion claims that anesthetic block procedures are the gold standard. [18] This would require a physician to inject one or both SIJs with an anesthetic to determine if the patient's pain is abolished or lessened as a result of the injection. The other opinion claims that there is no gold standard.[19] Anesthetic block procedures are considered effective if the patient's pain originates from intra-articular structures but not effective if their pain arises from extra-articular structures, such as accessory ligaments and muscle tissue that surrounds the joint.[19]

3.4 Biomechanics/anatomy

The sacroiliac joints involve the right and left ilium and their C-shaped articulations with the lateral sides of the sacrum.[20] Each iliac surface is lined with fibrocartilage and each sacral surface is lined with articular/hyaline cartilage.[20] Optimal SIJ function depends on optimal positioning and movement of six joints: both SIJ, the L5-S1 articulation, the pubic symphysis, and both hip joints (left and right acetabula and femoral heads). The SIJs are inherently stable and their design gives them the ability to safely transfer very high compressive loads under normal conditions.[20] Although it was once believed that no movement occurred at the SIJs, several research studies have since demonstrated that this is not the case.[21, 22] Patients undergoing a lumbar fusion, will likely have a resulting increase in SIJ motion and stress, as these joints are just distal to the fused segments. [23] Unilateral SIJ fusion has been documented to cause undesirable strain and load requirements on the contralateral SIJ.[22] The amount of motion that may occur at the SIJs depends on whether or not the joints are loaded, and on the position of the hip joints in their range of motion (ROM). Research study results have also depended on whether fresh cadavers were used.[22] SIJs that are loaded or in weight bearing are thought to move less than in non-weight bearing.[21] SIJ motion appears to be greater when the hip joints are at their end range, versus a neutral position.

According to research, the SIJs may function as hip joints to get needed motion for gait and other movements which results in SIJ ligament strain.[24] The innominate bone will generally displace in the same direction as the hip, and act as an extension of the femur when the hip is at its end ROM and the innominate through the SIJ will attempt to gain more hip motion.[24] A fresh cadaver study conducted within 24 hours of death of five donors reported sagittal plane motion of the SIJ between three to 17 degrees, and translation range was reported between four to eight millimeters (mm). [22] Authors of another study that did not use fresh cadavers reported SIJ rotation in a non-weight bearing position to be 2.5 degrees and 0.2 degrees in a weight bearing position.[21] Translation was reported as 1.6mm.[21]

A study using kinematic data with a magnetic tracking device reported that the right SIJ is capable of greater ROM than the L SIJ.[24] This study was done on 40 subjects including both females and males from 18-35 years who were pain free in their SIJs/low back and had no history of injury.[24] Sagittal plane motion was reported as 60% greater on the R than the L in a cadaver study using Computerized Tomography (CT) on subjects from 52-68 years. The average motion on the right was eight degrees and five degrees on the left.[22] No explanation for the increase in R sided motion was given.

It was once believed that an increase in bilateral laxity of the SIJs as a result of pregnancy from the release of the hormone relaxin was associated with SIJP. This belief however was disputed by a study by Damen who reported that increased motion/laxity of the SIJS is not related to pain for pregnant women.[25] He reported however that increased laxity of just *one* SIJ was related to pain. Pregnant women with "moderate to severe" SIJP/PGP had more laxity in one SIJ compared to the other SIJ based on Doppler imaging of vibrations in threshold units. The study was completed on 163 subjects.

Concepts referred to as form and force closure can aid in the stability of the SIJs.[13, 26] Form closure is stability achieved by virtue of the shape, structure and orientation of the bones that make up the joints. The R and L iliums interlock on either side, with the sacrum bone nestled in between. This osteological design contributes to the inherent stability of the joints. For optimal form closure however, there needs to be optimal position of each ilium on each side of the sacrum and/or each side of the sacrum on each ilium. Based on my 21 years of practice as a licensed physical therapist, some patients will complain that they feel their SIJ slipping, moving, rubbing or going out of place, usually on the right. These subjective reports may indicate that optimal form closure has been lost, at least temporarily.

Interventions to address positional faults of the SIJ include specific muscle activation using therapeutic exercises, muscle energy techniques and joint manipulation techniques. Joint manipulation techniques may improve pain and function however they do not change the position of the sacrum in relation to the ilium based on Roentgen Stereophotogrammetric Analysis (RSA).[27] The benefits of these interventions will be discussed in more detail toward the end of this chapter.

Force closure is the concept of compressive forces that are exerted across the joints to aid in stability.[13] SIJP has been associated with both insufficient force closure and *excessive* force closure coming from motor activation of lumbopelvic and surrounding musculature such as the pelvic floor.[28] Forces that are perpendicular to the joint surface have the most optimal angle of force to contribute to joint stability. These forces are often generated intrinsically by contracting muscle and can also be generated extrinsically by external supports such as a sacroiliac joint belt. There are several different muscles that act to compress and control the SIJs to enhance their stability and stiffness which allows for effective load transfer via the pelvis during a variety of functional tasks. Muscles that have been described as contributing to force closure include the gluteus maximus (GM), piriformis, and coccygeus of the pelvic floor, respiratory diaphragm, transverse abdominus (TA) and the internal oblique (IO).[12, 29 30 31] Those muscles that are transversely oriented such as the TA, IO, piriformis and coccygeus are positioned the best to contribute to increased SIJ ligament stiffness. When laxity of ligaments associated with the SIJs decrease and the stiffness increases, then force closure of the SIJs will increase. Richardson reported that independent contraction of the TA affects SIJ laxity/stiffness more than contraction (bracing) of all the abdominal muscles at once.[30]

The GM provides stability to the lumbopelvic region[13] and to the hip joints [32] and the deep fibers of the GM cross the SIJs. [33] The architecture of the piriformis lends itself to an angle of pull roughly transverse to the joint via its proximal attachment to the inferior lateral sacrum and the superior greater trochanter of the femur.[34] Even though the coccygeus is inferior to the SIJs, its line of pull from the proximal attachment site at the ischial spine to the distal attachment of the coccyx and anococcygeal ligament is transverse to the SIJs.[34]

The R and L respiratory hemi-diaphragms do not cross the SIJs however they are considered inner-core muscles. [13] If one hemidiaphragm pulls on the distal attachment site on the lumbar vertebrae more than the other, the entire sacrum could orient itself in contralateral rotation. The diaphragm and its position and contraction along with abdominal muscles influence the degree of intra-abdominal pressure (IAP) which can also aid in stability across the SIJs. Research by Hodges has elucidated the role of the diaphragm in increasing IAP prior to limb movement that occurs simultaneously with TA activation.[35] The respiratory diaphragm's contraction occurs before limb movement to aid in trunk stability. When demands are placed on the trunk such as the anticipation of fast upper extremity movement, the respiratory diaphragm is used more for stability of the trunk and for postural control than it is used for respiration. The diaphragm's primary role is for respiration and its role as a postural muscle or lumbar stabilizer is secondary.[35] When the diaphragm contracts too much, it can become more linear and loose its position and shape for the area of the diaphragm known as the zone of apposition (ZOA). The ZOA is the area of the diaphragm that encompasses the cylindrical portion of the diaphragm which corresponds to the portion directly apposed (adjacent) to the inner aspect of the lower rib cage.[36 37, 38] During exhalation, the ZOA should account for approximately 30% of the surface area of the diaphragm.[36] Importance of the ZOA is multifactoral. The ZOA is important because when the ZOA is decreased compared to optimal there is less descent of the dome of the diaphragm and less appositional diaphragm forces.[39] The diaphragm is therefore less effective during its inspiratory muscle action and has less ability to expand the lower rib cage.[40] Decreased ZOA will result in less IAP and may result in a short diaphragm.[41] Exercise tolerance has been reported to decrease with suboptimal (decreased) ZOA.[42]

There is a polyarticular chain of muscles where the diaphragm overlaps with the psoas muscle at the distal attachment of the diaphragm and the proximal attachment of the psoas.[34] The diaphragm can pull the lumbar spine up/cephalad/superior and forward/anterior and the psoas can pull the spine down/caudal/inferior and forward/anterior. (Figure 5) This situation would result in a decrease in IAP, an increase in lordosis and anterior pelvic tilt and lengthening of the abdominals.[41] This excessive pull on the diaphragm occurs with splinting or breath holding of the diaphragm and during situations of hyperinflation.[43, 44]

There is a relationship between suboptimal or faulty respiration, motor control strategies, posture and SIJP.[28] O'Sullivan et al. investigated the relationships between breathing and motor control strategies for patients with SIJP during an Active Straight Leg Raise (ASLR) test using real time ultrasound and spirometry. They reported that the subjects with SIJP have suboptimal breathing as evidenced by an increase in their respiration rate compared to controls. They also reported that subjects with SIJP had suboptimal core muscle function as evidenced by depression of the pelvic floor rather than optimal and expected pelvic floor elevation which was seen in the controls. Additionally diaphragm excursion was decreased compared to the controls. The authors noted that the subjects with SIJP had altered motor

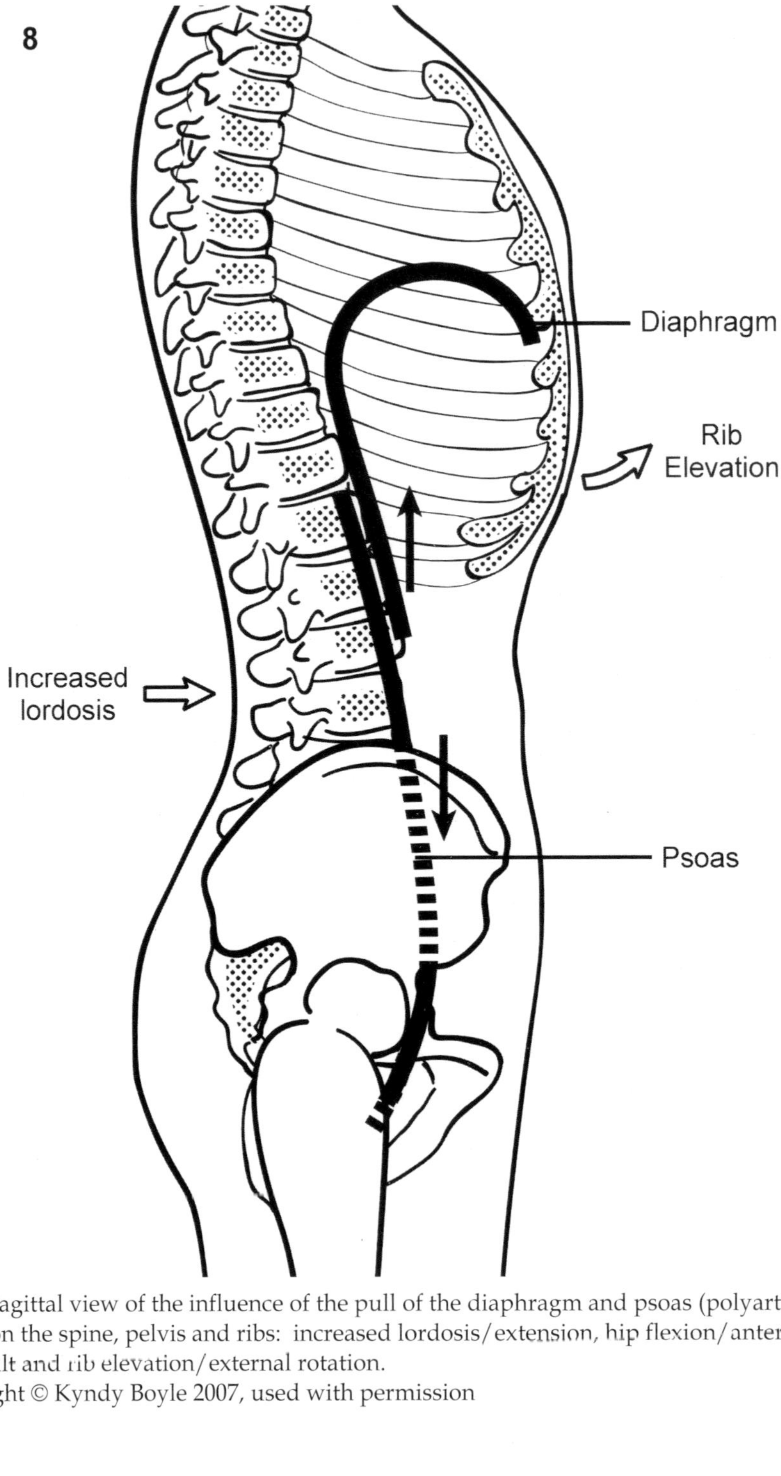

Fig. 5. Sagittal view of the influence of the pull of the diaphragm and psoas (polyarticular chain) on the spine, pelvis and ribs: increased lordosis/extension, hip flexion/anterior pelvic tilt and rib elevation/external rotation.
Copyright © Kyndy Boyle 2007, used with permission

responses during the ASLR as they attempted to compensate for their lack of ability to transfer load through their lumbopelvic region secondary to suboptimal form and/or force closure. When the ASLR was repeated with manual compression on the subjects with SIJP, their responses normalized: respiratory rate slowed, pelvic floor did not depress and their diaphragm had more excursion. O'Sullivan et al. described three possibilities for their findings. The first possibility was that subjects with SIJP and suboptimal form closure across one or both SIJs may have been a result of a lesion in their ligamentous system which required their diaphragm to be recruited to generate IAP which led to suboptimal respiration. The second possibility was the suboptimal force closure was a result of pain or a motor control deficit that lead to substitution strategies and splinting of the diaphragm which resulted in suboptimal respiration. The third possibility was reasoned as a possible compromise of *both* form and force closure mechanisms. The recommendations that O'Sullivan et al. make in conclusion of their study is that "intervention to integrate control of deep abdominals with the pelvic floor and diaphragm may be effective for patients with SIJP." The authors however do not give any examples of exercises that patients could do to achieve this aim.

A biomechanical theory to explain both R and L sided SIJP was developed by Ron Hruska PT. [45-48] His theory supports the concept of the SIJ functioning as a hip joint and also explains why the right SIJ may move more in the sagittal plane than the L SIJ. Through Hruskas 33 years of full time practice as a physical therapy clinician, he has recognized a common pattern of asymmetry that may contribute to a myriad of musculoskeletal conditions including SIJP/SIJD.[45] Other musculoskeletal conditions that the asymmetrical pattern may contribute to include thoracic outlet syndrome,[44] low back pain,[47, 49] sciatica,[46] trochanteric bursitis,[50] asthma[51], pelvic floor pain and proximal hamstring strain.[52] This pattern is called the Left Anterior Interior Chain (L AIC) pattern which gives focus to a polyarticular chain of muscles that is anterior to the spine and interior (deep) in the body, which includes the diaphragm and psoas.[45, 53 47] The belief is that this chain of muscles becomes imbalanced because of several factors such as the asymmetrical position of organs, asymmetrical forces exerted by the diaphragm and hemisphere dominance.[45] The pattern is thought to manifest in both right handed and L handed individuals. The liver which weights approximately 3.5 pounds in an average adult is on the right side of the body (unless an individual is born with their organs reversed). The liver hangs down from the diaphragm by the transverse and falciform ligaments which anchor the proximal attachment sites of the right hemi-diaphragm and help to preserve the area of the right hemidiaphragm known as the right ZOA. The absence of a liver on the L side of the body creates a situation where the L diaphragm is not as well anchored and therefore the area of the diaphragm known as the ZOA can become decreased, the L ribs may become more elevated/externally rotated relative the R side and the L abdominals may become more lengthened relative to the right side.[41, 45]

The influence of the asymmetrical pull of the hemi-diaphragms on the ribs can often be seen with visual observation of the anterior inferior rib angle which is often wider on the L than the R and the ribs may appear more protruded on the left side. [54] The asymmetrical distal attachment site of the L (anterior bodies of L1-2) versus R hemidiaphragm (anterior bodies of L1-3) and the inherent difference in the size of the large R central tendon versus the smaller L central tendon contribute to asymmetrical pull of the hemi-diaphragms on the spine. Asymmetrical hemidiaphragm on the spine could influence the SIJs along with many other areas of the body. This asymmetrical pattern when severe enough to be ten degrees or more of curvature is commonly known as idiopathic acquired scoliosis (IAS).[55] The L AIC pattern therefore compliments the common scoliosis pattern. The pattern of IAS is documented between 85-98% with right thoracic curves rather than left and possibly L lumbar curves rather than right.[56] The literature doesn't explain why the right thoracic curves are much more common than L thoracic curves; however the reasoning behind a L AIC pattern does. This reasoning includes the asymmetry of organ placement, asymmetrical pull of the hemi-diaphragms; lateralization of the brain and the direction of pelvic movement influences the direction of vertebral and rib movement. The greater pull of the left hemidiaphragm is thought to contribute to an asymmetrical lumbar-pelvic-sacral-femoral position. This position includes an anterior pelvic tilt and forward pelvic rotation on

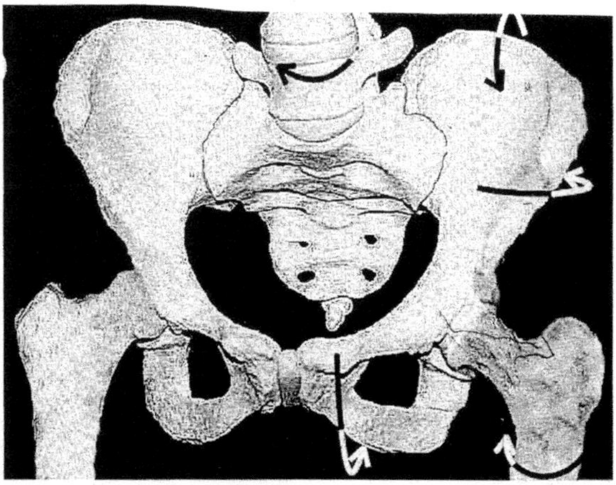

Anterior view of an anterior and forward positioned left innominate with accompanying right sacral torsion.

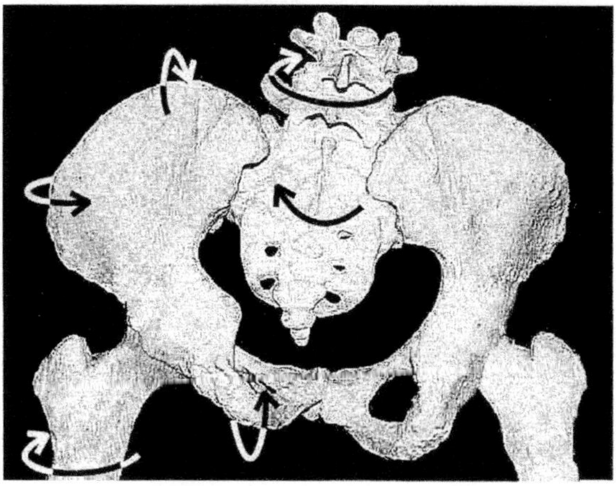

Posterior view of an anterior and forward positioned left innominate with accompanying right sacral torsion.

Note:
- Raised left ischium
- Right SI distraction
- Rotation of sacrum, L5 and L4 to the right
- "Out" flare of left innominate
- Closure of left obturator foramen

Fig. 6. Frontal plane anterior and posterior views of the lower lumbar-pelvic-sacral-femoral position in a Left Anterior Interior Chain Pattern (L AIC)
Copyright © Postural Restoration 2007, used with permission

the left side (i.e. left hemilordosis). Along with this position would be lower lumbar vertebrae and the sacrum oriented in right rotation. The right hip in a closed chain would therefore be in adduction and oriented in internal rotation. The left hip would be in abduction and either neutral in the hip joint (rather than rotated) or in compensatory external rotation to realign the foot in the sagittal plane. The pelvic position of left anterior pelvic tilt (sagittal plane) and forward rotation (transverse plane) compliments the position of right thoracic and left lumbar IAS. (Figure 6) A pelvic position of right APT and forward rotation would not direct the spine into left lumbar rotation or compensatory right thoracic rotation.

The IAS and L AIC patterns are supported by two Spine Journal articles. Kouwenhoven et al. used CT on 50 subjects to investigate whether or not an inherent pattern of asymmetry of the spine was present in individuals without diagnosed scoliosis..[57] He reported right rotation of lumbar-thoracic vertebrae (L5-T5) and L rotation of upper thoracic vertebrae (T3-4). The opposite pattern was reported in a separate study (N=37) where subjects with organ reversal (situs inversus totalis) were sampled and the same CT measurements were made.[58] This inherent pattern was left lumbar rotation (L5-T5) and R upper thoracic rotation (T3-4). These inherent patterns of spinal rotation were attributed to organ placement including the heart. Hruska's identification of the pattern has lead to development of conservative physical therapy management for a myriad of conditions that are believed to relate to it and this approach is called Postural Restoration.[45]

Clinicians trained in Postural Restoration often use the Ober's Test to assess triplanar pelvic position.[45] If the pelvis is neutral then the leg should be able to adduct at the hip joint below the horizontal. If the pelvis is not neutral (i.e. the acetabulum over the femoral head is not in an anatomical neutral position) then when the leg is moved by the clinician during the test, a bony block may be felt during the external rotation/abduction phase of the test and/or during the adduction phase of the test. The bony block may indicate an abutment of the femoral neck on the cotyloid rim of the acetabulum. An increase in either hip flexor tone may be felt by the clinician during the hip extension phase of the test or an increase in tone of the abductors during the adduction phase of the test are additional possible findings during the Ober's Test. A positive test on the left side is common for patients in a typical L AIC pattern and it is usually interpreted by the clinician as a left anterior tilt and/or left forward rotation of the pelvis.[46, 47, 50] A positive test on both the right and left sides is interpreted as a bilateral anterior pelvic tilt which is seen in patients with a Posterior Exterior Chain (PEC), which is discussed at the end of this section (page 14). This use of the test is relatively new and different from the traditional use which is to determine if there is shortness of the iliotibial band/tensor fascia latae.[59] Since the use of the Ober's Test by those clinicians trained in Postural Restoration is different in the reason to do the test, the interpretation of a positive test and in the intervention for a positive test, the Postural Restoration Institute™ began using a new name, the Adduction Drop Test (ADT) to avoid confusion. This ADT test is being used therefore as a reflection of triplanar position of the pelvis which does have some preliminary research support.[60, 61]

The L AIC pattern is thought to relate to SIJ instability in that the pattern leads to over use of the R leg for standing where the center of gravity (COG) is shifted to the right. The COG shifted right would place the R hip into adduction and oriented into internal rotation. The R adductor magnus may become over active (hypertonic) and short. In order to get more internal rotation at the hip in the position of relative hip IR (acetabulum over femur) the ilium would have to attempt forward motion which would cause tensile forces across the posterior SIJ. A gap or greater distance between the ilium and sacrum is seen on a MRI for a patient who was seeking physical therapy for her R SIJP. (Figure 7) Therefore, if the R SIJ begins to move too much it may become painful. If however the ligaments and muscles are stable and strong and continue to provide enough stability to the right SIJ to avoid pain, it is possible that the R hip joint itself may begin to move too much, but in a faulty position of the acetabulum over the femur. This situation may lead to anterior medial hip impingement commonly referred to as femoral-acetabular impingement (FAI).[62] It is possible as evidenced by my personal experience, to improve a patient's R SIJ stability with therapeutic exercise and then if discharged too early, the patient may begin to complain of R hip impingement.

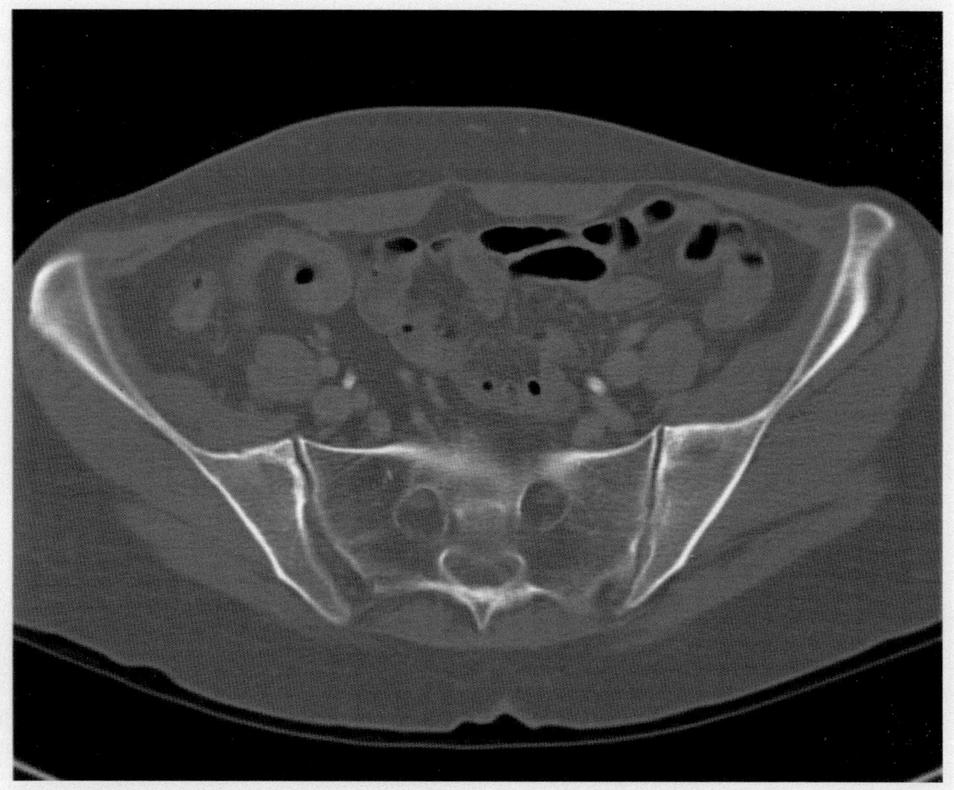

Fig. 7. Transverse plane view of the Sacroiliac Joints on Magnetic Resonance Imaging (MRI). The image shows a greater opening/gapping on the right side.
Copyright © Postural Restoration Institute™ used with permission, www.posturalrestoration.com

The pelvic position with this L AIC pattern is thought to result in part from the asymmetrical pull on the spine by the diaphragm and also from the weaker L abdominals which would result in an anterior tilt and forward rotation of the L innominate relative to the R and sacrum orientation to the right.[20, 45, 47] If the L femur stays neutral in the acetabulum when the pelvis goes anterior and forward it would appear to be oriented inward with toes pointing inward to the midline. This position often results in compensatory L hip external rotation (ER) to reorient the foot on the ground and the femur back into the sagittal plane.[45, 62, 63] When the L hip external rotators become over active because of this compensatory L hip position, the L hip is in abduction and external rotation (ER). The L ilium may begin to function as a L hip joint to increase the available hip ROM

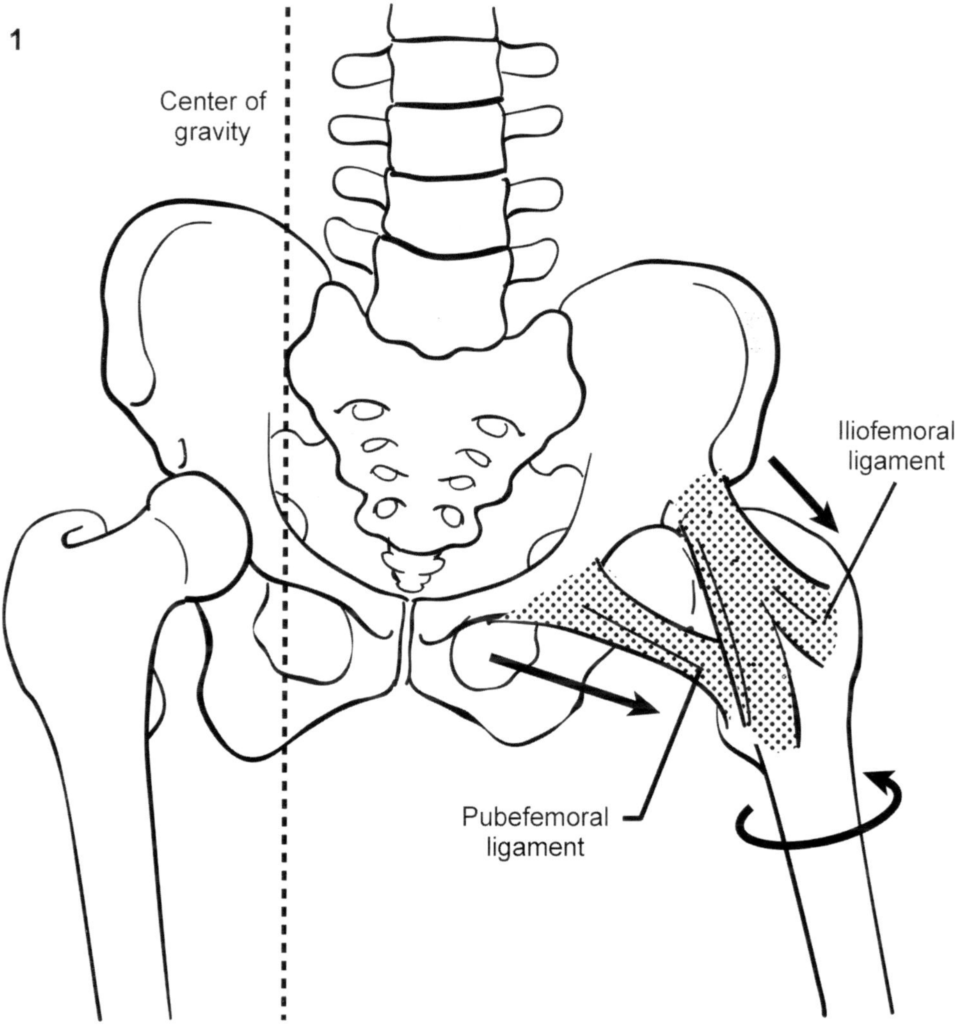

Fig. 8. Compensatory left hip external rotation (ER) associated with a L AIC pattern resulting in over lengthening/laxity of the iliofemoral and pubofemoral ligaments. The left femur (F) moves on the left acetabulum (A), therefore left FA ER.
Copyright © Kyndy Boyle 2007, used with permission

and the left SIJ may become unstable. If however, the excessive motion occurs at the hip rather the L SIJ, the anterior hip ligaments/capsule (pubofemoral and iliofemoral ligaments) may become stretched out and loose creating instability of the L anterior hip and may be associated with L anterior superior hip impingement.[64] (Figure 8)

A pattern that may overlay a L AIC pattern is called a Posterior Exterior Chain (PEC) pattern.[45, 48] The PEC terminology is used for a patient who has a bilateral anterior pelvic tilt and excessive lumbar lordosis as a result of over activity of muscles in the posterior back. The muscles that make up the PEC include the latissimus dorsi, quadrates lumborum, posterior intercostals, serratus posterior and ilocostalis lumborum.[48] These patients often have the inability to touch their toes, and/or reverse the extension/lordosis curvature of their spines. They may also lack the ability to do a full squat. Management of patients with a PEC pattern associated with SIJP and specific management and clinical reasoning for patients with SIJP on the right versus the left SIJ will be discussed toward the end of this chapter.

4. Traditional interventions for SIJP/SIJD

Interventions specifically for SIJP/SIJD (rather than general PGP) that appear in peer-reviewed literature include SIJ manipulation, muscle energy techniques, SIJ belt, patient education regarding the pain cycle, moist heat, soft tissue massage, electrical stimulation and therapeutic exercise including activation of the transverse abdominus, stretching exercises and aquatics. In spite of the prevalence of patients with SIJP/SIJD and the relatively long length of time of recognition of SIJ conditions, there is a paucity of published literature. Furthermore, published literature pertaining to the SIJs is primarily in the bottom half of the evidence pyramid. The good news however is that all of the listed interventions have shown to reduce pain and disability to varying degrees. The challenge is that the authors do not always describe the therapeutic exercise so the results are difficult to interpret and the studies are not replicable. With the exception of two randomized controlled trials (RCT), readers are not able to infer cause and effect with the existing studies. Lastly, Stuge believes that interventions should be based on a theoretical framework. [65]

A RCT published by Chiropractors investigated two different types of chiropractic manipulation for the SIJ: manual versus mechanical (with a piece of equipment). The Chiropractors studied 60 subjects using diagnostic criteria of a painful sulcus on palpation and a positive provocation test. They were treated for four visits over two weeks and function was measured with an Oswestry Disability Index (ODI) at the initial visit and three weeks post intervention. There were no differences between groups.[66] Stuge et al published the results of an RCT done on 81 subjects with PGP post partum with a positive ASLR and a positive provocation test. They studied two groups: the control group (CG) received "general interventions" that included massage, relaxation, joint mobilization, manipulation, electrical stimulation, hot packs and strengthening exercises. Specific parameters of the interventions including dosage and the specific exercises used were not described. The exercise group received all the treatments as the CG plus instruction in TA , multifidus, gluteus maximus (GM), latissimus dorsi (lats), obliques, erector spinae, quadratus lumborum (QL), hip adductors and hip abductor exercises. Again the specific ways the exercises were done including dosage parameters were not described. The outcome measure was taken at initial, 20 weeks, one year, and two years. The EG had superior outcomes for reducing pain as measured by the Visual Analog Scale (VAS), improved function as measured by the ODI, and improved quality of life as measured by the SF-36.[65]

Published case series have been reported with some improvements in pain and function. Osterbauer investigated chiropractic manipulation on ten subjects with positive provocation testing and were followed for 18 visits over six weeks.[67] The improvements in function (ODI) and pain (VAS) were reported at six weeks and one year. Hall was a physical therapist who reported on a case series of two who had a positive ASLR test and positive provocation tests. These subjects were managed with muscle energy techniques, TA and multifidus activation, isometric hip abduction/adduction, activation of lats, GM and abdominal crunches. They were also instructed in the use of a SIJ belt. These subjects were seen from five to seven visits over seven to ten weeks. Function significantly improved based on the ODI, however pain did not significantly improve using a numeric pain rating scale (NPRS).

O'Sullivan reported on a case series of nine subjects with SIJP with positive ASLR tests and provocation tests who were instructed in TA, IO and pelvic floor (PF) activation in a neutral spine in various positions: supine, sitting, sit to stand, standing, single leg stance and walking.[28] Outcomes included suboptimal movement of the pelvic floor, diaphragm and suboptimal respiration and disability. These outcomes were discussed earlier under the section of respiration and SIJP.

Two case studies were reported by O'Sullivan to highlight one patient with reduced force closure and one patient with excessive force closure. The female patient with R SIJP had reduced force closure based on a positive ASLR with breath holding and positive provocation testing. She was instructed in TA and pelvic floor activation without breath holding, while maintaining optimal spinal alignment and neutral posture in sitting, standing and lifting. She was also instructed in lunges, squats, aerobic exercise including bicycling and walking and patient education in the vicious pain cycle. At one year after discharge, O'Sullivan reported that she returned to work and to playing handball, however no formal outcome measures were used or reported. The other patient suffered from right more than left SIJP as a result of excessive force closure as measured by a negative ASLR, positive provocation testing and inability to relax her pelvic floor muscles based on an internal exam. This patient was educated in the vicious pain cycle and the need for pelvic floor muscle inhibition. She was instructed in relaxation strategies for muscles and anxiety in sitting, standing and activities of daily living (ADLs) including breathing and rest breaks. She was also referred to a psychologist and at one year, O'Sullivan noted that she experienced "little pain or disability." Again, no formal outcome measures were used or reported.

A case study published by Painter discussed a patient with a positive ASLR and positive provocation testing who was managed with pelvic floor and TA activation during ADLs, bridges, lunges, prone exercise over a physioball with alternating upper extremity flexion and lower extremity hip extension, abdominal crunches on a physioball, aquatic exercises and the use of a SIJ belt. The patient was seen for seven visits over three weeks and was reported to have returned to "full activity" with no "stress urinary incontinence" at six weeks. No formal outcome measure was used or reported.

A descriptive report was published by Sasso on 69 subjects with SIJ pain based on symptoms occurring in Fortin's area.[68] SIJ mobilizations were performed but not described, and strengthening of "muscular stabilizers and abdominals" were reported but not described in any detail. Patient education included instruction by the clinician in proper lifting technique and "activity modification." Outcomes were reported with the use of a survey at two years. Ninety-five percent of subjects reported their outcome as good or excellent and five percent reported their outcome as fair or poor.

The use of a SIJ belt has been used as one part of the intervention for reported patients/subjects with SIJP/SIJD to aid in force closure of the SIJ passively. One study included the investigation of the best placement of the SIJ belt to achieve the greatest decrease in SIJ ligamentous laxity. Placement just below the ASIS was reported as better than at the level of the pubic symphysis. [25] Damen also investigated how much force was best to decrease SIJ ligamentous laxity by using Doppler Imaging of Vibrations technology to assess ligamentous stiffness. Damen used a strain gauge in the belt for ten females 18-39 years of age without SIJP. Damen reported that either 50 Newtons or 100 Newtons achieved the same benefit.[25]

5. Specific Postural Restoration interventions for a PEC pattern relating to right and/or left SIJP

Postural Restoration therapeutic exercises (also known as non-manual techniques) can be used for all patients who suffer from pain in their right, left or bilateral SIJs. This chapter will include a description for management of patients who present with bilateral anterior pelvic tilt/PEC pattern followed by a description for management of patients who present with a L AIC pattern and right SIJP followed by those who present with compensation for a L AIC pattern and left SIJP. Clinical reasoning for a patient with a PEC pattern is to restore the ability of the patient to flex their spine and expand their posterior mediastinum as evidenced by the ability to easily touch their toes (without the use of a hamstring lengthening/stretching program) and the ability to fully squat comfortably while breathing. Exercises that may be used include a Standing Unresisted Wall Reach, Standing Resisted Wall Reach, Reverse Door Squat (with or without the assistance of a pole to hold on too) or a Wall Short Seated Reach. (Figures 9-12) The Unresisted Wall Reach may be enough to achieve spinal flexion and posterior mediastinum expansion, however some patients may need more abdominal recruitment to achieve the results, therefore the Resisted Wall Reach may be more beneficial. Some patients may have pain in their knee/s or back and therefore are unable to do either of the standing wall reach exercises or the squat exercise. In that case, the Wall Short Seated Reach may be a good option. Once the patient's sagittal plane motion and ability is restored, the patient is managed for the underlying L AIC pattern depending on the side of involvement.

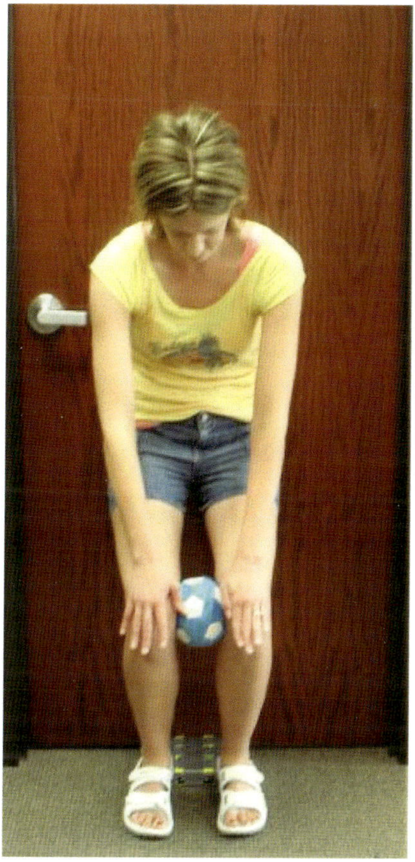

Fig. 9. Standing Un-resisted Wall Reach

1. Stand facing away from a wall and place your heels 7-10 inches away from the wall.
2. Stand up straight with a ball between your knees and feet shoulder width apart.
3. Bring your arms out in front of you as you round out your back, performing a pelvic tilt so your mid-back down is flat on the wall.
4. Squat down slightly as you squeeze the ball.
5. Keeping your mid-back down on the wall, inhale through your nose.
6. As you exhale through your mouth, reach your arms forward so your upper back comes off the wall (mid-back down should stay flat on the wall).
7. Hold your arms steadily in this position (reach), as you inhale through your nose again and expand your upper back (feel a stretch in your upper back).
8. Exhale and reach further forward.
9. Repeat this breathing sequence for 4-5 deep breaths.
10. Slowly stand up by pushing through your heels and slide up the wall, keeping your mid-back down on the wall.
11. Relax and repeat 4 more times.

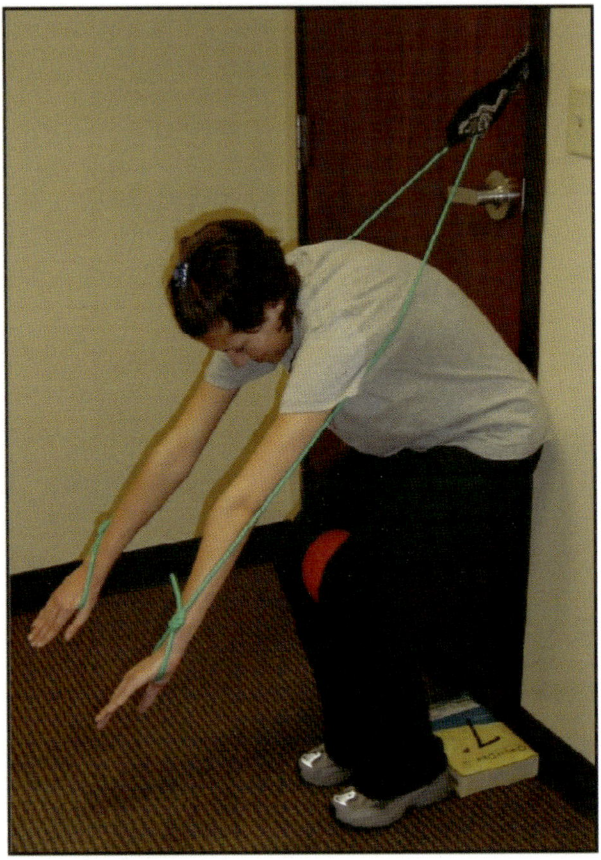

Fig. 10. Standing Resisted Wall Reach

1. Place tubing securely in door slightly below shoulder level.
2. Stand with your heels 7-10 inches away from the wall.
3. Stand up straight with a ball between your knees and feet lined up with each other.
4. Place your hands through the loops of the tubing with your palms facing down.
5. Straighten your arms out in front of you and round your back, engaging your abdominals.
6. Once you can feel your abdominals working begin to squat as you squeeze the ball.
7. Squat down until your bottom touches the wall (do not fall back into wall).
8. Inhale through your nose.
9. As you exhale through your mouth reach forward and downward as your back stays rounded.
10. Hold arms steadily in this position as you inhale again and expand your back.
11. Exhale and reach forward further with your arms.
12. Complete 2 more breaths in and out reaching further each time you exhale.
13. Stand up while keeping arms straight, back rounded, abdominals and inner thigh muscles engaged.
14. Relax and repeat 4 more times.

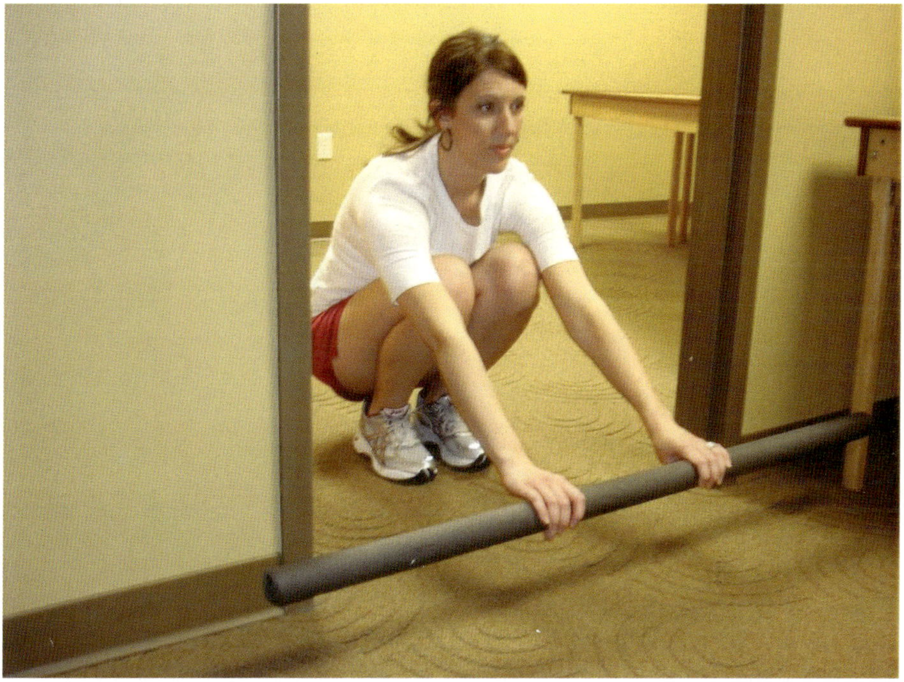

Fig. 11. Reverse Door Squat

1. Stand in front of an open doorway and place a wooden pole in front of the door frame at or below standing knee height.
2. Hold onto the pole and find the best functional squat position (bottom of pelvis to heel cords) while keeping your heels down and knees inside your elbows. You may need to stand back up and re-position your feet so you can get your bottom down as far as allowed.
3. Once you have positioned yourself in the most optimal squat position, take a deep breath in through your nose and fill the back of your chest wall with air while keeping your eyes up or level with the floor. Exhale through your mouth as you lean back until all your air is out. Repeat this sequence of inhalation and exhalation 3 to 4 more times always allowing your heel cords, front of your thighs/knees and your back muscles to relax and stretch.
4. After the fourth breath in, exhale and begin to stand up pushing down through your heels and keeping your back rounded while sliding the pole up the door frame as necessary to assist you in coming up.
5. Lower the pole and repeat the process 4 more times.
6. The goal is to perform the first 3 steps above with the pole at the level of your ankle, with your elbows straight, with your knees in your chest and with the bottom of your pelvis on your heel cords (PRI Squat Level Four or Five).

Once you've achieved the above goal, repeat the first three steps. After the fourth breathe in, reach forward with your hands as you exhale so that the pole loses contact with the door frame. As you exhale also begin to stand up pushing through your heels and continuing to reach forward so that the pole doesn't touch the door frame.

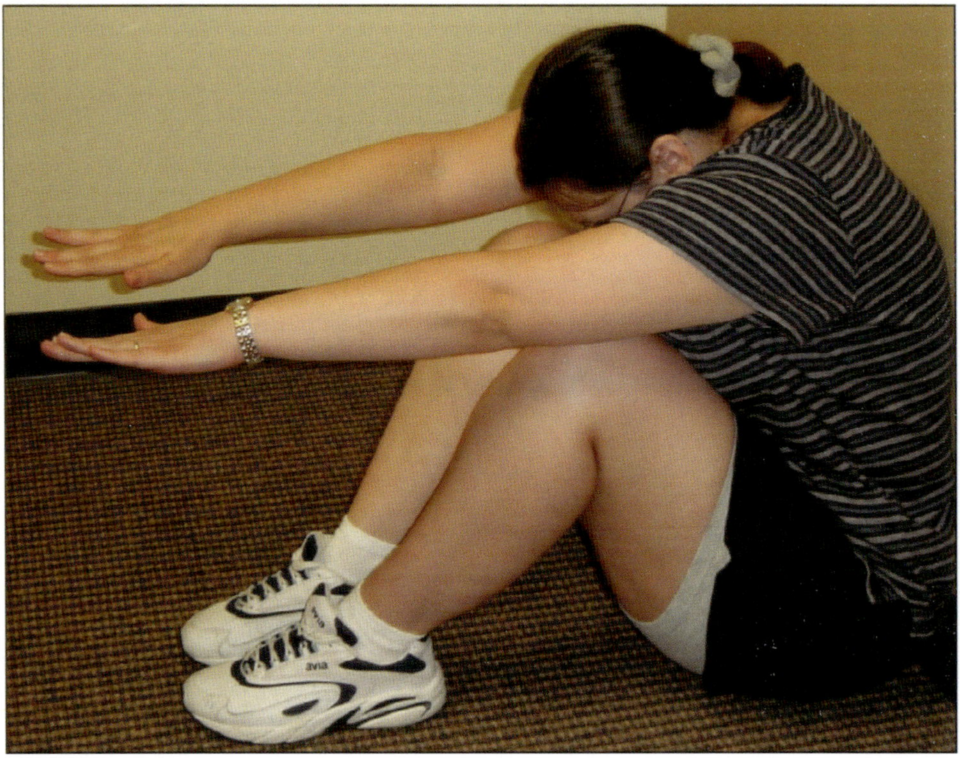

Fig. 12. Wall Short Seated Reach

1. Sit on the ground with your mid to low back flat against a wall and legs straight out in front of you.
2. Bring your knees as close to your chest as possible by bending your legs one at a time. Keep your knees together and feet slightly apart. Do not allow your legs to rotate outward.
3. Inhale through your nose.
4. Keeping your back on the wall from bra-line to belt-line, slowly exhale through your mouth and reach forward with both arms. Your arms may rest on your knees. Pause 3 seconds.
5. Maintaining the position, inhale again through your nose and concentrate on filling the back of your chest wall with air.
6. Exhale and reach forward further with your arms.
7. Continue in this manner for 4 breaths in and 3 breaths out pausing 3 seconds before each inhalation.
8. Relax and repeat 4 more times.

5.1 Right sacroiliac joint pain/dysfunction related to a left anterior interior chain pattern

Clinical reasoning used by clinicians trained in Postural Restoration to manage right SIJP/instability, is to optimize lumbar-pelvic-femoral position and train the patient to maintain it. This is achieved most commonly by therapeutic exercise instruction/prescription such as right GM activation in the transverse plane that emphasizes normal breathing through the exercise (to avoid breath holding/splinting of the diaphragm) and patient education in positional guidelines during activities of daily living (ADLs). The positional guidelines attempt to oppose the L AIC pattern (e.g. maintain weight over left leg, maintain desired hip positions) during common activities such as sit to stand, sleeping, standing etc. (Figures 13-15)

Therapeutic exercises that activate specific muscles on specific sides of the body and train a patient in different phases of gait to achieve for example, single leg stance control are often used. Exercises with the patient in a sidelying or supine position are usually done initially until motor control with the correct muscles is achieved. After the patient demonstrates mastery of correct position and muscle activation, exercises may be advanced to a standing position. These exercises are also designed for the patient to be able to eventually maintain stability without compensation. SIJP occurring on the right side is thought to occur because of too much motion across the posterior right SIJ. Based on the L AIC pattern, the right hip is often positioned in IR and adduction. Therefore, to achieve optimal lumbar-pelvic-femoral position the goal would be to achieve right hip ER, specifically right acetabulum over femur (AF) ER with concomitant left hip IR, specifically acetabulum motion over the femoral head (L AF IR). The right GM can be considered an important muscle for both form and force closure. The right GM can correct right hip IR in a transverse plane via its action as a powerful external rotator which may contribute to repositioning the sacrum from a position of orientation in right rotation toward neutral (i.e. form closure). The GM is also an effective muscle to restore force closure across the SIJ. There are currently no therapeutic exercises to activate the GM in the transverse plane in published literature relating to management of patients with SIJP outside of those related to Postural Restoration and developed by Ron Hruska PT.

The GM can be activated in the transverse plane in several patient positions: sidelying, supine hooklying and supine with the hips and knees at 90 degrees. In a sidelying position, the GM can be activated in the transverse plane against gravity with or without a band (fit loop) for resistance. (Figure 16) Sagittal plane position of the trunk/spine can be monitored to avoid excessive lumbar lordosis and the feet can rest over a small bolster and press against a wall to gain distal stability and to serve as a fulcrum for the motion and place the right hip into more IR which allows for more ER ROM during the movement of the right leg during the exercise. In a supine position, the right GM is again activated in the transverse plane usually with resistance (fit loop) around both femurs. (Figure 17) To avoid excessive lordosis or over activity of paraspinals the patient moves into a posterior pelvic tilt first with an exhalation and maintains that position throughout the exercise. The left hip can actively be moved into L AF IR which puts both the left and right hips into the desired positions based on the L AIC pattern. R AF ER is not only the desired position; it also shortens the GM positionally before further shortening through FA ER against the resistance of the fit loop. The supine 90/90 position is essentially the same as the supine hooklying position as the right GM is activated in the transverse plane against resistance after the patient moves into L AF IR and R AF ER with stability offered at the feet by the wall. (Figure 18)

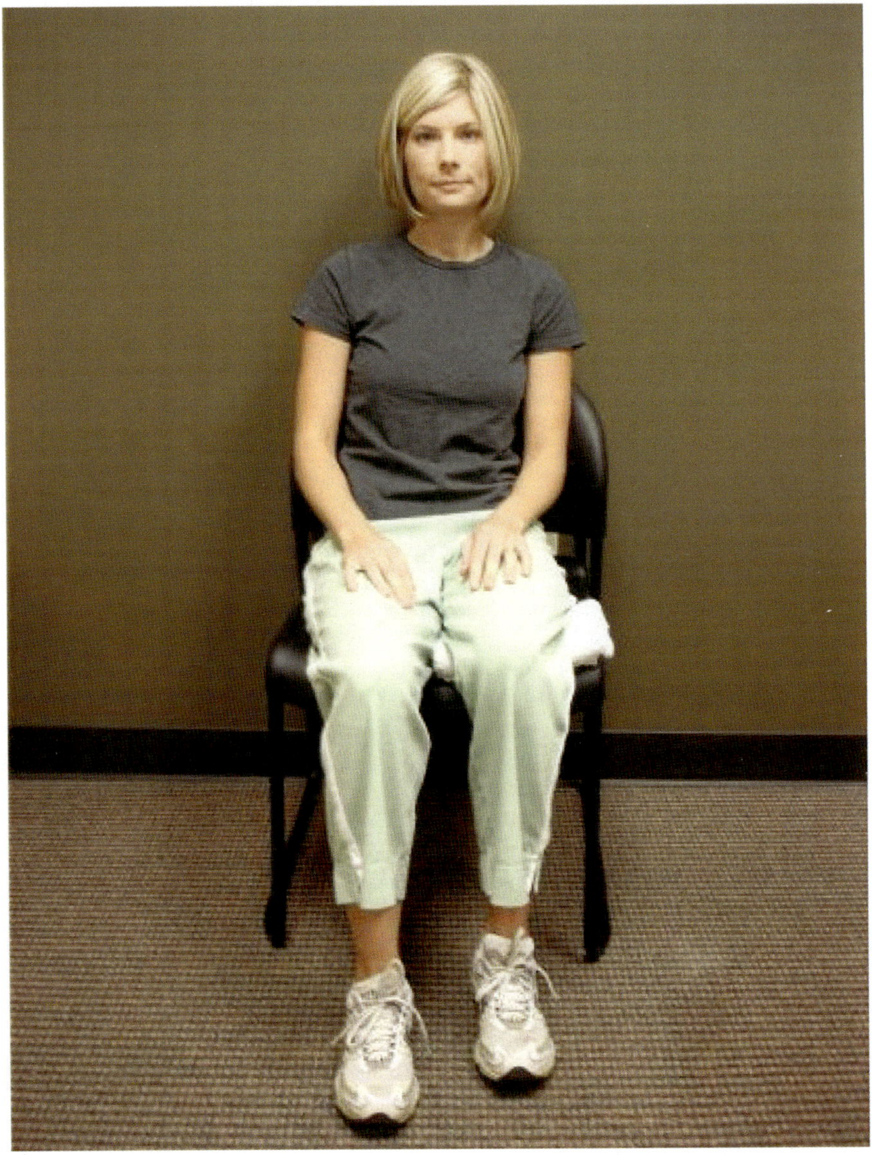

Fig. 13. Positional recommendations for sitting in a left hip (acetabulum over femur) internal rotation (L AF IR) position
When in a seated position attempt to keep your trunk rounded and your knees at or above hip level.
For increased comfort place a small bolster underneath your left thigh and shift your left knee back.

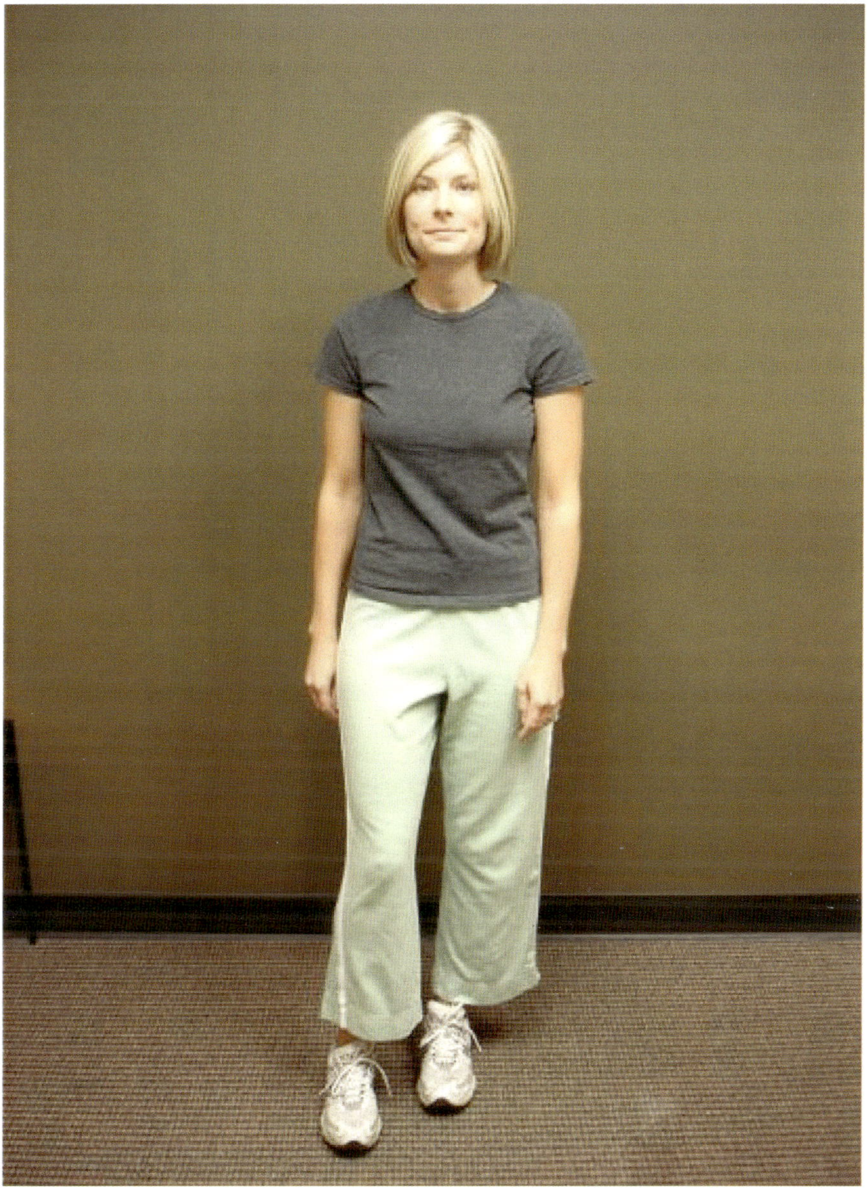

Fig. 14. Positional recommendation in a standing left hip (acetabulum over femur) internal rotation (L AF IR) position with center of gravity shifted to the left.
When standing, place your right foot ahead of your left and attempt to keep your body weight shifted to the left.

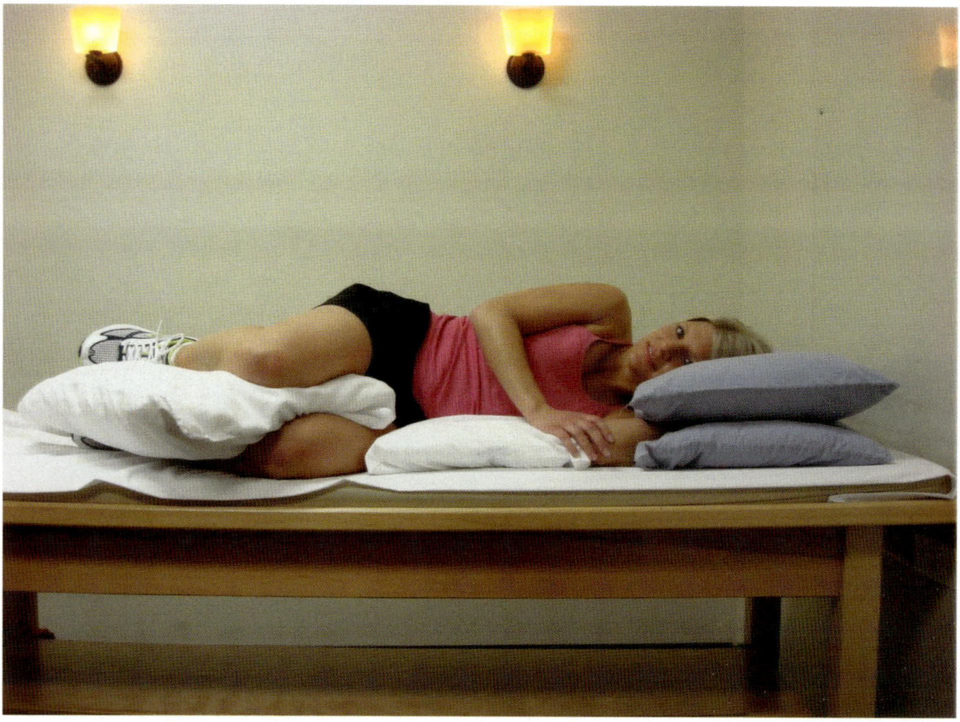

Fig. 15. Positional recommendations for sleeping with pillow support and L AF IR
Place a pillow between your legs when on either side. Place a pillow under your left side when lying on your left side. Use one-two pillows under your head to keep your head and neck relaxed.

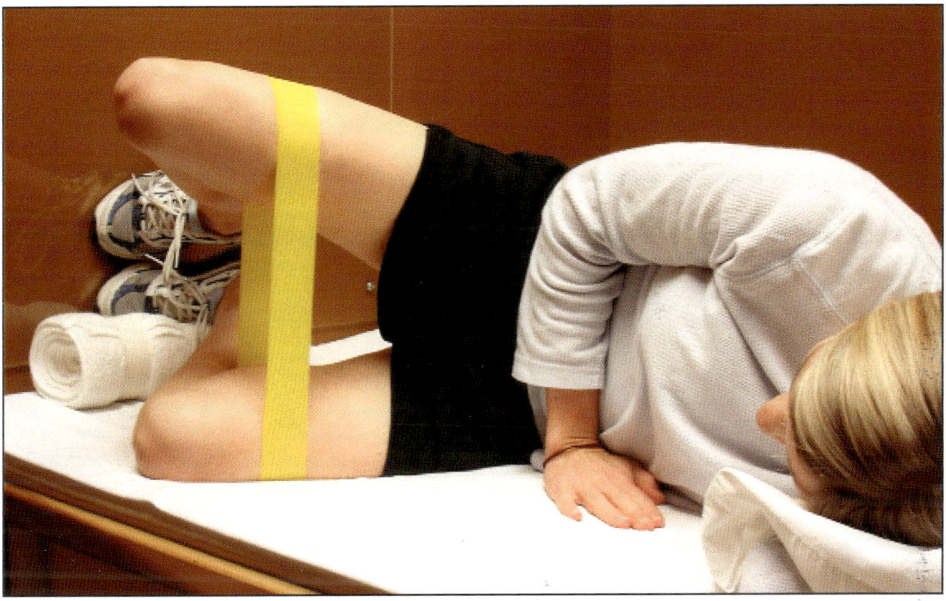

Fig. 16. Left Sidelying Right Glute Max

1. Lie on your left side with your hips and knees bent at a 60-90 degree angle.
2. Place your ankles on top of a 3-5 inch bolster and place your feet firmly on a wall.
3. Place tubing around both thighs slightly above your knees.
4. Shift your right hip forward until you feel a slight stretch or pull in your left outside hip.
5. Keeping your toes on the wall, raise your right knee keeping it shifted forward. You should feel your right outside hip engage.
6. Hold this position while you take 4-5 deep breaths in through your nose and out through your mouth.
7. Relax and repeat 4 more times.

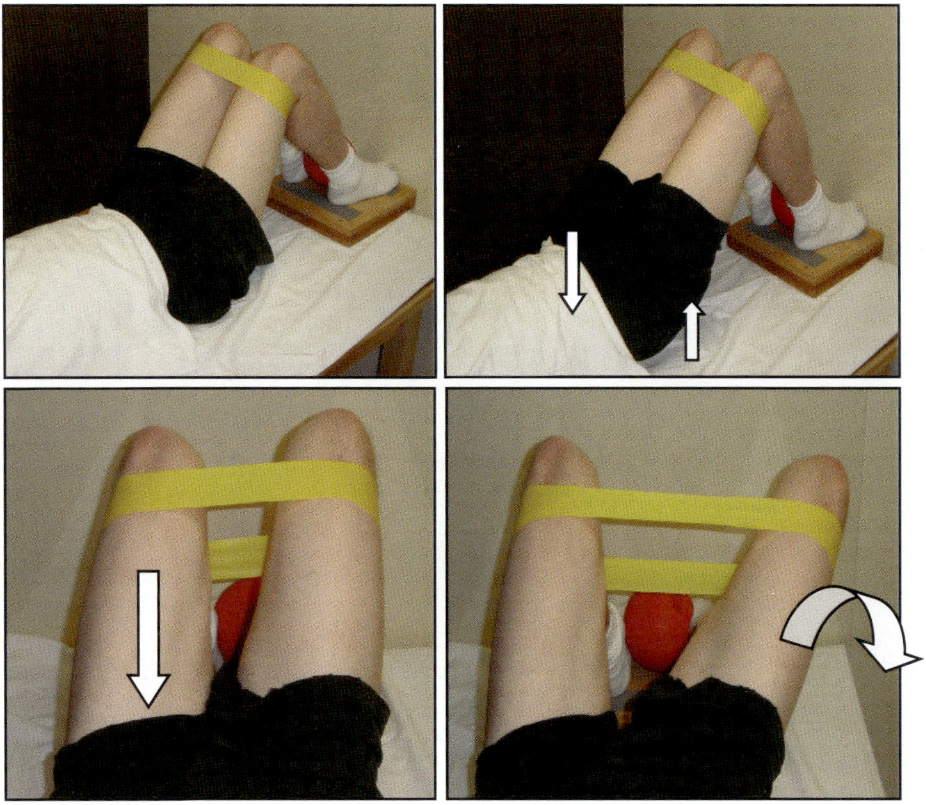

Fig. 17. Supine Hooklying Right Glute Max with R AF ER

1. Lie on your back and place your feet on a 2-inch block against the wall.
2. Place a band around your knees and a ball between your ankles.
3. Inhale through your nose and exhale through your mouth performing a pelvic tilt so that your tailbone is raised slightly off the mat. Keep your back flat on the mat.
4. Shift your left knee down. You should feel your left inner thigh engage.
5. Turn your right leg out. You should feel your right outside hip engage.
6. Hold this position while you take 4-5 breaths in through your nose and out through your mouth.
7. Relax and repeat 4 more times.

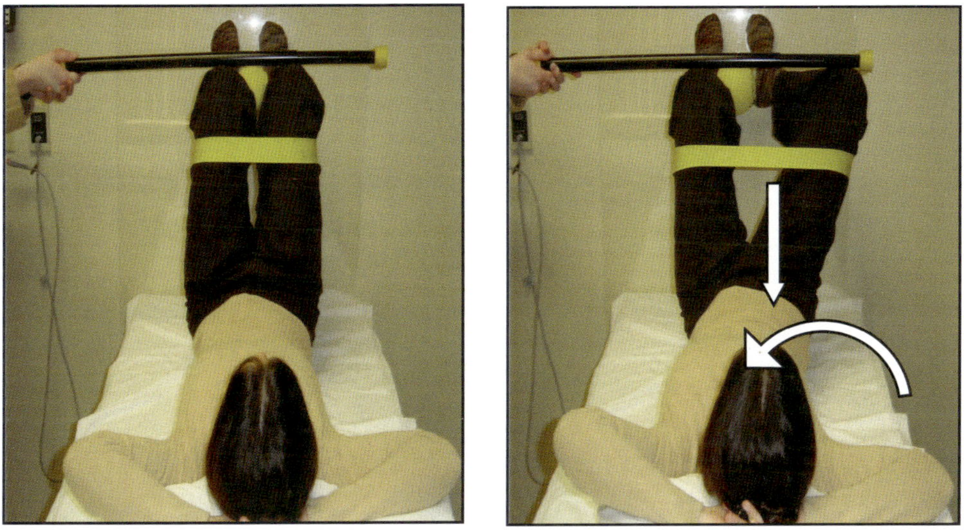

Fig. 18. Supine Right Glute Max with Right AF ER

1. Lie on your back with your feet on a wall and your knees and hips bent at a 90-degree angle.
2. Place tubing around your thighs (just below your knees) and a 4-5 inch ball between your ankles.
3. Inhale through your nose and exhale through your mouth performing a pelvic tilt so that your tailbone is raised slightly off the mat. Keep your back flat on the mat.
4. Maintaining a pelvic tilt, shift your left knee down as your left pelvis drops and your right pelvis raises and turns to the left. You should feel the muscles on the outside of your right hip engage.
5. Squeeze your left ankle into the ball feeling your left inner thigh engage.
6. Attempt to lift left heel off of the wall.
7. Hold position while you take 4-5 deep breaths in through your nose and out through your mouth. Relax and repeat 4 more times.

The L AIC pattern commonly involves over activity and possibly shortness of the right adductors which contribute to or are a result of the right hip IR/adduction seen with a L AIC pattern. If it is determined by the clinician that the adductors are over active/short a therapeutic exercise to inhibit/lengthen the right adductors may be prescribed. (Figure 19) An example of an upright exercise that facilitates activation of the R GM and a left hip position of L AF IR is the Single Leg Wall Left AF IR with Right Glute Max. This exercise is developed to oppose the typical L AIC pattern via activation of the R GM in a transverse plane, while weight bearing on the left leg in a hip position of L AF IR. (Figure 20) To summarize, management of R SIJP associated with a L AIC pattern includes a focus on R GM activation in a transverse plane with desired hip positions (R AF ER and L AF IR) that oppose the positions commonly seen in the L AIC pattern, and right adductor inhibition/lengthening as needed.

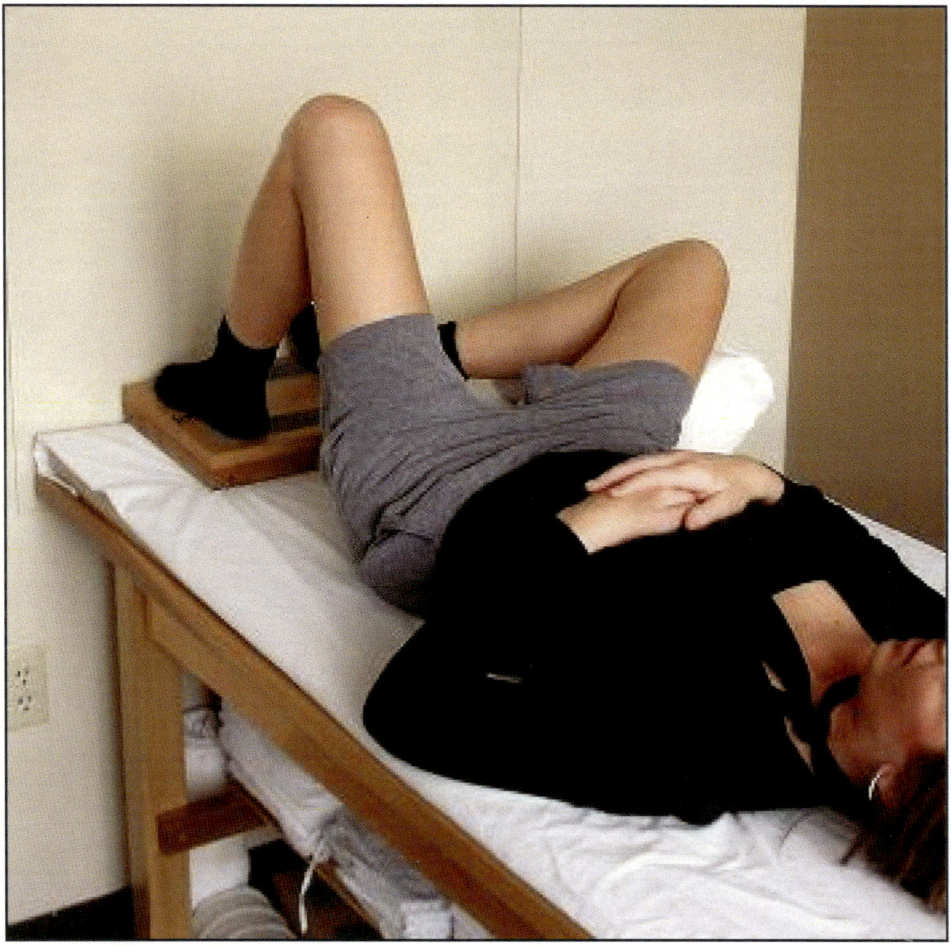

Fig. 19. Supine Hooklying Adductor Magnus Inhibition

1. Lie on your back with your feet on a 2-inch block.
2. Place a bolster or pillow of appropriate size on your right side.
3. Inhale through your nose and exhale through your mouth performing a pelvic tilt so that your tailbone is raised slightly off the mat. Keep your back flat on the mat.
4. Maintaining a pelvic tilt, let your right knee lower to the side until it reaches the bolster or pillows. You should feel a stretch across your right inner thigh.
5. Hold this position while you take 4-5 deep breaths in through your nose and out through your mouth.
6. Let your left knee drop down to meet your right.
7. Keeping both legs together, slowly bring them upright as one unit.
8. Relax and repeat 4 more times.

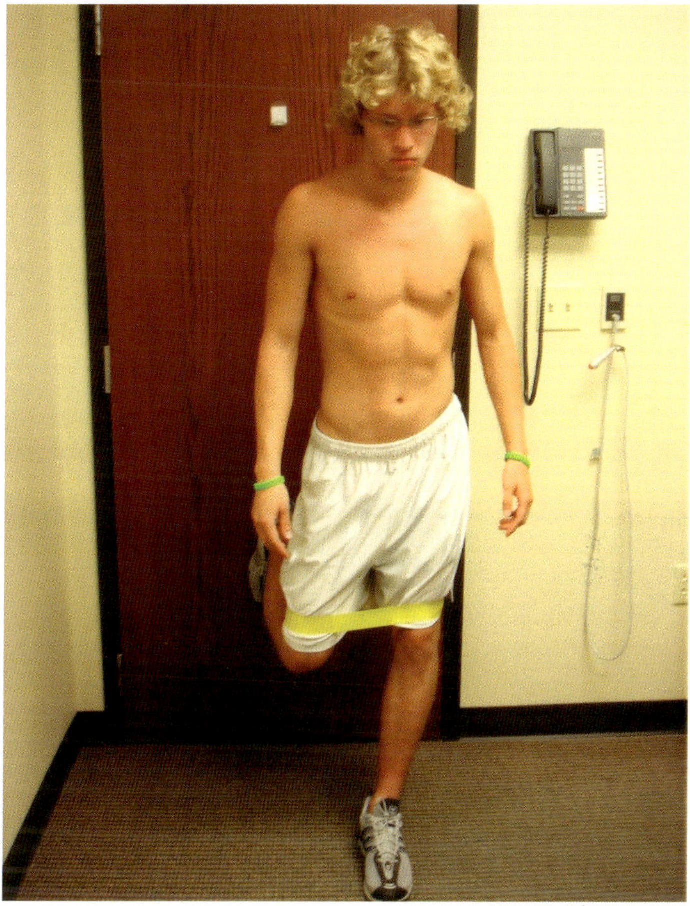

Fig. 20. Single Leg Wall Left AF IR with Right Glute Max

1. Place a band around both your legs slightly above your knees.
2. Stand facing away from a door. Place your right foot flat against the door by bending your right knee.
3. Align your knees together by adjusting your body's position and distance from the door.
4. Shift your right knee down towards the floor. Your right knee will be below the level of your left. You should feel your left outer hip engage.
5. While standing on your left leg, push your right foot firmly into the door as you maintain steady control and balance of your trunk.
6. Turn your right knee outward. You should feel your right outside hip engage along with your left outside hip.
7. Balance in this position while you take 4-5 deep breaths in through your nose and out through your mouth.
8. Relax and repeat 4 more times.

5.2 Left sacroiliac joint pain/dysfunction related to a left anterior interior chain pattern

Clinical reasoning for L SIJP/SIJD related to a L AIC pattern is similar to that of the R SIJ but rather than the strongest focus being on the R GM, the focus is on addressing the left hip/femur ER that is thought to occur as a result of compensation for the asymmetrical pelvic position. Left hip IR may be a challenging position for a patient to achieve if they have over active/strong and perhaps short left hip external rotator muscles holding them into hip ER and strong/over active right adductors holding them in right IR or a position of COG shifted right. Patients however require left hip IR for early stance phase of gait which requires them to shift their left acetabulum over the left femoral head. Compensation for the inability to get L AF IR may result in too much motion occurring in the L SIJ which may contribute to L SIJ instability. Intervention then would focus on training the left hip to IR via motion of the left acetabulum to move over the left femur (AF IR) and to activate left hip IR muscle such as the anterior gluteus medius (ant glut med) and the ischiocondylar (IC) portion of the left adductor magnus (AM). There are no known published articles relating to management of patients with SIJP that describe exercises or the importance of exercises that activate the adductors or anterior gluteus medius with the exception of one published case study that used Postural Restoration exercises.[47] Additionally, there is one poster presented and abstract published including a case series of patients with SIJP where Postural Restoration exercises were prescribed.[69, 70]

If the pattern has been present for a long time, the L posterior capsule/ischiofemoral ligament may become adaptively short. This would require stretching/lengthening of the posterior hip ligament to allow for the L AF IR position and proper seating of the left femoral head into the acetabulum. An exercise called the Right Sidelying Left Adductor Pull Back[48] done in right sidelying facilitates the desired hip positions (L AF IR and concomitant R AF ER), stretches the left ischiofemoral ligament/posterior capsule and activates left hip IR muscle i.e. adductors. (Figure 21) Resistance can be used to facilitate recruitment of the left hamstrings/adductors if desired, however that requires an individual to hold the band and may not be feasible for many patients.

A Left Sidelying Knee to Knee exercise[46-48] takes advantage of gravity when activating left hip IR muscles (adductor magnus and anterior glut med) while also activating the R GM in a transverse plane to anchor the left hemipelvis back to the L and discourages over activity of paraspinals and an excessive lordotic position. (Figure 22) Another exercise to activate the left anterior gluteus medius against resistance while having the hip internally rotate (femur on acetabulum or "FA IR") is the Supine Hooklying Right Glute Max with Left Glute Med. (Figure 23) The Left Sidelying Left Flexed Adduction with concomitant Right Lowered Extended Abduction[71] exercise integrates L abdominal wall activation along with L hip IR muscle (ant glut med and IC AM) with right GM and glut med in a position of right hip and knee extension as used in a R stance phase of gait. (Figure 24) This exercise may help to neuromuscularly reeducate the patient's left leg to rotate internally rather than externally while in a right stance phase of gait. Lastly, an exercise designed to activate the left internal oblique and transverse abdominus while also activating the right GM and L IC AM in a position of left stance phase of gait is the Left Sidelying IO/TA and Left Adductor with Right Glute Max. (Figure 25) This exercise may help to neuromuscularly reeducate the patient's left leg to rotate internally rather than externally while in a left stance phase of gait, while keeping the COG shifted left and the abdominal wall muscles on.

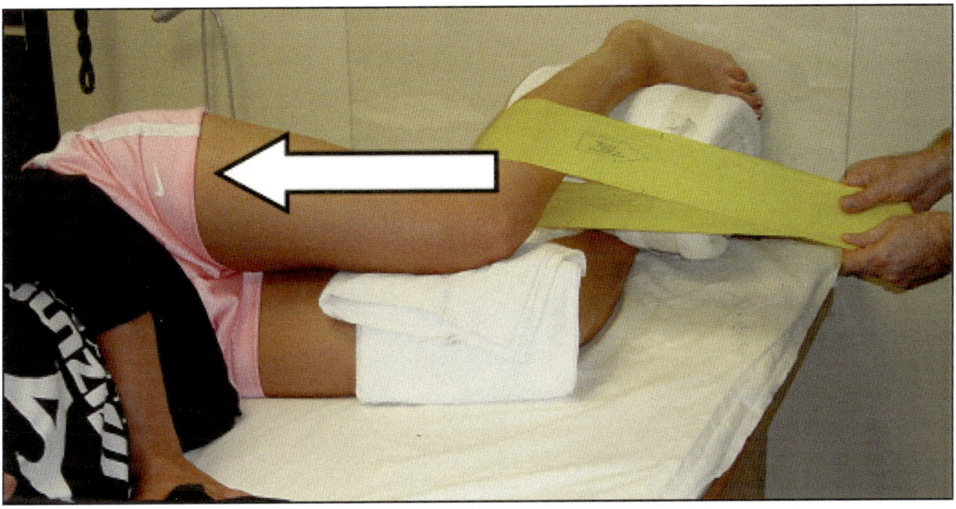

Fig. 21. Right Sidelying Left Adductor Pull Back

1. Lie on your right side with your toes on a wall, ankles and knees together and your back rounded. Place a pillow under your head and keep back and neck relaxed.
2. Place a bolster of appropriate size between your feet and a towel between your knees. Your left knee should be lower than your left hip and ankle.
3. Place tubing around your left leg just below your knee for resistance. Have another person hold the other end to provide resistance.
4. Push your bottom foot into wall.
5. Begin by inhaling slowly through your nose as you "pull back" your left leg.
6. Exhale through your mouth as you squeeze your left knee down into the towel for 3 seconds.
7. Inhale again as you "pull back" your left leg further. You should begin to feel your left inner thigh engage.
8. Exhale and squeeze your left knee down.
9. Continue the sequence until you have completed 4-5 breaths in and out. Attempt to pull back your left leg further each time you inhale.
10. Relax your knees back to the starting position and repeat the sequence 4 more times.

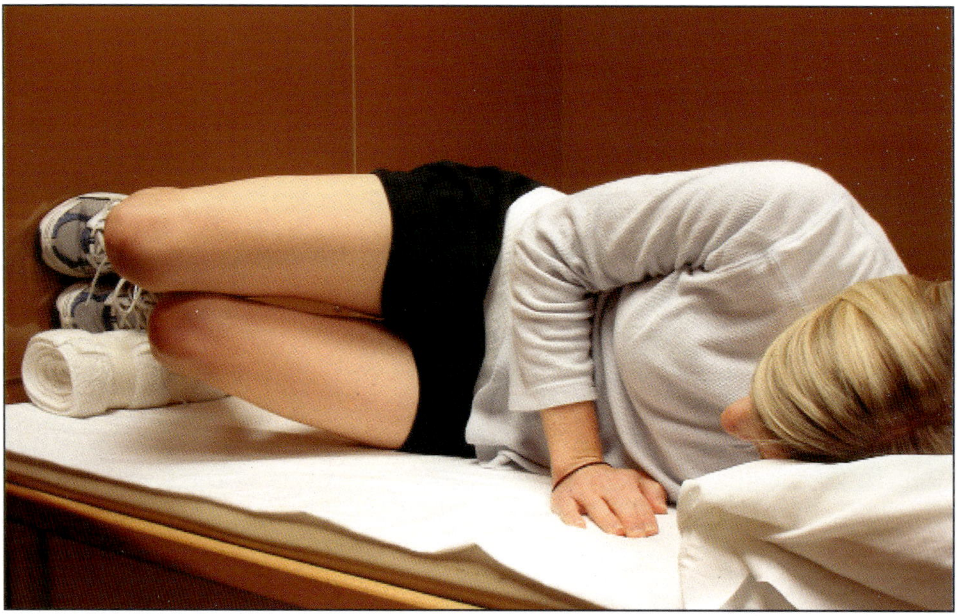

Fig. 22. Left Sidelying Knee to Knee

1. Lie on your left side with your toes on the wall, knees together and back rounded.
2. Place a bolster underneath your ankles.
3. Push your bottom toes into the wall.
4. Lift up or turn "out" your upper thigh.
5. Then lift up or turn "in" your lower thigh. You should feel your left inner thigh engage.
6. Hold your legs together while you take 4-5 deep breaths in through your nose and out through your mouth.
7. Relax and repeat 4 more times.

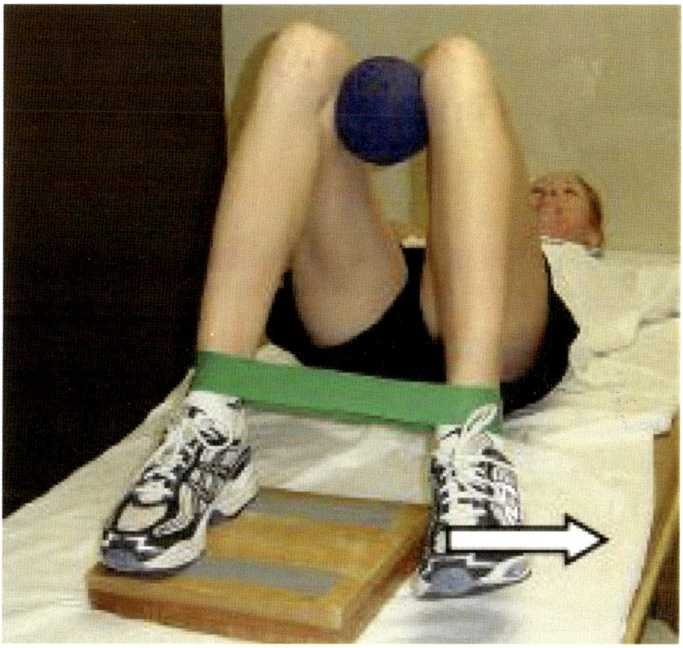

Fig. 23. Supine Hooklying Right Glute Max with Left Glute Med

1. Lie on your back with your feet on a 2-inch block and your knees bent.
2. Place a ball between your knees and a band around your ankles.
3. Inhale through your nose and then exhale through your mouth performing a pelvic tilt so that your tailbone is raised slightly off the mat. Keep your back flat on the mat.
4. Shift your right knee down towards you so that your right knee is slightly below your left. You should feel your right inner thigh engage.
5. Now lift your left foot off of the block. You should feel the back of your right leg and outside hip engage.
6. With your left foot off of the block turn your left ankle out to the side. You should feel your left outer hip engage.
7. Hold this position while you take 4-5 deep breaths in through your nose and out through your mouth.
8. Relax and repeat 4 more times.

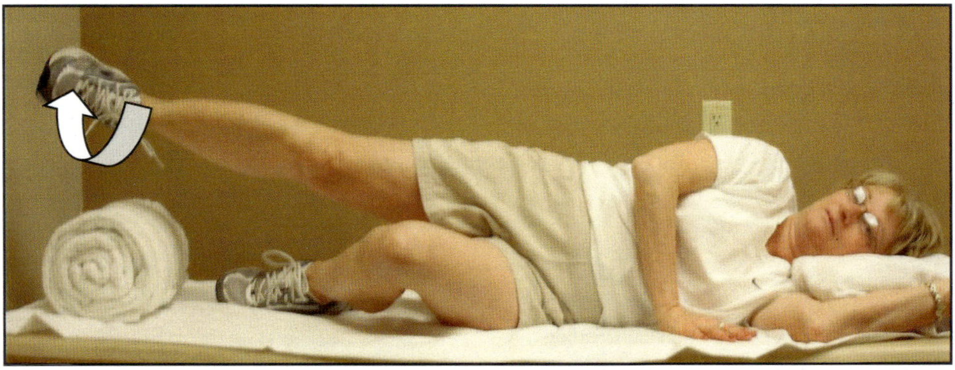

Fig. 24. Left Sidelying Left Flexed Adduction with Concomitant Right Lowered Extended Abduction

1. Lie on your left side and place a 2-3 inch bolster under your left abdominal wall and 1-2 pillows under your head so that your neck is slightly side bent to the right.
2. Place a bolster of appropriate size under your right ankle so that your right leg is level with your trunk and bend your left knee.
3. Inhale through your nose and as you exhale through your mouth reach down with your right foot.
4. Push your left hip down firmly into the mat and try to arch your left abdominal wall. You should feel your left abdominal wall engage.
5. With your left abdominal wall engaged and your right leg reaching down, push the outside border of your left foot down into the mat and "turn" your left knee up. You should feel your left inner thigh engage.
6. With your left inner thigh engaged, turn your right toes out and attempt to pick your right leg off of the bolster. You should feel your right outer hip engage.
7. Hold this position while you take 4-5 deep breaths in through your nose and out through your mouth.
8. Relax and repeat 4 more times.

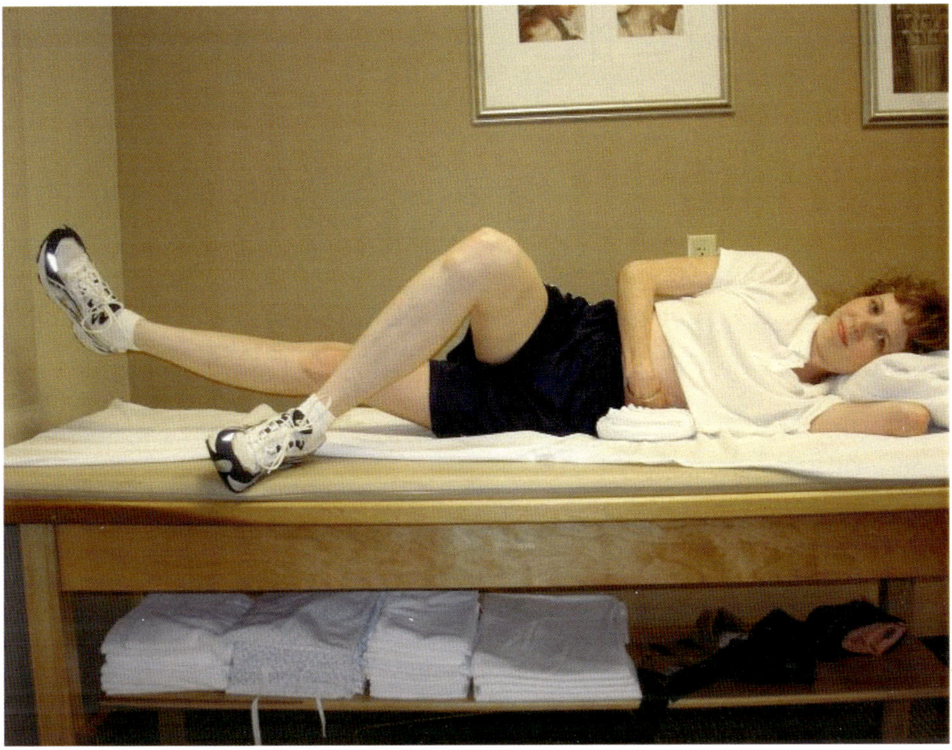

1. Lie on your left side with your left leg straight.
2. Place a 2-3 inch towel under your left side and 1-2 pillows under your head so that your neck is slightly side bent to the right.
3. Bend your right leg and cross it over your left leg.
4. Place your right foot slightly ahead of your left knee and drop the inside of your right foot toward the mat so that you can feel the arch of your foot push into your shoe.
5. Push your left hip down into the mat, bring your right knee forward and arch your left abdominal wall over the bolster. With your right hand you should feel your left abdominal wall engage. Do not engage your neck.
6. Keeping your right arch in contact with the mat, turn your right knee out. You should feel your right outside hip engage.
7. Keeping your left hip down and right knee turned out, turn your left toes up towards the ceiling and pick your entire leg up. You should feel your left inner thigh engage.
8. Hold this position while you take 4-5 deep breaths in through your nose and out through your mouth.
9. Relax and repeat 4 more times.

Fig. 25. Left Sidelying IO/TA and Left Adductor with Right Glute Max
Copyright © Postural Restoration Institute™ used with permission
www.posturalrestoration.com

6. Published case studies involving Postural Restoration for L AIC patterns

A recent case study was published describing PR management for a 65 year old female with L SIJP/SIJD, and painful intercourse.[47] Left hamstrings were activated to restore optimal sagittal plane pelvic position because of the anterior tilt of the left innominate. L AF IR position was achieved and left IR muscle was activated (anterior glut med and L IC AM). R GM was activated to help train the patient to keep her L acetabulum over her L femur (L AF IR). She had a remarkable decrease in her pain from an 8/10 to a 0/10 and an increase in her function as measured by a change from an Oswestry Disability Index (ODI) score of 20% to 0%.[47] A case series was presented at an international meeting on four patients with SIJP.[69] There were two patients with right SIJP and two with left SIJP from 30-54 years of age. They had duration of pain from two weeks to three years, and were seen between two to seven visits over 2.5 to 3.5 weeks. The improvement in function based on the ODI change score ranged between 16-33%, with a mean of 26% and an average percent improvement in function of 85%. The Patient Specific Functional Scale (PSFS) was also used to measure function and the change scores ranged from 3.0-7.3 and a mean of 5.2.[72] Both the ODI and PSFS exceeded the minimally clinical important difference (MCID) of 10 for the ODI and 2 for the PSFS.[72, 73] Currently a RCT is underway to investigate outcomes related to pain and function comparing traditional intervention to postural restoration exercises for patients with sacroiliac joint pain. This data however is not yet published. There are four other case studies relating to a L AIC pattern where a Postural Restoration approach was used however these were not specifically for patients with SIJP, but rather LBP,[46] Thoracic Outlet Syndrome,[44] Asthma[51] and Trochanteric Bursitis.[50]

In summary, disorders involving the SIJs are relatively common and can be diagnosed using subjective history elements (pain arising from long term sitting, pain located over one SIJ (Fortin's Finger Test) and possibly into the buttock (Fortin's Area) and special tests for load transfer (ASLR) and pain provocation (e.g. posterior shear, compression). Motion palpation tests should be avoided as their reliability is poor. The Ober's Test or Adduction Drop Test may be helpful in determining the presence of pelvic asymmetry and/or ipsilateral hip flexor tone and/or adductor tone. There is motion in the SIJs, and asymmetrical laxity is associated with PGP rather than generalized bilateral SIJ laxity. Motion in the sagittal plane is greater in the R SIJ than the L SIJ. The concepts of form and form closure are important to integrate into clinical reasoning for patients with SIJP/SIJD. Force closure may be reduced *or excessive* in patients with SIJP/SIJD. There is a paucity of research, particularly higher levels of research to substantiate interventions for these conditions. Many lower levels of research i.e. case reports and descriptive studies do not describe the exercises used in enough detail to apply them to patient management or to replicate the studies. This chapter offered a theoretical framework and biomechanical rationale for the management of patients with right and/or left SIJP as it relates to an underlying postural pattern of asymmetry referred to as a Left Anterior Interior Chain (L AIC) pattern. Unique Postural Restoration therapeutic exercises with face validity to address the theoretical framework were also presented and described. These exercises focused on right gluteus maximus activation in the transverse plane for right SIJP/SIJD and on left anterior gluteus medius and ischiocondylar adductor magnus activation for left SIJP/SIJD. Peer reviewed and published data to highlight a theoretical framework for therapeutic exercise management of SIJP is currently lacking. Randomized controlled trials are needed to substantiate the effectiveness of all interventions used to manage patients with SIJP/SIJD and to compare interventions to determine which are most efficacious.

7. References

[1] Paris SV. Introduction to spinal evaluation and manipulation. 3rd ed. St. Augustine: Patris Press 1997.
[2] Vleeming A, Albert HB, Ostgaard HC, et al. European guidelines for the diagnosis and treatment of pelvic girdle pain. Eur Spine J 2008;17:794-819.
[3] Schwarzer AC CNA, N Bogduk. The Sacroiliac Joint in Chronic Low Back Pain. Spine 1995;20(1):31-7.
[4] Maignes JY, Aivaliklis A, Pfefer F. Results of Sacroiliac Joint Double Block and Value of Sacroiliac Pain Provocation Tests in 54 Patients With Low Back Pain. Spine 1996;21:1889-92.
[5] Ostgaard HC, Andersson GBJ, Karlsson K. Prevalence of back pain inpregnancy. Spine 1991;16(549-552).
[6] van Kessel-Cobelens AM, Verhagen AP, Mens JM, Snijders CJ, Koes BW. Pregnancy-related pelvic girdle pain: intertester reliability of 3 tests to determine asymmetric mobility of the sacroiliac joints. J Manipulative Phys Ther 2008;31(2):130-6.
[7] van der Wurff P, Hagmeijer RHM, Meyne W. Clinical tests of the sacroiliac joint: a systematic methodological review. Part 1: reliability. Manual Therapy 2000;5(1): 30-6.
[8] Szadek KM. Diagnostic validity of criteria for sacroiliac joint pain: a systematic review. . J Pain 2009 10(4):354-68.
[9] Young S, Aprill C, Laslett M. Correlation of clinical examination characteristics with three sources of chronic low back pain. Spine 2003;3:460-5.
[10] Fortin JD, Falco FJ. The Fortin finger test: an indicator of sacroiliac pain. Am J Orthop 1997 26:477-80.
[11] Fortin JD, Dwyer AP, West S. SIJ: pain referral maps upon applying a new injection/arthrography technique. Part II: Clinical evaluation. Spine 1994;19:1483-9.
[12] O-Sullivan PB. Altered Motor Control strategies in Subjects With Sacroiliac Joint Pain During the Active Straight-Leg-Raise Test. Spine 2002;27(1):E1-E8.
[13] Lee D. The Pelvic Girdle an approach to the examinat in and treatment of the lumbopelvic-hip region. 3rd ed. New York, NY: Churchhill Livingstone, 2004.
[14] Laslett M, Young SB, Aprill CN, McDonald B. Diagnosing painful sacroiliac joint: a validity study of the McKenzie evaluation and sacroiliac provacation tests. Aust J Physiother 2003;49(2):89-97.
[15] Stuber KJ. Specificity, sensitivity and predictive values of clinical tests of the sacroiliac joint: a systematic review of the literature. J Can Chiropr Assoc 2007;51:30-41.
[16] Sizer PS, Phelps V, Thompsen K. Disorders of the sacroiliac joint. 2 2002;1:17-34.
[17] Freburger JK RD. Using Published Evidence to Guide the Examination of the Sacroiliac Joint Region. Physical Therapy 2001;81(5):1135-43.
[18] Maignes JY AA, Pfefer F. Results of Sacroiliac Joint Double Block and Value of Sacroiliac Pain Provocation Tests in 54 Patients With Low Back Pain. Spine 1996;21:1889-92.
[19] Cohen SP. Sacroiliac joint pain: a comprehensive review of anatomy, diagnosis, and teatment. . Anesth Analg 2005;101:1440-53.

[20] Levangie P. The Vertebral Column. Joint Structure and Function A Comprehensive Analysis. Philadelphia: FA Davis Co., 2005:173-6.
[21] Sturesson B, Uden A, Vleeming A. A radiostereometric analysis of movements of the sacroiliac joints during the standing hip flexion test. Spine 2009;25(3):364-8.
[22] Smidt G, Wei S, McQuade K, Barakatt E, Sun T, Stanford W. Sacroiliac motion for extreme hip positions: a fresh cadaver study. Spine 1997;22(18):2073-82.
[23] Ivanov AA, Kiapour A, Ebraheim NA, Goel V. Lumbar fusion leads to increases in angular motion and stress across sacroliacjoint: a finite element study. Spine 2009;34(5):E162-9.
[24] Bussey MD, Bell ML, Milosavljevic S. The influence of hip abduction and external rotation on sacroiliac motion. Man Ther 2009(5):1-6.
[25] Damen L, Spoor CW, Snijders CJ, Stam HJ. Does a pelvic belt influence sacroiliac joint laxity? Clinical Biomechanics 2002;17(7):495.
[26] Vleeming A, Stoeckart R, Volkers ACW, Snijders CJ. Relation between form and funciton in the sacroiliac joint. 2: Biomechanical aspects. Spine 1990;15(2):133.
[27] Tulberg T, Blomberg S, Branth B, Johnsson R. Manipulation does not alter the position of the sacroiliac joint. A roentgen stereophotogrammetric analysis. Spine 2008;31(2):123-7.
[28] O'Sullivan PB. Diagnosis and classification of pelvic girdle pain disorders Part 1: A mechanism based approach within a biopsychosocial framework. . Man Ther 2007;12:86-97.
[29] Snijders CJ VA, Stoeckart R. Transfer of Lumbosacral Load to Iliac Bones and Legs. Clinical Biomechanics 1992;8:285-94.
[30] Richardon CA, Snijders CJ, Hides JA, Damen L, Pas MS, Storm J. The relation between the transversus abdominis muscles, sacroiliac joint mechanics and low back pain. Spine 2002;27(4):399-405.
[31] Pool-Goudzwaard AL, Marijke CPH, ten Hove S, et al. Relations between pregnancy-related low back pain, pelvic floor activity and pelvic floor dysfunction. Int urogynecol J 2005;16:468-74.
[32] Sahrmann SA. Diagnosis and Treatment of Movement Impairment Syndromes. St. Louis: Mosby, 2002.
[33] Gibbons S. The integration of the psoas major and the deep sacral gluteus maximus muscles into the lumbar cylinder model. In: World Congress on Manual Therapy, 2005.
[34] Moore KL, Dalley AF. Clinically Oriented Anatomy. 5 ed. Philadelphia, PA: Lippincott Williams and Wilkins, 2006.
[35] Hodges PW, Butler JE, McKenzie DK, et al. Contraction of the human diaphragm during rapid postural adjustments. J Phys 1997;505(2):539-48.
[36] De Troyer A, Estenne M. Functional Anatomy of the Respiratory Muscles. Clin Chest Med 1988;9(2):175-93.
[37] Mead J. Functional significance of the area of apposition of diaphragm to rib cage. Am Rev Respir Dis 1979;11:31.
[38] Reid WD, Dechman G. Considerations when testing and training the respiratory muscles. Phys Ther 1995;75(11).
[39] DeTroyer A, Estenne M. Respiratory Anatomy of the Respiratory Muscles. Clin Chest Med 1988;9(2):175-93.

[40] Loring SH, Mead J. Action of the diaphragm on the rib cage inferred from a force-balance analysis. J Appl Physiol 1982;53(3):756-60.

[41] Boyle K, et al. The Value of Blowing Up a Balloon. N Am J Sports Phys Ther 2010;5(3):179-88.

[42] Lando Y, Boiselle PM, Shade D, et al. Effect of Lung Volume Reduction Surgery of Diaphragm Length in Severe Chronic Obstructive Pulmonary Disease. Am J Respir Crit Care Med 1999;159(3):796-805.

[43] Cassart M, Pettiaux N, Gevenois PA, et al. Effect of Chronic Hyperinflation on Diaphragm Length and Surface Area. Am J Respir Crit Care Med 1997;156:504-8.

[44] Robey JH, Boyle KL. Bilateral functional thoracic outlet syndrome in a collegiate football player. N Am J Sports Phys Ther 2009;4(4):170-81.

[45] Boyle K. Ethnography of the postural restoration subculture: a posture based approach to patient/client management [Dissertation]. Fort Lauderdale, FL: Nova Southeastern University, 2006.

[46] Boyle K, Demske J. Management of a Female with Chronic Sciatica and Low Back Pain: A Case Report. Physiother Theory Pract 2009;25 (1):44.

[47] Boyle K. Postural Restoration Management of a Female with Left Low Back Pain and Sacroiliac Joint Pain: A Case Report. Physiother Can 2011;63(2):154-63.

[48] Hruska R. Myokinematic Restoration An Integrated Approach to Treatment of Patterned Lumbo-Pelvic-Femoral Pathomechanics [Course manual]. Elon, NC: PRI, 2005.

[49] Boyle K. Conservative Management for patients with low back pain: a case series. JOSPT 2008;38(1):A67.

[50] Boyle K, et al. Management of a woman diagnosed with trochanteric bursitis with the use of a Protonics® neuromuscular system. Journal on the Section of Women's Health 2003;27(1):12-7.

[51] Coughlin KJ, Hruska RJ, Masek J. Cough-Variant Asthma: Responsive to Integrative Management and Postural Restoration. Explore 2005;1(5):377-9.

[52] Boyle K, Rane S. Postural Restoration management of a Female with Right Pelvic and Proximal Hamstring Pain. In: WCPT-AWP & IAP Congress; 2009 Mumbai, India, 2009

[53] Ebmeier J, Hruska R. Postural Restoration Institute Web site. 2010 [cited 2010 1-28-2010]; Available from: www.posturalrestoration.com

[54] Hruska R. Postural Respiration An Integrated Approach to Treatment of Patterned Thoraco-Abdominal Pathomechanics. Chandler, AZ: Postural Restoration Institute, 2007.

[55] Reamy BV, Slakely JB. Adolescent Idiopathic Scoliosis:Review and Current Concepts. American Family Physician 2001;64:111-6.

[56] Song K, Herring JA. Early recognition and assessment of idiopathic scoliosis. J Musculoskel Med 1993;10(4):63-76.

[57] Kouwenhoven JM, et al. Analysis of preexistent vertebral rotation in the normal spine. Spine 2006;31(13):1467-72.

[58] Kouwenhoven JW, et al. The relation between organ anatomy and pre-existent vertebral rotation in the normal spine. Spine 2007;32(10):1123-8.

[59] Kendall FP, et al. Muscles Testing and Function with Posture and Pain. 5th ed. Philadelphia: Lippincott Williams and Wilkins, 2005.

[60] Tenney R, Boyle K, Debord A. Influence of Hamstring and Abdominal Muscle Activation on a Positive Ober's Test in Subjects with Lumbo-pelvic Pain. Physiother Can 2011:in review.
[61] Boyle K, Albarran I. The Influence of Hamstring Activation on the Outcome of a Postive Ober's Test. In: APTA Annual Conference San Antonio,Texas, 2008.
[62] Masek J. Soccer Hip Impingement as it Relates to Postural Restoraiton Part III: Management Considerations. In: Perofrmance Soccer Conditioning, 2007:1-4.
[63] Boyle K. Management of patients with sacroiliac joint pain: what's old, what's new, what's in, what's out. In: Combined Sections Meeting APTA; 2010; San Diego, CA, 2010.
[64] Hruska R. Impingement and Instability [course manual]. Lincoln, NE, 2009.
[65] Stuge B, Bragelien V, Laerun E. The efficacy of a treatment program focusing on specific stabilizing exercises for pelvic girdle pain after pregnancy: a two-year follow-up of a randomized clinical trial. Spine 2004;29(10):E197-E203.
[66] Shearar KA, Colloca CJ, White HL. A randomized clinical trial of manual versus mechanical force manipulation in the treatment of sacroiliac joint syndrome. J Manipulative Phys Ther 2005;28(7):493-501.
[67] Osterbauer PJ, DeBoer KF, Widmaier R. Treatment and biochemical assessment of patients with chronic sacroiliac syndrome. J Manipulative Phys Ther 1993(16):82-90.
[68] Sasso RC, Ahmad RI, Butler JE, Reimers DL. Sacroiliac joint dysfunciton: a long-term follow-up study. In: www.orthobluejournal.com, 2001:457-60.
[69] Boyle K, Tenney R, Robey J, Gross M. Postural Restoration Management for Patients with Sacroiliac Joint Dysfunction: A Case Series. In: World Congress Physical Therapy; 2011; Amsterdam, Netherlands, 2011.
[70] Boyle K, Tenney R, Robey J, Gross M. Postural Restoration Management for Patients with Sacroiliac Joint Dysfunction: A Case Series. Physiotherapy 2011;97(1):eS1-eS1638, RR-PO-205-20.
[71] Hruska R. Advanced Integration [Course manual]. Lincoln, NE: Postural Restoration Institute, 2004.
[72] Stratford P GC, Westaway M, Binkley J. Assessing disability and change on individual patients: a report of patient specific measure. Physiotherapy Canada 1995;47(4): 258-63.
[73] Ostelo RWJG, deVet HCW. Clinically important outcomes in low back pain. Best Pract Res Clin Rheumatol 2005;19(4):593-607.

Permissions

The contributors of this book come from diverse backgrounds, making this book a truly international effort. This book will bring forth new frontiers with its revolutionizing research information and detailed analysis of the nascent developments around the world.

We would like to thank A.A. Norasteh, PhD P.T, for lending his expertise to make the book truly unique. He has played a crucial role in the development of this book. Without his invaluable contribution this book wouldn't have been possible. He has made vital efforts to compile up to date information on the varied aspects of this subject to make this book a valuable addition to the collection of many professionals and students.

This book was conceptualized with the vision of imparting up-to-date information and advanced data in this field. To ensure the same, a matchless editorial board was set up. Every individual on the board went through rigorous rounds of assessment to prove their worth. After which they invested a large part of their time researching and compiling the most relevant data for our readers. Conferences and sessions were held from time to time between the editorial board and the contributing authors to present the data in the most comprehensible form. The editorial team has worked tirelessly to provide valuable and valid information to help people across the globe.

Every chapter published in this book has been scrutinized by our experts. Their significance has been extensively debated. The topics covered herein carry significant findings which will fuel the growth of the discipline. They may even be implemented as practical applications or may be referred to as a beginning point for another development.

The editorial board has been involved in producing this book since its inception. They have spent rigorous hours researching and exploring the diverse topics which have resulted in the successful publishing of this book. They have passed on their knowledge of decades through this book. To expedite this challenging task, the publisher supported the team at every step. A small team of assistant editors was also appointed to further simplify the editing procedure and attain best results for the readers.

Our editorial team has been hand-picked from every corner of the world. Their multi-ethnicity adds dynamic inputs to the discussions which result in innovative outcomes. These outcomes are then further discussed with the researchers and contributors who give their valuable feedback and opinion regarding the same. The feedback is then collaborated with the researches and they are edited in a comprehensive manner to aid the understanding of the subject.

Apart from the editorial board, the designing team has also invested a significant amount of their time in understanding the subject and creating the most relevant covers. They scrutinized every image to scout for the most suitable representation of the subject and create an appropriate cover for the book.

The publishing team has been involved in this book since its early stages. They were actively engaged in every process, be it collecting the data, connecting with the contributors or procuring relevant information. The team has been an ardent support to the editorial, designing and production team. Their endless efforts to recruit the best for this project, has resulted in the accomplishment of this book. They are a veteran in the field of academics and their pool of knowledge is as vast as their experience in printing. Their expertise and guidance has proved useful at every step. Their uncompromising quality standards have made this book an exceptional effort. Their encouragement from time to time has been an inspiration for everyone.

The publisher and the editorial board hope that this book will prove to be a valuable piece of knowledge for researchers, students, practitioners and scholars across the globe.

List of Contributors

Akira Minematsu
Kio University, Japan

E. Latorre Marques
Spanish Working Group of COST B13 Program, Dep. of Anesthesiology, "Miguel Servet" Hospital, School of Medicine, University of Zaragoza, Spain

Hiroharu Kamioka
Department of Physical and Health Education, Faculty of Environmental Science, Tokyo University of Agriculture, Japan

Takuya Honda
Department of Physical and Health Education, Graduate School of Education, the University of Tokyo, Japan

Jadranka Stričević and Majda Pajnkihar
Faculty of Health Sciences, University of Maribor, Maribor, Slovenia

Zvone Balantič
Faculty of Organisational Sciences, University of Maribor, Kranj, Slovenia

Zmago Turk and Dušan Čelan
University Clinical Center Maribor, Maribor, Slovenia

J. Nicholas Penney
Centre of National Research on Disability and Rehabilitation Medicine, University of Queensland, Australia

Carine Vossen, Helen Vossen, Wiesje van de Wetering, Marco Marcus, Jim van Os and Richel Lousberg
Maastricht University Medical Centre, the Netherlands

Christophe Demoulin
Department of Motricity Sciences, Liege University and Liege University Hospital Centre (CHU), Belgium

Marcia Miller Spoto
Nazareth College of Rochester, USA

Johnson Olubusola Esther
Department of Medical Rehabilitation, Obafemi Awolowo University, Ile-Ife, Nigeria

A.I. Cuesta-Vargas, M. González-Sánchez, M.T. Labajos-Manzanares and A. Galán-Mercant
Department of Psychiatry and Physiotherapy, University of Malaga, Spain

Krzysztof Radziszewski
Clinic of Rehabilitation, Military Hospital in Bydgoszcz,
Department of Clinical Fundamentals of Physiotherapy, Collegium Medicum in Bydgoszcz, Nicolaus Copernicus University, Poland

Erik J. Groessl and Douglas Chang
VA San Diego Healthcare System, USA
University of California San Diego, USA

Marisa Sklar
SDSU/UCSD Joint Doctoral Program in Clinical Psychology, USA

A. Luque-Suárez, E. Díaz-Mohedo, I. Medina-Porqueres and T. Ponce-García
Physiotherapy Department, Malaga University, Spain

Kyndall Boyle
Appalachian State University, USA